Blueprints

CLINICAL CASES
IN PSYCHIATRY

Check Out all the Titles in This Great Series!

Blueprints

CLINICAL CASES

SECOND EDITION

PSYCHIATRY

Jennifer Hoblyn, MD, MRCPsych, MPH
Palo Alto Veterans Affairs Health Care System, Palo Alto, California
Department of Psychiatry and Behavioral Sciences,
Stanford University School of Medicine

Judith Neugroschl, MD
Assistant Professor
Director, Geriatric Psychiatry Fellowship
Director, Medical Student Education in Psychiatry
Director Geriatric Psychiatry Clinic
Department of Psychiatry
Mount Sinai School of Medicine

Asher B. Simon, MD
Assistant Professor of Psychiatry
Medical Director, Continuing Day Treatment Program
Mount Sinai School of Medicine

Aaron B. Caughey, MD, PhD (Series Editor)
Assistant Professor
Department of Obstetrics & Gynecology
University of California, San Francisco

 Wolters Kluwer | Lippincott Williams & Wilkins
Health
Philadelphia • Baltimore • New York • London
Buenos Aires • Hong Kong • Sydney • Tokyo

Acquisitions Editor: Donna Anastasi Duffy
Managing Editor: Stacey L. Sebring
Marketing Manager: Jennifer Kuklinski
Production Editor: Kevin P. Johnson
Creative Director: Doug Smock
Compositor: International Typesetting and Composition

WM
18.2
H683p
2008

Second Edition

Library of Congress Cataloging-in-Publication Data

Hoblyn, Jennifer.
  Blueprints clinical cases in psychiatry / Jennifer Hoblyn, Judith Neugroschl, Asher B. Simon. — 2nd ed.
      p. ; cm.
  Includes bibliographical references and index.
  ISBN 1-4051-0496-1
  1. Psychiatry—Case studies.   I. Neugroschl, Judith.   II. Simon, Asher B.   III. Title.
    [DNLM: 1. Mental Disorders—Examination Questions.   2. Case Reports—Examination Questions.   WM 18.2 H683b 2008]
    RC465.H59 2008
    616.890076—dc22

                                                                    2007033286

DISCLAIMER

Care has been taken to confirm the accuracy of the information present and to describe generally accepted practices. However, the authors, editors, and publisher are not responsible for errors or omissions or for any consequences from application of the information in this book and make no warranty, expressed or implied, with respect to the currency, completeness, or accuracy of the contents of the publication. Application of this information in a particular situation remains the professional responsibility of the practitioner; the clinical treatments described and recommended may not be considered absolute and universal recommendations.

The authors, editors, and publisher have exerted every effort to ensure that drug selection and dosage set forth in this text are in accordance with the current recommendations and practice at the time of publication. However, in view of ongoing research, changes in government regulations, and the constant flow of information relating to drug therapy and drug reactions, the reader is urged to check the package insert for each drug for any change in indications and dosage and for added warnings and precautions. This is particularly important when the recommended agent is a new or infrequently employed drug.

Some drugs and medical devices presented in this publication have Food and Drug Administration (FDA) clearance for limited use in restricted research settings. It is the responsibility of the health care provider to ascertain the FDA status of each drug or device planned for use in their clinical practice.

To purchase additional copies of this book, call our customer service department at **(800) 638-3030** or fax orders to **(301) 223-2320**. International customers should call **(301) 223-2300**.

Visit Lippincott Williams & Wilkins on the Internet: http://www.lww.com. Lippincott Williams & Wilkins customer service representatives are available from 8:30 am to 6:00 pm, EST.

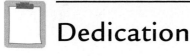

Dedication

We would like to dedicate this book to our families—Ian, Patrick, Angus and Flora; Ari, Jacob, Jonah, Gerry and Seth; and Katy; for all of their love and patience.

      Jennifer, Judith, and Asher

I dedicate this book to my parents, Bill and Carol, who have committed their professional lives to the mental and social well being of children.

      Aaron

Preface

Blueprints Clinical Cases in Psychiatry provides a comprehensive array of clinical cases from across the large spectrum of psychiatric disorders. It has been designed to complement the clinical education received during the third and fourth years of medical school and is not meant to cover all aspects of clinical management in psychiatry; it is an aid for preparation for clinical rotations and examinations. The specific design of the cases is meant to take the student through the clinical experience, parallel to the manner in which patients actually present. Because each diagnosis is not revealed immediately, the cases lead students to think through clinical presentations as they unfold. Once the diagnosis is made, the cases continue on to the treatment of the illness and other management issues. The book is organized by age group and by place of contact (e.g., Emergency Room, inpatient consultation, office). This was done to foster skills in critical diagnostic reasoning.

DIAGNOSTIC FRAMEWORKS IN PSYCHIATRY

Psychiatric diagnoses are formulated in accordance with the multiaxial scheme of the Diagnostic and Statistical Manual of Mental Disorders Fourth Edition (DSM-IV-TR). The American Psychiatric Association developed this text in 1994 for use in clinical work, education, and research. The term "mental disorder" is defined as a **"clinically significant psychological or behavioral condition that causes distress or disability in an individual or increased risk of disability, loss of important freedom, pain, or death."** Importantly, it is not merely an understandable response to an event such as death. The DSM is categorical in nature and divides mental disorders into groups according to defining features and criteria. Because the etiology of most psychiatric illnesses is not well defined, the DSM defines illnesses by symptom clusters, not by etiology. The categories, therefore, may not be discrete entities, and even those patients who have the same disorder may present in a heterogeneous manner. Though necessarily somewhat abstract and arguably artificial in its groupings, it is a highly useful, comprehensive, and widely employed system of classification, providing for clearer communication among practitioners.

The DSM provides for a "multiaxial" diagnosis, in appreciation of the fact that psychiatric illnesses are complex and have multiple influences. **Axis I** refers to clinical disorders or conditions requiring clinical attention; additionally, course specifiers (e.g., degree of remission or severity) may be used. **Axis II** refers to personality disorders and mental retardation. **Axis III** is used for general medical conditions. **Axis IV** includes psychosocial and environmental problems and stressors. **Axis V** allows for a quantifiable (i.e., numeric) assessment of the patient's overall global functioning. (Adapted from American Psychiatric Association: Task Force on DSM-IV. In: *Diagnostic and Statistical Manual of Mental Disorders DSM-IV.* 4th ed. Washington, DC: American Psychiatric Association, 1994.)

CASE FORMAT

The cases have been specifically designed to take students through the clinical experience of evaluating and treating patients presenting with a variety of chief complaints representing the common reasons patients seek psychiatric help. Below is a description of the specific design of the cases and suggestions for how to use/read each section.

Title/CC: The case titles and chief complaints (CC) are based on common presenting signs or symptoms. Our intent is that you will begin with a broad differential diagnosis.

HPI: The history of present illness (HPI) is the initial descriptive history in paragraph form. In addition to the presenting history and the course of symptoms, it usually includes a review of pertinent symptoms, both positive and negative. At the end of the HPI, you should be thinking about a more specific differential diagnosis, what would be anticipated on the mental status and physical exams, and which diagnostic tests should be ordered. Some of these items have been formalized in the thought questions.

PPHx: Usual items of import in past psychiatric history include (i) previous psychiatric admissions, diagnoses, medications used, and responses to same; (ii) previous suicide attempts and the circumstances surrounding them; (iii) previous substance dependence or abuse and treatments; (iv) legal problems arising from previous psychiatric illnesses or substance-related occurences, including episodes of violence. Only pertinent positives and negatives will be presented.

Past Medical/Surgical History/Medications: The past medical and surgical history along with medications and allergies are meant to further inform the HPI. It is important to consider how one's baseline medical status in conjunction with medications impacts the differential diagnosis and eventual treatment plans.

Family History: Of relevance here is any psychiatric illness in family members, diagnoses, and previous treatment responses if known.

Social History: Important assessments include functional capacity (including previous or present highest level of functioning), educational attainments, occupational and marital status, position in and current relationships within family, as well as current alcohol, nicotine, or substance use.

VS/PE: The vital signs (VS) and physical exam (PE) are meant to further clarify the differential diagnosis from the patient's presentation. In these cases, usually only the pertinent positive and negative findings are mentioned. They should be utilized to further narrow the differential diagnosis and revise the previous list of diagnostic tests you were considering. The physical examination may reveal signs of comorbid disease or clues to aid in current diagnoses, such as needle marks in a substance user.

MSE: The mental status exam is a part of the exam that is uniquely elaborated in psychiatry. A full mental status exam includes a description of appearance, relatedness, psychomotor agitation or retardation, speech, mood, affect, thought process, thought content, perception, insight into illness, judgment, and a measure of cognition such as a mini-mental state exam.

Labs/X-ray: Only pertinent positives and negatives are recorded. The common abbreviations are used, as well as the standard format for the complete blood count (CBC) and electrolyte panels.

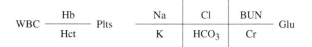

Thought Questions and Answers: These open-ended questions are meant to stimulate your thinking of diagnosis, pathophysiology, and treatment as you work through the cases. It is intended that you read the question and then spend some time reflecting on possible answers prior to continuing the case. We suggest actually writing down your answers or, if working in a group, discussing possible answers. Answers immediately follow sets of thought questions, so try not to read ahead. The thought questions are often after the HPI or the PE, but are used throughout the cases on many occasions to help stimulate clinical thinking.

Case Continued: This section usually gives further diagnostic information and may reveal the final diagnosis, or at least offers further information that can lead you to clarify considerations of treatment.

Multiple Choice Questions: There are four in-service or board-style multiple choice questions following each case. They are designed to be completed at the end of the case and the answers reviewed at that point. The answer section often provides more in depth discussions of some of the issues raised in the cases.

Review Q&A: At the end of the text, after the 60 cases, you will find an additional 100 board-style multiple choice questions followed by answers and explanations.

Finally, we have done our utmost to exclude any errors, but, as you will appreciate in any text, some inaccuracies may have slipped in. We welcome any constructive comments or suggestions, so that future editions may be improved.

> Jennifer Hoblyn, MD, MRCPsych (UK), MPH
> Judith Neugroschl, MD
> Aaron B. Caughey, MD, MPP, MPH
> Asher Simon, MD

Reviewers

Heidi Ashih, M.D., Ph.D., M.S.
Clinical Fellow, Psychiatry
Harvard Medical School

Rashida, M. Gray
4th Year, University of Illinois at Chicago

Kathleen A. Hecksel
4th Year, Mayo Clinic College of Medicine
Mayo Medical School

Christiane Kubit
Medical University of Ohio

Alexander C. Tsai
PGY-II, University of California at San Francisco

Contents

Abbreviations/Acronyms

AA	Alcoholics Anonymous
ABG	arterial blood gas
ACTH	adrenocorticotropic hormone
AD	Alzheimer disease
ADHD	attention-deficit/hyperactivity disorder
ADLs	activities of daily living
afib	atrial fibrillation
AIDS	acquired immunodeficiency syndrome
AIMS	Abnormal Involuntary Movement Scale
All	allergies
ALT	alanine aminotransferase (SGPT)
ANC	absolute neutrophil count
APP	Alzheimer precursor protein
AST	aspartate aminotransferase (SGOT)
BDD	body dysmorphic disorder
β-hCG	beta human chorionic gonadotropin
BID	*bis in die* (two times a day)
BP	blood pressure
BPD	borderline personality disorder
BPH	benign prostatic hypertrophy
BUN	blood urea nitrogen
BZD	benzodiazepine
C-BASP	cognitive-behavioral analysis system of psychotherapy
CBC	complete blood count
CBT	cognitive behavioral therapy
CC/ID	chief complaint/identification
CD	conduct disorder
CDD	childhood disintegrative disorder
cGMP	cyclic guanosine monophosphate
CHF	congestive heart failure
Cl	chloride
CNS	central nervous system
CO_2	carbon dioxide
COPD	chronic obstructive pulmonary disease
CPAP	continuous positive airway pressure

CPK   creatine phosphokinase
CPS   chronic paranoid schizophrenia
Cr   creatinine
CRF   corticotropin-releasing factor
C-section cesarean section
CSF   cerebrospinal fluid
CT   computed tomography
CV   cardiovascular
CVA   cerebrovascular accident
CVD   cardiovascular disease
DDAVP   1-desamino-8-D-arginine vasopressin (desmopressin)
DevHx   developmental history
DNR   do not resuscitate
DSM-IV-TR *Diagnostic and Statistical Manual of Mental Disorders Fourth Edition, Text Revision*
DST   dexamethasone suppression test
DTs   delirium tremens
DWI   driving while intoxicated
ECG   electrocardiogram
ECT   electroconvulsive therapy
ED   emergency department
EEG   electroencephalogram
EMG   electromyogram
EMS   emergency medical service
EPSE   extrapyramidal side effects
ER   emergency room
ESP   extrasensory perception
EtOH   ethyl alcohol/ethanol
Ext   extremities
FBI   Federal Bureau of Investigation
FDA   Food and Drug Administration
FHx   family history
FISH   fluorescence in situ hybridization
5HIAA   5-hydroxyindoleacetic acid
5HT   5-hydroxytryptamine
GABA γ-aminobutyric acid
Gen   general
GGT γ-glutamyltransferase
GI   gastrointestinal
Glu   glucose
Hbg   hemoglobin
Hc   homocysteine
HCl   hydrochloric acid
Hct   hematocrit

HEENT	head, eyes, ears, nose, throat
HIV	human immunodeficiency virus
HPA	hypothalamic-pituitary-adrenal
HPI	history of present illness
HR	heart rate
IADLs	instrumental activities of daily living
ICU	intensive care unit
IDDM	insulin-dependent diabetes mellitus
IM	intramuscular
IQ	intelligence quotient
IRS	Internal Revenue Service
IV	intravenous
K	potassium
LAAM	L-α-acetyl-methadol
labs	laboratory tests
lb	pounds (weight)
LDL	low-density lipoprotein
LFT	liver function test
LH	leuteinizing hormone
LSD	lysergic acid diethylamide
MAOI	monoamine oxidase inhibitor
MCV	mean corpuscular volume
MDD	major depressive disorder
meds	medications
MHPG	3-methoxy-4-hydroxyphenylglycol
MI	myocardial infarction
MMA	methylmalonic acid
MMSE	Mini-Mental State Examination
MR	mental retardation
MRG	murmurs, rubs, and gallops
MRI	magnetic resonance imaging
MSE	mental status exam
MSLT	multiple sleep latency test
mTHF	methyltetrahydrofolate
MWF	married white female
MWM	married white male
Na	sodium
NAD	no apparent distress
neg	negative
Neuro	neurologic
NKDA	no known drug allergies
NMDA	N-methyl-D-aspartate
NMS	neuroleptic malignant syndrome
NOS	not otherwise specified

NSAID	nonsteroidal anti-inflammatory drug
NTD	neural tube defects
OCD	obsessive-compulsive disorder
OCPD	obsessive-compulsive personality disorder
OD	overdose
ODD	oppositional defiant disorder
OSA	obstructive sleep apnea
PCP	phencyclidine
PD	personality disorder
PE	physical examination
PERRLA	pupils equal, round, reactive to light and accommodation
PET	positron emission tomography
PFC	prefrontal cortex
PKU	phenylketonuria
PMDD	premenstrual dysphoric disorder
PMHx	previous medical history
PMR	psychomotor retardation
PMS	premenstrual syndrome
PO	*per os* (by mouth)
pos	positive
PPHx	previous psychiatric history
PRN	*pro re nata* (as needed)
PSHx	previous surgical history
PTA	posttraumatic amnesia
PTSD	posttraumatic stress disorder
QD	*quaque die* (every day)
QHS	*quaque hora somni* (at bedtime, every night)
QID	*quater in die* (four times a day)
RA	room air
REM	rapid eye movement
ROS	review of systems
RPR	rapid plasma reagin (test for syphilis)
RR	respiratory rate
RR&R	regular rate and rhythm
rT_3	reverse triiodothyronine
SDA	serotonin-dopamine antagonist
SGOT	serum glutamic oxalo-acetic transaminase
SGPT	serum glutamic pyruvic transaminase
SHx	social history
SLE	systemic lupus erythematosus
SMA7	serum chemistries: Na, K, Cl, HCO_3, BUN, Cr, Glu
SNRI	serotonin-norepinephrine reuptake inhibitor
SNS	sympathetic nervous system

SSRI	selective serotonin reuptake inhibitor
SWF	single white female
SWM	single white male
T_3	triiodothyronine
T_4	thyroxine
TBI	traumatic brain injury
TCA	tricyclic antidepressant
Temp	temperature
TENS	transcutaneous electrical nerve stimulation
TFT	thyroid function test
THF	tetrahydrofolate
TIA	transient ischemic attack
TID	*ter in die* (three times a day)
TSH	thyroid-stimulating hormone
UA	urinalysis
UTI	urinary tract infection
Utox	urine toxicology
VDRL	Venereal Disease Research Laboratories (test for syphilis)
VS	vital signs
WBC	white blood cells
WDWN	well-developed, well-nourished
WNL	within normal limits

Blueprints

CLINICAL CASES
IN PSYCHIATRY

I

Adult Patients Who Present in the Office or Inpatient Psychiatry

"I Don't Feel Like Myself"

CC/ID: 20-year-old single white male who, as a Junior, presents to his college mental health clinic complaining of a month of "not feeling like myself . . . wanting to sleep all the time."

HPI: Mr. R awakens early in the morning but, still fatigued, stays in bed staring at the ceiling. He describes poor appetite, energy, and concentration, does not enjoy anything, and is feeling passively suicidal. He has been able to do the reading for his classes, but barely, feeling as though he cannot retain anything he reads. He has failed to hand in two short papers because "I just couldn't." He states that he doesn't have any plans to kill himself, but if he didn't wake up tomorrow, that would be "a relief." He is an English major and describes that at baseline he has no difficulty writing or concentrating—"I used to love this stuff, but now I just can't do anything right."

Mental Status Exam: *General:* he is mildly disheveled, unshaven, and his hair is not brushed. He is sitting in a chair with shoulders hunched, making poor eye contact, and is psychomotorically retarded. *Speech:* somewhat slow, with low volume, and lacks normal prosody; his speech latency is increased. *Mood:* initially described as "bad" which, upon further clarification, is "empty . . . sad . . . numb . . . frustrated." *Affect:* dysphoric and painful, constricted, and congruent. *Thought process:* linear and goal directed, though occasionally he struggles to find the best way to describe his emotional experiences. *Thought content:* manifests ruminations and preoccupations about his worthlessness and how his life is "going nowhere." No delusional material is elicited. Though he is experiencing passive suicidal ideations, he has no active ideation, intent, or plan. He denies perceptual changes and does not appear distracted or preoccupied with internal stimuli. *Cognition:* grossly intact for knowledge, memory, and abstraction, as well as orientation to time and place. *Insight:* fair (he knows that he needs help, but he thinks that everything is hopeless and nothing will actually help) and his social judgment is intact.

THOUGHT QUESTIONS

■ How are diagnoses organized in psychiatry?

■ How was his exam described? What is the "mental status exam"?

DISCUSSION

Psychiatric diagnoses are formulated in accordance with the multi-axial scheme of the Diagnostic and Statistical Manual of Mental Disorders Fourth Edition, Text Revision (DSM-IV-TR). The American Psychiatric Association developed this for use in clinical work, education, and research in 1994 to allow for uniformity in psychiatric evaluation and communication between colleagues.

A "mental disorder" is a "clinically significant psychological or behavioral condition that causes distress or disability in an individual, or increased risk of disability, loss of important freedom, pain, or death." It is not merely an understandable response to an event such as the death of a loved one.

The DSM-IV-TR divides mental disorders into groups according to defining features and criteria. Because the etiology of most psychiatric illnesses is not well defined, in the DSM illnesses are represented by symptom clusters rather than etiologies. The categories, therefore, may not actually represent discrete entities, and individuals with the same diagnosis may actually be etiologically heterogeneous. That said, the DSM represents a comprehensive and widely used system of statistical and phenomenological classification. The DSM provides for a "multiaxial" diagnosis, in appreciation of the fact that psychiatric illnesses are complex and have multiple influences (Table 1-1).

The specialized exam in psychiatry is called the **mental status exam,** although in certain settings, psychiatrists are still expected to do physical and neurological exams in the assessment of their patients. The mental status exam is an primarily objective **cross-sectional** (i.e., snapshot) evaluation that is organized by psychological faculty (i.e., emotional, cognitive, perceptual, motor functioning). In it, each aspect of a patient's presentation is broken down into component parts; for example, speech is distinguished from syntax and the form of one's thinking, which is further distinguished from the content of what one is thinking, and so on (Table 1-2).

TABLE 1-1   The five Axes of DSM-IV-TR

Axis	Definition	Examples
Axis I	Disorders or conditions requiring clinical attention (course specifiers, such as degree of remission or severity, may be used)	Major depression, bipolar disorder, schizophrenia
Axis II	Personality disorders and mental retardation	Antisocial personality disorder, dependent personality disorder, mental retardation
Axis III	General medical conditions	Hypertension, cerebrovascular accident, gout
Axis IV	Psychosocial and environmental problems and stressors (the severity is often included)	Divorce, death of spouse, occupational problems, legal problems
Axis V	Global assessment of functioning (100 point scale, broken down into 10 categories)	91–100: superior functioning, no symptoms 61–71: some mild symptoms or difficulties, but generally functioning pretty well 21–30: behavior considerably influenced by delusions, serious impairment in communication or judgment

TABLE 1-2   Elements of the Mental Status Examination

- Appearance
- Activity and behavior
- Attitude, cooperation, and relatedness
- Speech
- Mood / Affect
- Thought process
- Thought content
- Suicidality, homicidality
- Perception
- Insight, judgment, impulsivity
- Concentration, memory, cognition, +/− MMSE

Many disorders have classic presentations on mental status exam. The man described above has a classic episode of major depressive disorder. Not only do his symptoms reflect this (e.g., depressed mood, decreased sleep, energy, appetite, and concentration), but his exam is also consistent with a major depression. After one month of treatment with an antidepressant and a course of psychotherapy, his exam is as follows: Well-groomed, calm, and cooperative, with good eye contact, and no psychomotor agitation or retardation. His speech is of normal volume, rate, and tone and without increased latency. His mood is "much better," and his affect is more neutral and reactive. His thought process is linear and goal directed, and his thought content is no longer ruminative. He is hopeful and has no suicidal or homicidal ideations. He denies perceptual changes. His cognitive functioning is intact. His insight is good and his judgment is intact. He reports that he was able to finish his term paper last night.

CASE CONTINUED

A patient with mania may provide another classic case example. In this disorder the exam might be as follows: This 31-year-old woman is dressed in a low-cut gold lamé blouse and floral scarf, wearing a great deal of hastily applied makeup. She is psychomotorically agitated, frequently standing, walking, and then sitting down. She manifests a seductive demeanor throughout the interview, though interspersed with some hostility. Her speech is pressured and rapid. Her mood is described as "excellent, fantastic, stupendous, and fabulous," Her affect is expansive and elated. Her thought process is rapid with flight of ideas. Her thought content manifests grandiose delusions (e.g., she thinks that she has been chosen to "go to the UN with Bono to deliver her theory for world peace"). She denies suicidality or homicidality ("Everyone should just live forever.") She has no hallucinations or other altered perceptions. Her insight is poor, thinking that nothing is wrong. Her judgment is impaired, having impulsively spent $5000 on new clothing for travel to the United Nations, having had sex with three strangers in the last 2 days, and having been brought in by the police because she was singing and starting to disrobe at the central fountain in Lincoln Center in New York. She is cognitively intact, although extremely distractible.

In doing a mental status exam, there are number of terms that make effective communication about a patient and his or her condition possible. A list with embedded glossary is below.

Glossary

Appearance

Actual and apparent ages
Grooming, hygiene
Attire
Body habitus
Physical "abnormalities"
Tattoos, scars, body piercings, etc.
Jewelry and cosmetics

Attitude, cooperation, and relatedness
Relatedness: ability to display normal human reciprocal interaction (well, fair, poor, odd)
Eye contact: continuous, good, intermittent, fleeting, absent
Attentiveness to interviewer: bored, distractible, waxing/waning, preoccupied
Attitude/Demeanor:

- Passive—taking no part; offering no opposition; submissive

- Dependent—relies excessively on examiner for support or aid

- Indifferent—lack of concern, interest, or feeling

- Hostile—unfriendly; adverse; antagonistic

- Suspicious—mistrusting; questions motives

- Manipulative—artful management or control by shrewd use of influence or handling

- Dramatic—vivid; highly emotional; action-oriented

- Others; seductive; cooperative; calm; eager; defensive; antagonistic; childish; sullen; withdrawn

Psychomotor behavior
Agitation: excessive bodily movements; hand wringing; pacing
Retardation: slowness of bodily movements
Abnormal movements: tremors; stereotypies; involuntary movements; tics; movements associated with tardive dyskinesia; etc.

Speech
Volume
Rate: slow; fast; pressured
Rhythm/Prosody: fluctuation in tone of speech; inflection
Articulation: clarity
Spontaneity: degree of engagement
Latency: interval to answer or connect sentences

Mood

The patient's subjective experience of her or his internal feeling state (self-described).

Parameters include *quality* (i.e., depressed; anxious; elated) and *intensity* (adjective qualifier); it is important to ask more about mood than the patient's one-word answer.

Affect (Figure 1-1)
The external appreciation of the patient's affective state (i.e., how mood is shown to examiner).
Quality: What is it? For example; depressed; anxious; neutral; etc.
Quantity: How expressive are the person's states of emotional expression? For example, expansive (broad range of emotion); full range (normal); constricted (decreased range); blunted (more decreased); flat (absolute inexpressiveness); etc.
Stability: Does it shift? For example, labile (rapidly changing); reactive (normal); fixed (not changing); etc.
Appropriateness: Is it consistent with what the patient is thinking about?

Thought process (Figure 1-2)

The organization, coherence, quantity of associations, and flow of ideas; the route the patient takes from one thought to another.

Linear: goal-directed

Circumstantial: ideas clearly linked; indirect and overly detailed with irrelevant additions; eventually wanders back to original point

Tangential: ideas linked; never gets back to original point

Flight of ideas: ideas linked but with rapid shifts in topic; associations are still evident both to patient and examiner

Loose associations: syntax is intact; links between ideas or contiguous thoughts are illogical or nonsensical to examiner but make sense to the patient

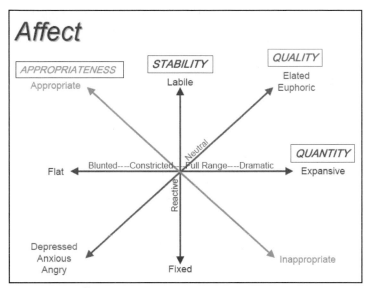

FIGURE 1-1.   Affect.

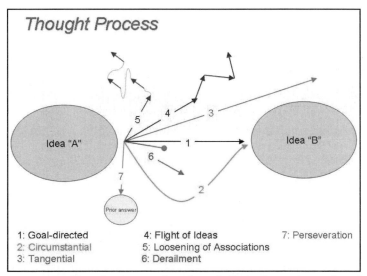

FIGURE 1-2. Thought process (numbers indicate increasing order of pathology).

Derailment: syntax intact, but speech shifts topic strangely; no meaningful connections, even to patients themselves

Thought blocking: sudden cessation in a train of thought that the patient cannot explain

Retardation: very slow thinking may impede reaching goal

Word salad: words intact; no syntax; seemingly random words produced in sequence

Clang associations: speech constructed on the basis of sound, not meaning, syntax, or logical flow

Echolalia: automatic repetition of someone else's speech

Perseveration: automatic repetition of a response despite change in questioning; involuntary pathological persistence of a single response or idea (different than preoccupation)

Neologisms: made up words or phrases that have idiosyncratic meanings for patients

Thought content

Helplessness/Hopelessness

Rumination/Preoccupation: voluntarily repetitive and often circular speculations; excessive worrying

Obsession: recurrent, persistent, unwanted, uncontrollable thought that cannot be eliminated; usually recognized by the patient as irrational or absurd

Overvalued idea: idea that preoccupies a person and alters behavior; less firmly held than delusions (e.g., superstitions)

Idea of reference: incorrect interpretation of incidents and events as having direct reference to one's self (e.g., TV is talking to me); a delusion of reference is held with delusional conviction

Delusion: fixed false belief; out of keeping with educational and cultural background; specify type (e.g., paranoid, religious, grandiose, guilty, jealous, etc.)

Hyperreligiosity: detrimental excessive concern with spiritual and religious matters; not necessarily of delusional nature

Phobia: marked and persistent fear that is experienced as unwanted and excessive; clearly circumscribed

Poverty: decreased content; also known as impoverished

Suicidality or homicidality: Clarify ideation, intent, plan, action

Perception

Illusion: misinterpretation in context of a real stimulus (e.g., towel on door is initially mistaken for intruder)

Hallucination: sensory perception in the absence of an actual external stimulus; specify type and content (e.g., auditory, visual, olfactory, gustatory, tactile)

Hypnagogic hallucination: occurs in semiconscious state at verge of sleep

Hypnapompic hallucination: occurs in semiconscious state at verge of awakening

Depersonalization: person has feeling that his or her actions seem automatic, mechanistic

Derealization: external world seems like a dream; disconnected

Micropsia: seeing things as smaller than they are

Hyperesthesia: perceptual experiences seem more intense (e.g., louder, brighter)

Déjà vu: feeling of familiarity

Insight/Judgment

Insight: awareness of illness, symptoms, limitations, level of functioning, need for treatment

Judgment: ability to survey situations and make reasonable decisions; encompassing judgment about social, financial, planning, and other issues; includes impulse control and engagement in dangerous behaviors

Intellectual/Cognitive functioning

Folstein's Mini-Mental State Exam (MMSE) covers orientation to time, place, immediate and delayed recall, naming, repeating, copying, attention, and concentration. Even if MMSE is not conducted, orientation to person (self and examiner) and long-term memory should be assessed in the interview.

QUESTIONS

1-1. Which of the following is a disorder of the form of thought?
A. Delusion
B. Hallucination
C. Tangentiality
D. Lability
E. Preoccupation

1-2. Ms. G. is a 21-year-old woman who presents on exam with psychomotor agitation, pressured speech, flight of ideas, and grandiose delusions. Given these findings on mental status exam, the first item on your differential diagnosis is
A. Schizoaffective disorder
B. Schizophrenia
C. Brief psychotic disorder
D. Schizophrenifrom disorder
E. Bipolar disorder

1-3. Mr. P. is a 57-year-old man who presents for his monthly medication appointment and manifests the following MSE: fairly groomed, guarded, poor eye contact, mood "okay" and not further specified, affect blunted, speech goal directed, some thought blocking, poverty of content, denies hallucinations but some paranoid delusions. Given these findings on mental status exam, what is the first item on your differential diagnosis?
A. Major depression
B. Schizoaffective disorder
C. Schizophrenia
D. Bipolar disorder
E. Adjustment disorder with depressed mood

1-4. Ms. W. is a 24-year-old woman who is sitting in the emergency room and looks scared. On exam she is cooperative, but has some psychomotor agitation, is picking at the sheets, and describes feeling like bugs are crawling over her. She is paranoid and very anxious that people are trying to hurt her. Given her presentation, the most likely etiology of her symptoms is
A. Major depression with psychotic features
B. Schizophrenia
C. Schizoaffective disorder
D. Substance use
E. Mania

ANSWERS

1-1. C. Tangentiality is a disorder of the form of thought, marked by the patient's inability to focus on his or her ultimate idea or goal. Though the syntax of the thoughts makes sense and the ideas are linked, the patient seems to veer off target and never returns to his or her original point. Tangentiality is more pathological than circumstantiality (which can be normal), and less so than flight of ideas and loosening of associations. Hallucinations are disorders of perception. Delusions and preoccupations are disorders of thought content. Lability is a disorder of affect.

1-2. E. This mental status presentation is classic for bipolar disorder, which would be at the top of the differential. Depending on the delusions, and whether she had psychotic symptoms for 2 weeks in the absence of mood symptoms, this could be schizoaffective disorder. The other diagnoses are possible and would be clarified on careful history and time course. Brief psychotic disorder requires at most 1 month of psychotic symptoms followed by full resolution, schizophreniform disorder 1 to 6 months of symptoms, and schizophrenia requires at least 6 months of psychotic symptoms.

1-3. C. This is a classic description of someone with schizophrenia who is suffering from predominantly negative symptoms. Although poor grooming and eye contact can be seen in major depression, the presence of thought blocking, poverty of content, and delusions, as well as the mood being "okay" do not point to depression. He has no clear mood symptoms at present, making schizoaffective and bipolar-depressed less likely. A complete history would clarify the extent that these other syndromes should be included in the differential.

1-4. D. Though these symptoms may be present in multiple different syndromes, substance intoxication always needs to be ruled out prior to diagnosing a non-substance-induced condition. In this case, the patient's symptoms of formication (the sensation that bugs are crawling over one's body) and persecutory delusions are most commonly seen in the context of cocaine or amphetamine intoxication, and are commonly found together with anxiety and agitation. While somatic delusions may be present in a psychotic depression, they are generally focused on a belief that one's body is rotting or not functioning well, and they are usually associated with significantly depressed mood, social withdrawal, and other signs of depression.

SUGGESTED READINGS

Diagnostic and Statistical Manual of Mental Disorders, Fourth Edition, Text Revision. Washington, DC, American Psychiatric Association, 2000.

Manley MRS. Psychiatric interview, history, and mental status examination, In: Sadock BJ, Sadock VA, eds. *Kaplan & Sadock's Comprehensive Textbook of Psychiatry.* 7th ed. Philadelphia: Lippincott Williams & Wilkins; 2000.

Sims ACP. *Symptoms in the Mind: An Introduction to Descriptive Psychopathology.* 3rd rev ed. London: Saunders; 2003.

"I'm Tired All the Time"

CC/ID: 46-year-old man complaining of increased difficulties, including daytime sleepiness, poor concentration, and impaired ability to do his job.

HPI: O.W. is obese at 380 pounds, and he stands 5 feet 9 inches tall. He says his wife thinks that his personality has changed, with increased irritability. He has become afraid to drive his car, as he has fallen asleep at the wheel a couple of times. This is a major concern because he has a significant freeway commute to work. His wife also complains that his snoring has become significantly worse and she is threatening to move downstairs so she can sleep. He has also noticed that he is getting headaches in the morning, and this is associated with his becoming more forgetful and very sleepy in the afternoons. He notes that these difficulties are getting him down, though he denies frank anhedonia or depressed mood for significant periods of time. He enjoys his work and time with his family, but he is worried about his relationship with his wife and his future career prospects.

PPHx: No past psychiatric history

PMHx: Treated for hypertension for the past 10 years; blood pressure is fairly well maintained.

Meds: Lisinopril 20 mg po qd

Allergies: NKDA

FHx: Obesity and NIDDM

SHx: Married, two children aged 8 and 10. Works as a forklift driver in a large warehouse facility. Denied ever smoking; drinks "three or four" beers every evening. His wife works part-time as a school receptionist.

Labs: CBC and serum chemistries (including liver function) are within normal limits.

MSE: *General:* obese man, appears older than stated age, appropriately dressed in casual attire. Good eye contact, rapport, and well-related. No abnormal movements appreciated, no PMA/R. *Speech:* normal rate, volume, and tone. *Mood:* described as "OK," though upon further inquiry he describes moderate frustration. Affect anxious and constricted. *Thought process:* logical and goal directed. *Thought content:* denied SI/HI/PI/AH/VH. *Insight/ judgment:* good. *Cognitive function:* MMSE score 28/30, missing 2 points on serial 7's.

THOUGHT QUESTIONS

- What is probably going on with this man?
- How is the diagnosis made definitively?
- What treatments are available for this disorder?

DISCUSSION

Epidemiological studies have reported that about 5% of the population has moderate or severe sleep apnea. **Apnea is defined as the complete cessation of airflow for at least 10 seconds.** Associated findings include decreased blood oxygen saturation as well as sleep fragmentation on EEG. Risk factors for sleep apnea include **male gender** (M:F ~ 3:1), **family history, increased age, obesity, certain craniofacial features** (maxillary and mandibular abnormalities, small chins, and high, narrow palates), and **ethnicity** (increased rates in African Americans, East Asians, Mexicans, and Pacific Islanders). Consumption of **alcohol** in the evening may exacerbate symptoms. **Hypothyroidism** may also be a risk factor. Individuals with obstructive sleep apnea (OSA) may complain about **cognitive and performance difficulties, which may be directly related to the level of hypoxemia**. Cognitive functions that may be affected include **attention, information processing, memory, and executive functioning** (task planning and completion). Both fragmented sleep patterns and nocturnal hypoxemia/hypercarbia contribute to these deficits in cognition and performance. Treatment with continuous positive airway pressure (CPAP) may improve these deficits. About 80% of patients with OSA report cognitive impairments and daytime sleepiness, and almost 50% report personality changes, both toward the more irritable and the more depressive ends. Sleep apnea is a major element in the differential diagnosis of major depressive disorder, specifically that marked by cognitive abnormalities and anergia. Impaired attention and concentration may affect work performance and lead to increased accidents, adding to the impairment in the individual's quality of life. Clinicians may have a duty to report an individual who is unfit to drive due to falling asleep, depending on individual state legislation. Patients with OSA have a two- to fourfold increased risk of motor vehicle accidents. Patients need to be educated about the increased risk of driving while sleepy and should use rest stops, caffeine, and naps to avoid such difficulties. Obesity can lead to the development of sleep apnea, hypertension, and type II diabetes; however, there may actually be an association between sleep apnea and the development of both glucose intolerance and insulin resistance.

If suspected in history and evaluation, the diagnosis of sleep apnea is confirmed by a sleep study/polysomnography, which shows evidence of complete or partial obstruction of the pharynx during sleep, causing apneic episodes, marked by oxygen desaturations five or more times per hour on the respiratory disturbance index. The loudness and disturbance caused by associated snoring or snorting can cause partners to sleep separately resulting in marital discord. Partners may actually notice the apnea episodes and be frightened by them. The sleep of OSA sufferers may be very restless, tossing and turning and sweating a lot. Up to a third of patients may actually complain of choking feelings or difficulty breathing which interferes with sleep. Nocturnal dyspnea may also be caused by cardiac failure, which may coexist with OSA. Other relatively common symptoms in OSA include bruxism, dry mouth (with increased need to drink fluids at night), nocturia, and reflux.

Table 2-1 lists the treatments for OSA. Pharmacological stimulants can be effective for daytime drowsiness, but there is concern about the potential of abuse and side effects. Modafinil is a wakefulness-promoting agent with an unknown mechanism of action, which is effective in increasing daytime alertness, attention (vigilance), and memory performance; importantly, it appears to lack the peripheral sympathomimetic effects observed with amphetamines. The gold standard of treatment for OSA remains CPAP by nasal mask. Side effects may include feelings of claustrophobia, skin rash, nasal congestion, nosebleeds, and even aerophagy. Very rare more dangerous side effects include pneumothorax, pneumocephaly, subcutaneous emphysema, and raised intraocular pressure. CPAP should be used cautiously after facial surgery or neurosurgery. Side effects may decrease patient's compliance with the CPAP and should be minimized if possible (Figures. 2-1 and 2-2).

TABLE 2-1   Treatments of Sleep Apnea

Behavioral	Weight loss
	Smoking cessation
	Sleep hygiene
	Avoid sleep deprivation
	Sleep in lateral recumbent position and avoid supine
	Avoid alcohol, barbiturates, hypnotic sedatives, and opiates
Mechanical	Continuous positive airway pressure
	Nasal dilators
	Head of bed elevation
Pharmacological	Hormone replacement therapy
	Adjunctive oxygen therapy
	Protriptyline (TCA)
	SSRIs
	Buspirone (serotonin agonist)
	Modafinil
Surgical	Correction of craniofacial abnormalities

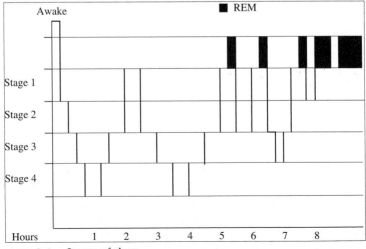

FIGURE 2-1.   Stages of sleep

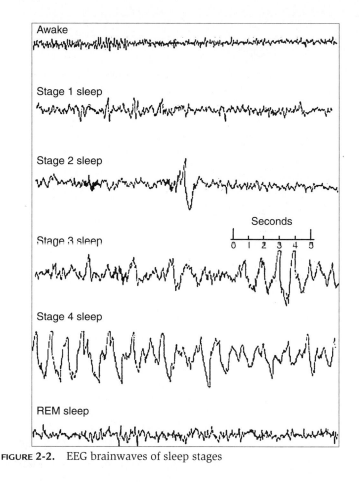

FIGURE 2-2. EEG brainwaves of sleep stages

CASE CONTINUED

You refer Mr. W for polysomnography, which confirms the diagnosis of sleep apnea. You counsel both his wife and him about the dangers of driving while sleepy, and provide information about sleep hygiene and behavioral interventions. You encourage him to persist with the CPAP machine and to lose weight. When he returns in 6 months, he has lost 20 pounds, his concentration and daytime sleepiness have improved, and his wife sends her thanks.

QUESTIONS

2-1. M.J. is an 18-year-old African-American man who has presented to your clinic with complaints of daytime sleepiness. He almost wrecked his car when he feel asleep at a traffic light. Which of the following symptoms or tests will aid you in your diagnosis?

A. Catalepsy
B. Catatonia
C. Normal MSLT results
D. Sleep paralysis
E. Visual hallucinations

2-2. Which of the following is a treatment for the above condition and its associated symptoms?

A. Nortriptyline
B. Pemoline
C. Scheduled naps
D. Benzodiazepines
E. Psychosurgery

2-3. Which of the following psychiatric disorders is correctly matched with its associated changes in sleep?

A. Depression | Increased stages 3 and 4, decreased REM latency
B. Anxiety | Decreased stages 1 and 2
C. Alzheimer's disease | Increased REM and stages 3 and 4
D. Alzheimer's disease | Decreased REM and stages 3 and 4
E. Creutzfeldt Jakob | Triphasic waves

2-4. The parents of a 6-year-old present to the clinic asking for your advice. Their son has been a normal child but recently has been experiencing episodes during which he appears to be waking up in a nightmare. This has happened several times over the past month. During these episodes he is difficult to wake, is obviously terrified, and is screaming loudly. What advice do you give them?

A. Nightmares are very common and occur early in the sleep cycle.
B. Night terrors are less common and occur early in the sleep cycle.
C. Night terrors do not run in families.
D. Nightmares occur late during REM sleep.
E. Night terrors occur during REM sleep.

ANSWERS

2-1. D. The classical tetrad of symptoms in narcolepsy include cataplexy (sudden loss of muscle tone, may cause falling to the floor), sleep paralysis, an abnormal Multiple Sleep Latency Test (MSLT), and hypnagogic (going to sleep) or hypnopompic (waking up) hallucinations. The MSLT is an EEG performed during the day, which shows the subject entering REM sleep within 10 minutes of falling asleep, and is virtually diagnostic of this condition. Sleep paralysis is described as an unpleasant experience where the individual is actually awake but unable to move. Only a quarter of patients with narcolepsy have the classic tetrad of symptoms. The onset of symptoms is usually between 10 and 20 years of age.

2-2. C. Scheduled naps have been shown to be helpful in the treatment of narcolepsy. Nortriptyline is not used, but clomipramine or selective serotonergic reuptake inhibitors (SSRIs) have been used to treat cataplexy. Pemoline is a stimulant used to treat attention deficit hyperactivity disorder; it has shown liver toxicity. Pharmacological stimulants used to treat narcolepsy include caffeine, methylphenidate (Ritalin), dextroamphetamine (Dexedrine), and modafinil (Provigil). Neither benzodiazepines nor psychosurgery is used to treat this condition.

2-3. D. Alzheimer disease is associated with several changes in sleep pattern and architecture, including increased sleep fragmentation, decreased stages 3 and 4 sleep, and decreased REM. These are accompanied with generalized decreases in sleep efficiency. Depression is associated with reductions in stages 3 and 4 sleep and decreased REM latency (i.e., REM occurs earlier in the night). Anxiety and panic disorders may be associated with increased sleep latency (i.e., taking longer to fall asleep), increases in the lighter stages 1 and 2 of sleep, and decreased sleep efficiency. These patients may also have difficulty staying asleep and may have multiple awakenings during the night. Those with alcohol dependence may have increased REM sleep and increased delta activity on EEG. Triphasic waves are seen most commonly in hepatic encephalopathy, and they are not associated with sleep.

2-4. B. Along with sleepwalking, both nightmares and night terrors are parasomnias. Night terrors run in families and occur in about 3% of children, usually between the ages of 4 and 7 years. They occur during non-REM stage 4 sleep, early in the night, usually within the first couple hours of sleep. During such an episode, the child is difficult to arouse and may be obviously terrified, thrashing about and screaming. Treatment usually involves reassurance, but if the condition persists, a behavioral intervention such as a waking schedule may be needed. Nightmares are fairly common and usually occur late in sleep, during REM, and the child is easily roused. Treatment consists of reassurance and supportive measures. Sleepwalking, like night terrors, occurs during non-REM stage 4, usually early in the night, during the first couple of hours of sleep. However, somnambulism can occur in both children and adults. Individuals do not remember these episodes (as with night terrors), and treatments include safety precautions and avoiding being deprived of sleep.

SUGGESTED READINGS

Ng A, Gotsopoulous H, Darendeliler AM, Cistulli PA. Oral appliance therapy for obstructive sleep apnea. *Treat Respir Med.* 2005;4(6):409–422.

Pagel JF. Nightmares and disorders of dreaming. *Am Family Physician.* 2000;61(7):2037–2042.

Raizen DM, Thorton MBA, Pack AI. Genetic basis for sleep regulation and sleep disorders. *Semin Neurol.* 2006;26 (5): 467–483.

Saunmäki T, Jehkonen M. A review of executive functions in obstructive sleep apnea syndrome. *Acta Neurol Scand* 2007;115:1–11.

"He Seems Like a Different Person"

CC/ID: 46-year-old married male who presents to your office with his wife who notes that he has seemed like a different person lately.

HPI: A.S. describes feeling a little **depressed** lately (past 3 months) and reports **anhedonia,** loss of interest in usual activities, **poor energy,** and **loss of concentration and libido.** About 1 year ago, he was involved in a motor vehicle accident in which he received a **traumatic brain injury (TBI)** with loss of consciousness, a fractured pelvis, and several fractured ribs. In the emergency room, he had a Glasgow Coma Scale score of 10, and he was unconscious for about 2 days, followed by posttraumatic amnesia that lasted for about 24 hours. His recovery has been slow, and he continues to attend outpatient physical therapy. Additionally, he has been experiencing generalized tonic-clonic **seizures** which now appear to be under control with medication. His wife complains that his **personality and behavior have changed,** and that he is becoming more difficult to live with. She further describes that he has become very **irritable,** with poor concentration, and she's not sure how he is ever going to return to work. This is causing financial hardship, as she does not work outside the home. He has fallen out with several of his close friends and even with two of his siblings, which is very unlike his old self. He spends most of his time sitting in front of the television watching sports but **does not seem to remember** the outcomes a short time later when asked.

SHx: A.S. worked as a salesman for a large agricultural machinery company and traveled much prior to his accident. Currently he is receiving state disability payments. He is married and has two daughters, aged 12 and 10. He has a college education. He does not drink or smoke and has never taken any illicit substances.

Meds: Acetaminophen/hydrocodone (500 mg/5 mg), one tablet every 6 hours as needed for pain, phenytoin 200 mg po BID

Allergies: NKDA

PMIIx.   Apart from MVA, no significant illness.

FHx: Father was an alcoholic who died at 56 from a stroke. His mother is alive and well, as are his four siblings.

Labs: Phenytoin level 11 (range 10–20)

MSE: *General:* appears stated age; hygiene, eye contact, and rapport are all fair. Appears irritable when his wife tries to contribute information. No gross abnormalities of movement are noted and his gait is normal. *Speech:* mildly dysarthric at times. *Mood:* "A little depressed . . . I'm okay, though." *Affect:* constricted, neutral. *Thought process:* slow and circumstantial at times. *Thought content:* denies any psychotic symptoms or thoughts of harming himself or others. *Insight:* limited into his level of impairment. *Judgment:* impaired. *Cognitive:* 27/30 on the Mini-Mental State Exam, missing 1 point for date, 1 on short-term recall, and 1 on attention and concentration.

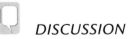

THOUGHT QUESTIONS

- What has happened to this man?
- What are the psychiatric comorbidities associated with TBI?
- What can you do to help?

DISCUSSION

TBIs are a major cause of morbidity and mortality in the United States. Head injuries are frequently classified and assessed in the ER by the **Glasgow Coma Scale,** which incorporates measures of eye opening, verbal response, and best motor responses; 13 to 15 is considered mild, 9 to 12 is moderate, and 3 to 8 is severe. Head injuries result from many different types of mechanical forces at work during an impact: static and dynamic loading, acceleration (rotational and translational), strain, and coup-contrecoup. On a cellular level, the membrane lipid bilayer may be disrupted, impairing axonal transport; oxidation may induce genes that alter nerve growth factors and amyloid precursor proteins; and glutamate induces excitotoxicity and calcium entry into cells causing **cell death** (apoptosis). Free radicals are released, macrophages accumulate, and programmed cell death occurs. Arterial hypotension and intracranial hypertension may lead to a **decrease in cerebral perfusion.** The resulting injuries may be ischemic, diffuse axonal, or vascular edematous in nature. There may also be **hemorrhaging** into the ventricles, the brain parenchyma, and the extradural, subdural, or subarachnoid spaces. The effects of TBI are greater on the developing brain (those under 5 years) than the older brain, and **75% of preschool-aged brain-injured children may be unable to work as adults.** Language disorders develop more commonly in children with TBI. **IQ may be permanently reduced** (performance more than verbal), and math skills appear to be impaired more than spelling or reading skills. Other functions that may be impaired include both **executive functioning** (ability to plan/sequence tasks and regulate behavior) and visual perception. **Memory is usually the most affected cognitive function,** with recent memory affected more than distant or remote memory (Ribot's law). Explicit memory is affected more than implicit memory, and patients also tend to report experiencing an increased subjective loss compared to objective findings of those close to them. Anterograde amnesia usually persists longer than retrograde amnesia. Subtle changes may require a specialized neuropsychological battery to be detected. Brain imaging such as PET or SPECT may show decreases in metabolism or perfusion not detected by other imaging methods.

Psychiatric comorbidities include (see Table 3-1 for correlation with location of injury):
1. **Depression:** Increased risk with left-sided lesions. Not predicted by severity of illness. Inversely related to level of social supports. Increased risk of suicide.
2. **Mania:** A type of secondary mania, not associated with particular lesions. Less common than depression. Clinically looks like classical mania seen in bipolar disorder and is treated in the same manner.
3. **Anxiety disorders:** Those who develop acute stress disorder are at increased risk of developing posttraumatic stress disorder (PTSD). Risk of developing PTSD is also related to premorbid functioning and coping skills. May not have flashbacks. Right hemisphere lesion reported to be more associated with anxiety disorders than are left-sided lesions.
4. **Psychosis:** No association with lesion location. Tends to be paranoid in theme, with hallucinations.

TABLE 3-1   Frontal Lobe Disorders After TBI

Location of Injury	Symptoms and Signs
Orbitofrontal	*Disinhibition syndrome:* behavioral disinhibition, with acquired sociopathy, with impulsive and inappropriate behaviors and a lack of affective regulation
Mediofrontal	*Apathetic syndrome:* amotivational syndrome, inattention to environment, a lack of intentional behavior, and even akinetic mutism
Dorsolateral	*Disorganized syndrome:* inflexible, rigid thinking with perseverative answers, difficulty integrating sensations into a whole, difficulty switching cognitive sets, and poor self monitoring

5. **Personality changes:** May develop antisocial or borderline traits. Difficult to measure. Gross personality changes most common, and include irritability.
6. **Aggression:** More likely with frontal injuries. Increased risk in those with premorbid substance abuse or premorbid aggressive/impulsive tendencies.

 CASE CONTINUED

You take a comprehensive history and assess both cognitive and neurological functioning. Computed tomography (CT) scan reveals **frontal encephalomalacia** with some spike and wave activity on EEG. You arrange for the patient to undergo a comprehensive neuropsychological assessment and refer him to a specialized brain injury rehab program. You advise his wife to obtain support from friends and family or a local support group for caregivers of individuals with TBIs, to try to minimize caregiver stress. For treatment of his depressive symptoms and irritability, you start him on a low dose of citalopram, which he tolerates well and is doing better at followup.

QUESTIONS

3-1. His wife asks, "Will he always be like this?" Which of the following factors is associated with a better outcome after head injury?
   A. An initial Glasgow Coma Scale score of 8
   B. Posttraumatic amnesia lasting 1 to 7 days
   C. High level of premorbid functioning

    D. Recovery level at 1 month
    E. Apolipoprotein E4

3-2. The incidence of TBIs per year in the United States is approximately
    A. 5 million
    B. 2 million
    C. 1 million
    D. 500,000
    E. 100,000

3-3. Which of the following is most likely following a closed head injury?
    A. Seizure disorder prevalence of approximately 20%
    B. Seizure disorder prevalence of approximately 15%
    C. Damage to the frontal lobes and the temporal tips
    D. Damage to the cerebellum
    E. Damage to the occipital poles

3-4. Which of the following best describes the treatment of psychiatric comorbidities in patients with TBIs?
    A. Antidepressants do not affect the seizure threshold.
    B. SSRIs may make patients more agitated.
    C. Phenytoin increases the plasma level of fluoxetine.
    D. Fluoxetine decreases the level of phenytoin.
    E. Levels do not need to be checked more often than in usual clinical practice with non-TBI patients.

ANSWERS

3-1. C. Higher levels of premorbid functioning and an absence of premorbid psychiatric conditions are associated with better outcome post head injury. Children with learning disorders and adults with a history of substance abuse have a worse prognosis. A Glasgow Coma Scale score of 8 reflects a severe injury and resultant poorer prognosis. The length of posttraumatic amnesia (PTA) predicts the return to independent functioning: PTA <1 hour implies a slight concussion, and individuals usually return to work within 4 to 6 weeks; PTA between 1 and 24 hours indicates a moderate concussion with a return to work in 1 to 2 months; PTA between 1 and 7 days indicates a severe concussion and a return to work between 2 and 4 months; PTA over a week indicates a very severe concussion, and it may take up to 8 months for the individual to return to work. The recovery level at 3 months has been reported to predict future recovery, with the majority of recovery occurring at 6 months, even in those with severe head injuries. After brain trauma there is increased expression of amyloid precursor protein and increased deposition of amyloid beta peptide, so those individuals with ApoE4 and a head injury actually have a poorer outcome.

3-2. B. There are approximately 2 million TBIs annually in the United States and between 50,000 and 55,000 deaths per year.

3-3. C. The areas most likely to be injured during a closed head injury include the frontal poles, temporal lobes (particularly the lateral and inferior surfaces), and the cortex next to the sylvian fissures. The prevalence of seizure disorders after a closed head injury is approximately 5%, but this increases to 30% after an open head injury.

3-4. B. SSRIs may cause increased agitation or even induce mania in some individuals with TBI. With TBI patients, as with geriatric patients, it is best to start with low doses and increase slowly. Use medications with low anticholinergic profiles to avoid additive problems (e.g., interacting with other antimuscarinic agents or inducing delirium). Head injury itself may induce enzyme induction, and medication levels may have to be followed more closely in TBI patients; this is of particular relevance for anticonvulsant agents. Carbamazepine, phenytoin, and phenobarbital may induce the metabolism of some antidepressants, and carbamazepine induces its own metabolism. Fluoxetine inhibits the metabolism of phenytoin, causing increased plasma levels. If depression is severe, ECT may be used.

SUGGESTED READINGS

Rao V, Lyketsos CG. Psychiatric aspects of traumatic brain injury. *Psychiatr Clin North Am.* 2002;25(1):43–69.

Lee HB, Lyketsos CG, Rao V. Pharmacological management of the psychiatric aspects of traumatic brain injury. *Int Rev Psychiatry.* 2003;15:359–370.

Handel SF, Ovitt L, Spiro JR, Rao V. Affective disorder and personality change in a patient with traumatic brain injury. *Psychosomatics* 2007;48:1 67–70.

NIH. Diagnosis and treatment of attention deficit hyperactivity disorder (ADHD). NIH Consensus Statement, 1998.

"We're Losing Our Son"

CC/ID: 22-year-old college student who has just been admitted to psychiatry with his first episode of psychosis. The reliability of the history obtained from the patient appears questionable.

HPI: C.Q.'s parents reported that about 6 months ago he began to withdraw, spending more and more time alone in his room. Although while growing up he was always a quiet boy, with only a couple of close friends, over the past few months he stopped interacting with them as well. Additionally, his attention to hygiene has become quite impaired, and he has refused to have his hair or nails trimmed. Prior to admission he had become very agitated, and one evening when his father had entered his room to ask him to come down to supper, he physically attacked his father with a penknife. His parents called 911 and he was placed on a psychiatric hold, due to a present danger to others and severe personal disability. During the interview, he refuses to answer questions targeting hallucinations, delusions, mood, suicidality, or homicidality. However, his parents note that he has been seen talking to himself and frequently looking over his shoulder. He has not mentioned suicidality to them. Since admission he has been isolated and withdrawn and has shown little interaction with his peers. He does not attend groups, preferring to stay in his room staring at the wall. He has been adherent to and appears to be tolerating medications well without any significant side effects.

PPHx: None

PMHx: Infectious mononucleosis at age 19; treated for fungal toenails.

Meds: Risperidone 2 mg BID, Lorazepam 2 mg po q 6 hours prn agitation; both begun after admission

Allergies: NKDA

FHx: Paternal uncle institutionalized with schizophrenia

SHx: Youngest of five children. Normal birth; achieved milestones appropriately; described as a quiet child. Graduated from high school; currently attending local junior college taking business courses. Not currently involved in any romantic relationships. Denies any substance or alcohol abuse, but smokes one pack of cigarettes per day.

MSE: *General:* thin, pale, unshaven. Eye contact intense at times. Rapport fair though limited. *Motor:* no abnormal movements noted. *Speech:* monotonous. *Mood:* "I don't feel anything." *Affect:* blunted. *Thought process:* slowing, blocking. *Thought content:* impoverished. Denies thoughts of harming himself, but he is still experiencing thoughts of harming his father whom he believes is "Satan himself." He believes he is being "watched," even while in the hospital. *Perception:* denies hearing voices or having visions but appears to be responding to internal stimuli during interview, staring at the wall above your head. When asked if he is looking at anything, he replies "nothing." *Insight and judgment:* significantly impaired.

Labs: UTox negative; CBC, TFTs, and chemistries all within normal limits

THOUGHT QUESTIONS

- His parents visit you and are concerned about the possible side effects of antipsychotics. What do you tell them?
- They ask you if he could be prescribed clozapine, a medication that helped his uncle. What do you tell them?
- The bioavailablity of antipsychotics may be affected by which metabolic factors?

DISCUSSION

Antipsychotics are generally divided into two main catagories: typical and atypical (Tables 4-1 and 4-2). The side effects of the low-potency drugs include **anticholinergic** effects (blurred vision, mydriasis, confusion, constipation, retention, and ECG changes), **antiadrenergic** effects (orthostatic hypotension), and **antihistaminergic** effects (sedation). Side effects of high-potency antipsychotics include acute **dystonia**, **parkinsonism** (cogwheel rigidity, tremor, and bradykinesia), **akathisia,** and hormone changes (elevated prolactin, galactorrhea,

TABLE 4-1   Typical Antipsychotics

Low Potency	Mid Potency	High Potency
Chlorpromazine (Thorazine) Thioridazine (Mellaril)	Molindone (Moban) Loxapine (Loxitane)	Fluphenazine (Prolixin) Haloperidol (Haldol) Perphenazine (Trilafon) Trifluoperazine (Stelazine) Pimozide (Orap)

and decreased testosterone). Mid-potency drugs have side effects somewhere in the middle. Other side effects of typical antipsychotics include bone marrow suppression **(agranulocytosis),** retinitis pigmentosa (Mellaril), **seizures** (less likely with molindone), skin changes (dermatitis, photosensitivity, hyperpigmentation with chlorpromazine), and **weight gain.** Both thioridazine and pimozide carry warnings about **QT prolongation.** Overdoses with these medications are rarely fatal. Signs and symptoms of overdose include hypotension, decreased deep tendon reflexes, mydriasis, extrapyramidal symptoms, and elevated heart rate. Severe overdose can lead to seizures, delirium, respiratory depression, or coma. Neuroleptic malignant syndrome has been reported with every antipsychotic medication, including the atypicals.

TABLE 4-2   Review of the Receptor Profile of the Atypical Antipsychotics

Atypical Antipsychotic	Receptor Activity
Aripiprazole (Abilify)	Partial agonist of D_2 and 5-HT_{1A} Antagonist of α_1 and 5-HT_{2A}
Clozapine (Clozaril)	Antagonist of α_1, 5-HT_{2A}, D_1, D_3, and D_4
Olanzapine (Zyprexa)	Antagonist of α_1, 5-HT_{2A}, D_1, D_3 and D_4, H_1, muscarinic M_1–M_5
Quetiapine (Seroquel)	Antagonist of α_1, α_2, D_1 and D_2, H_1 and 5-HT_2 and 5-HT_6
Risperidone (Risperdal)	Antagonist of α_1, α_2, D_2, H_1, and 5-HT_{2A} and 5-HT_6
Zisprasidone (Geodon)	Antagonist of α_1, D_2, D_3 and D_4, H_1, 5-HT_{1D}, 5-HT_{2A} and 5-HT_{2C} Agonist of 5-HT_{1A} and also acts as an SNRI

Atypical antipsychotics include aripiprazole (Abilify), clozapine (Clozaril), quetiapine (Seroquel), olanzapine (Zyprexa), risperidone (Risperdal), and zisprasidone (Geodon). Aripiprazole is a partial D_2 agonist. The other agents are also referred to as serotonin-dopamine antagonists (SDAs). Table 4-2 presents a review of the receptor profiles of atypical antipsychotics. Although risperidone is as potent a D_2 blocker as haloperidol, it is less likely to cause extrapyramidal symptoms (EPS), particularly at doses at or less than 6 mg per day; this reduction in EPS is hypothesized to result from a concurrent blockade of specific serotonin as well as dopamine receptors. Other side effects of **risperidone** include nausea, weight gain, orthostatic hypotension, and sedation. **Olanzapine** is associated with sedation, dizziness, dry mouth, weight gain, tremor, and elevated triglycerides, blood sugars, and transaminases. **Quetiapine** is thought to be the least likely of the atypicals to cause EPS but is associated with constipation, weight gain, and sedation, and may cause a transient elevation in transaminases. **Ziprasidone** is associated with dizziness, headache, nausea, and sedation. It may also produce a potentially fatal prolongation of the QT interval on ECG. Due to its multiple adverse side effects **clozapine** is reserved for use in treatment-resistant schizophrenia, in which patients have failed at least two or three other antipsychotic regimens. Patients on clozapine treatment must demonstrate good adherence and are required to follow up with weekly blood monitoring to check for the development of agranulocytosis, which occurs in 1% of patients on this therapy. Additionally, there is a dose-dependent reduction in the seizure threshold. Of note, **atypical antipsychotics have been found to occasionally result in a metabolic syndrome** (obesity, diabetes, and hyperlipidemia), with olanzapine and clozapine highly represented in those drugs leading to this side effect (Table 4-2).

All antipsychotics are metabolized by the liver **P450 cytochrome** system. Various medications or substances may induce or inhibit their metabolism (Table 4-3). Between 3% and 10% of Caucasians genetically have poor or no 2D6 activity; these poor metabolizers are at greater risk of sustaining drug interactions. Older persons also have reduced P450 activity and should initially be prescribed lower doses. Factors that affect P450 metabolism include ethnicity, age, liver function, kidney function, coadministered medications, comorbid medical illness, diet (fruit juices, cruciferous vegetables such as broccoli, and some teas), pregnancy, and smoking. Smoking actually induces cytochrome enzymes and can cause levels of antipsychotics to fall (Table 4-3).

TABLE **4-3** Review of the P450 Cytochrome Enzymes

Cytochrome	Substrates/Inhibitors
1A2	Substrates: caffeine, tricyclic antidepressants, erythromycin, haloperidol, theophylline, naproxen, acetaminophen, propranolol, verapamil, clozapine, mirtazapine, warfarin Inhibitors: grapefruit juice, fluvoxamine
2D6	Substrates: codeine, dextromethorphan, beta blockers, haloperidol, chlorpromazine, thioridazine, perphenazine, risperidone, TCAs, mirtazapine, fluoxetine, citalopram, paroxetine, venlafaxine, flecainide, propafenone, mexiletine, procainamide, bupropion metabolites Inhibitors: fluoxetine, sertraline paroxetine
3A4	Substrates: terfenadine, astemizole, triazolam, midazolam, alprazolam, diazepam, mirtazapine, cyclosporine, haloperidol, diltiazem, verapamil, felodipine, cisapride, pimozide, fentanyl, erythromycin, tricyclic antidepressants, codeine, granisetron, hydrocortisone, ethinyl estradiol, testosterone, carbamazepine, glyburide, ketoconazole, lovastatin, HIV protease inhibitors, tamoxifen Inhibitors: grapefruit juice, fluvoxamine, sertraline, paroxetine, ketoconazole astemizole
2C19	Substrates: coumadin, phenytoin, tertiary TCAs, possibly bupropion metabolites Inhibitors: fluoxetine, fluvoxamine, omeprazole

 ### CASE CONTINUED

You meet with the patient's parents to answer their questions and obtain further collateral information. You provide them with printed information about schizophrenia and arrange to meet with them again to answer further questions and help in discharge planning. You also encourage them to attend a local support group for family members of individuals suffering from schizophrenia. Unfortunately C.Q. displays only a partial response after 6 weeks of medication and manifests significant negative symptoms; you decide to change to aripiprazole, which is titrated to 20 mg daily with some improvement. He is discharged to a vocational rehabilitation program with outpatient followup.

QUESTIONS

4-1. Which of the following statements is correct concerning P450 interactions?

A. There is no concern about fatal outcomes.
B. Nicotine does not affect P450 enzymes.
C. Ketoconazole causes decreased levels of terfenadine.
D. Ketoconazole causes increased levels of terfenadine.
E. Erythromycin causes decreased levels of pimozide.

4-2. Which of the following is a potentially fatal side effect of clozapine?
A. Hypertension
B. Stevens-Johnson syndrome
C. Myocarditis
D. Dry mouth
E. Weight loss

4-3. Which of the following is a common side effect of aripiprazole (Abilify)?
A. Fever
B. Tremor
C. Anxiety
D. Akathisia
E. Rash

4-4. Which of the following side effects from atypicals is correctly matched with its first-line treatment?

A. Sialorrhea	systemic atropine
B. Sialorrhea	clonidine
C. Agranulocytosis	epoetin
D. Seizures	continue medication, add anticonvulsant
E. Hyperprolactinemia	add dopamine agonist

ANSWERS

4-1. D. Ketoconazole inhibits 3A3/4, causing an increase in the levels of terfenadine, which may result in fatal cardiac arrhythmias. Certain macrolide antibiotics (e.g., azithromycin, clarithromycin, erythromycin) are contraindicated in patients taking pimozide as they inhibit its metabolism (P450 3A3/4), and deaths from cardiac arrhythmias have been reported. Cigarette smoking induces the metabolism of various antipsychotics, including clozapine. Interestingly, it is not the nicotine that is at fault, but rather other constituents of cigarette smoke; thus, nicotine replacement strategies (e.g., transdermal nicotine) do not tend to affect drug metabolism. When compared with more high-potency antipsychotics, low-potency medications are more likely to cause potentially fatal ECG changes.

4-2. C. There are several potential serious side effects reported with the use of clozapine (Clozaril). Hematologic effects include agranulocytosis (in up to 1.3%), eosinophilia, leucopenia, and neutropenia. Other side effects include hypotension, tachycardia, sweating, rash (not Stevens-Johnson syndrome), constipation, nausea, vomiting, dizziness, sedation, tremor, vertigo, myocarditis, seizures, weight gain, and sialorrhea (drooling). Baseline lab tests include WBC and absolute neutrophil count (ANC), with weekly WBCs for the next 6 months. If the WBC has been greater than or equal to 3500/mm^3 and ANC greater than or equal to 2000/mm^3, then counts can be checked every 2 weeks. Clozapine should be avoided in patients with myeloproliferative disorders or severe seizure disorders.

4-3. D. Akathisia not uncommonly occurs during treatment with aripiprazole. Other side effects include anxiety, dizziness, vomiting, headache, and sedation. Fever, rash, blurred vision, and tremor are more rare side effects of aripiprazole.

4-4. B. Sialorrhea is a common side effect resulting from treatment with clozapine and is not only very troublesome for patients, but may also place them at increased risk of aspiration. Treatment options may include clonidine, benztropine, or low-dose TCAs (amitriptyline or clomipramine). Though anticholinergic agents (benztropine) are commonly used as first-line treatments, atropine should generally be avoided as it may seriously exacerbate the anticholinergic side effects of clozapine. Weight gain is also a serious problem for many patients and is more likely to occur with clozapine and olanzapine. If possible, it is advisable to switch patients to risperidone, quetiapine, or zisprasidone, which are less likely to cause weight gain. Additionally, patients should be encouraged to partake in regular exercise, avoid sedentary activities, and eat healthy food. If the side effect of seizures should occur, then the offending medication should be stopped. If another medication choice is possible, this new medication should be tried. However, if the patient responds only to the offending medication, it may be slowly reintroduced only when therapeutic serum levels of anticonvulsants have been achieved. Hyperprolactinemia is caused by antagonism of the tuberoinfundubular D$_2$ receptors and is most likely to occur with risperidone or high-potency typical antipsychotics. It can result in galactorrhea, gynecomastia, amenorrhea, and impotence. First-line treatment is to change medications to a different atypical which is less likely to cause hyperprolactinemia (e.g., quetiapine, clozapine, olanzapine). Though they may be helpful in treatment-refractory hyperprolactinemia, the use of dopamine agonists may exacerbate psychotic symptoms.

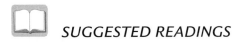 *SUGGESTED READINGS*

Sullivan PF, Owen MJ, O'Donovan MC, et al. Genetics. In: Lieberman J, Stroup T, Perkin D, eds. *Textbook of Schizophrenia*. Washington, DC: American Psychiatric Publishing, Inc.; 2006;39–53.

CASE 5

"I've Been Having Trouble Sleeping for the Last 10 Years"

CC/ID: 52-year-old single man employed as partner in a large New York City law firm, who presents following a referral from his psychotherapist for psychopharmacological evaluation.

HPI: D.G. has been experiencing insomnia for the past 10 to 12 years, but only recently, on advice from his therapist (of 5 years), did he entertain the notion of referral for medication treatment of this symptom, which he describes as follows: Initially he describes his insomnia as an isolated symptom: $1^{1}/_{2}$ hours to fall asleep; waking up three to four times per night and falling back asleep after 10 minutes; no early morning awakening. This has been his nightly routine for the past 10 to 12 years and is associated with significant daytime fatigue. Additionally, he notes a conditioned phobic-like response to the idea of going to sleep—**tension and worry-ridden thinking that he will not be able to fall asleep**. He has taken behavioral steps suggested by his therapist to improve his sleep hygiene but has not experienced any relief. His internist has prescribed him zolpidem (Ambien), which offered only a few hours of relief, and lorazepam (Ativan), which allows him to sleep for 6 hours. However, he is concerned about becoming addicted to the latter medication and is currently seeking a second opinion. He denies any symptoms consistent with a major depression (e.g., no change in mood, appetite, interest, guilt, suicidality) and denies feelings of autonomic arousal (e.g., heart palpitations, shaking, trembling).

PMHx: D.G. is in good physical health.

PPHx: Psychotherapy with psychologist for the past 5 years. Medications as in HPI. No history of antidepressant treatment. No history of suicide attempts or deliberate self-harm.

Substance Hx:　Social alcohol. No other drugs. Never experimented with drugs.

Meds:　　　　Lorazepam 2 mg po qhs prn insomnia; uses approximately 3 times/week

SHx:　　　　　D.G. was born into a wealthy suburban family in New England, the second of two boys. He was raised by his mother and a governess and had little contact with his financier father who traveled a great deal for work. He describes his childhood as "privileged but relatively constricted because **I always had to watch out to not upset my mother and make her sick**." He had many friends in high school and attended an Ivy League college and law school. His brother is successful in business. He has never been married and has no children, though he states that he is interested in both. He **spends most of his free time working** and is highly esteemed within the legal community.

FHx:　　　　　Mother has history of multiple psychosomatic illnesses (multiple chemical sensitivity syndrome, tension headaches, chronic fatigue syndrome).

MSE:　　　　*General:* Well groomed, tall, thin, attractive man with firm handshake. Impeccably clothed in professional attire. Well-related, calm, and cooperative. *Motor:* relatively fidgety and appears tense both in his face and bodily musculature. *Speech:* deliberate and normal in rate, rhythm, and volume. *Mood:* described as euthymic, though affect clearly manifests a worried expression with nervous laughter after many responses. *Thought process:* no formal thought disorder; process is deliberate and to the point. *Thought content:* remarkable for **minimizing problems** other than insomnia, as well as a great **lack of interest in discussing his emotional reactions to things.** No psychosis or obsessions are evident, nor is suicidality or homicidality. *Insight and judgment:* intact. *Cognition:* intact.

THOUGHT QUESTIONS

- What else is important to know about his presentation?
- Why is this symptom appearing now?

CASE CONTINUED

In any psychiatric presentation, beyond the presenting symptom and complaints, it is **always important to evaluate a psychiatric**

review of symptoms. This part of the assessment is even more important in patients who minimize their symptoms and limit themselves to a single complaint.

Initially, D.G. denies anxiety and depression symptoms when they are phrased as "how are you feeling . . . are you anxious . . . are you sad?" However, when asked if he worries excessively, he comments that he does worry a lot, but his job is so stressful that it is adaptive and part of his routine. He feels he would not be so successful were he not to worry about his cases. He does note, though, that he **wishes he could just "turn my mind off"** when going to bed, but "this is how I've always been and it works for me." When it was noted that he appears tense, he looked surprised and said, "Am I? I guess I am. How do you like that?" He then describes experiencing **daily muscle tension for many years with accompanying end-of-day headaches and excessive fatigue**. However, at the mention of each symptom, he proceeds to minimize its significance. While initially he denies an obvious precipitant for this sleep routine, upon deeper psychological examination he notes with surprise that it coincided with his promotion to partner, "Now I have to work even harder. When am I going to meet someone and be able to start a family?"

THOUGHT QUESTIONS

- What is the differential diagnosis?
- What are the psychological factors involved in this patient's presentation?
- How should he be treated?

DISCUSSION

While the differential in this case involves multiple other anxiety disorders, depression, dysthymia, and primary insomnia, the constellation of symptoms of insomnia, muscle tension, easy fatigability, and excessive worry determine that this patient has been suffering from **generalized anxiety disorder** (GAD) for several years. However, the significant symptomatic, syndromal, and epidemiological overlap between GAD and major depressive disorder (MDD) clearly necessitate pursuing questions related to parsing out comorbidity. While he clearly is not depressed (as per his symptom history), **a diagnosis of primary insomnia is only ruled out by**

virtue of performing a psychiatric review of systems, which leads to the diagnosis of GAD. It is not uncommon for such patients to be relatively inhibited regarding their emotions, both in terms of presenting them to others as well as in experiencing them themselves. Their worry seems to serve to protect them from actually experiencing anxiety. It keeps them cognitively focused on external concerns rather than on their responses to events and stimuli; they are all "in their head" rather than their experiential bodies. Thus these patients are frequently not in touch with their own emotional lives and reactions. In simple terms, their in-their-head worrying serves as a type of distraction from their greater fears of experiencing other symptoms of anxiety. A similar statement could be made regarding this patient's mother, who suffered from numerous psychosomatic illnesses, which also serve to minimize the affective experience of anxiety at the expense of physical symptoms. Thus, it is not surprising that he **limited his presenting symptom to insomnia, a sanctioned and tangible complaint that for him is rather safe.** Supporting this interpretation, while growing up he was made to limit his emotional expressiveness in order to not upset his mother's fragile health.

Additionally, it is possible that he is currently in the midst of a conflict over his desire to work hard for continued financial success and his desire to slow down to develop a relationship and raise a family. Rather than experience the anxiety caused by this conflict, he worries about his work, meeting someone, and how they can be combined.

When he was presented with the psychiatrist's assessment, he was appalled that he was found to be suffering from a true disorder, and he initially refused the treatment recommendations. However, with the psychiatrist's explanation of the nature of the disorder and the facility of its treatment, the patient agreed to a trial of antidepressant medication. He remains concerned that he will become addicted to the medication; this is a common worry in patients with GAD (Table 5-1).

TABLE 5-1   Phenomenology of Worry

GAD	Panic Disorder	MDD
Preoccupied with multiple excessive worries that are constant and nagging; possibly limited insight into the pathological nature of their concerns. Occasionally, such worries drive financial and work-related successes at the expense of personal emotional and relationship development.	Preoccupied with worry about having a future panic attack and avoiding situations that can precipitate a panic attack. Worry is discrete and limited to the panic concerns.	Worry may occur, but is usually secondary to low self-esteem and negative feelings about oneself. Focus is on negative view of self rather than on worry-driven concern over the future.

QUESTIONS

5-1. GAD is most commonly comorbid with which disorder?
A. Panic disorder
B. Major depressive disorder
C. Posttraumatic stress disorder
D. Bipolar disorder
E. Substance dependence

5-2. Which of the following neurobiological markers manifest in generalized anxiety disorder rather than panic disorder?
A. Hyperactivity of the amygdala
B. Hypoactivity of the reticular activating system
C. Consistent basal ganglia dysfunction
D. Hyperactivity of the prefrontal cortex
E. Discrete lesions present on MRI

5-3. Patients with GAD commonly present for psychiatric treatment of their
A. Excessive worry
B. Muscle tension
C. Dysphoric mood
D. Insomnia
E. Phobic symptoms

5-4. Which of the following medications is best used in the maintenance treatment of GAD?
A. Anticonvulsants
B. SSRIs
C. Benzodiazepines
D. Antipsychotics
E. Buproprion

ANSWERS

5-1. B. The comorbidity of MDD with GAD can approach 50%. Thus, it is generally the rule rather than the exception that these two conditions occur together. Substance abuse is less of a concern with GAD, as these patients worry excessively, and as such, tend to shy away from medications and drugs, though alcohol may be more accepted. Patients with panic disorder manifest excessive worry, but it is limited to their concern over having future panic attacks. Likewise, patients with PTSD experience near-constant anxiety, but this too can be traced back to specific and discrete concerns, as opposed to the free-floating nature of the worry in GAD.

5-2. D. The symptoms of panic disorder are neurobiologically manifest in an overactive fear system, with amygdalar hyperactivity and prefrontal cortical (PFC) hypoactivity; essentially, the regulating influence of the PFC is unable to restrain subcortical fear centers. In contrast, GAD manifests an overactive prefrontal cortex leading to symptoms of cognitive worry. Interestingly, physiological markers such as heart rate and skin conductance display hyperarousal in panic disorder (in line with an overactive fear network) and hyporesponsivity in GAD. Basal ganglia dysfunction may occasionally be present but has not been a consistent finding, as it has in obsessive compulsive disorder. Neither syndrome includes discrete lesions on MRI.

5-3. D. For many years, patients with GAD may experience their worry as adaptive and reality based. Only when suffering becomes evident or discrete associated symptoms begin to cause impairment do they reluctantly present for treatment. Even then they may minimize the excessive nature of their worry, seeking help only with their insomnia. The more intangible and "everyday" symptoms of muscle tension and irritability likewise receive short shrift as far as these patients are concerned.

5-4. B. Nearly every class of available antidepressants is effective in the treatment of GAD, including SSRIs, SNRIs, MAOIs, and TCAs. An exception to this is buproprion (an NDRI) which has as a side effect of worsening anxiety. While benzodiazepines are clearly palliative in GAD, they should be neither a first line choice nor generally used for maintenance as significant side effects are present (e.g., dependence, memory impairment, sedation). Another medication approved for use in GAD is buspirone, a partial agonist at the 5-HT_{1A} receptor. Anticonvulsants and antipsychotics have little to no role in the maintenance treatment of GAD.

SUGGESTED READINGS

Focus on generalized anxiety disorder, *J Clin Psychiatry.* 2001;62(11).

Borkovec TD, Newman MG. Worry and generalized anxiety disorder. In: Bellack AS, Hersen M., eds., *Comprehensive Clinical Psychology*. Oxford: Pergamon. 1998;6:439–459.

Mathew SJ, Mao X, Coplan JD, et al. Dorsolateral prefrontal cortical pathology in generalized anxiety disorder: a proton magnetic resonance spectroscopic imaging study. *Am J Psychiatry.* 2004 Jun;161(6):119–121.

Ballenger JC, Davidson JR, Lecrubier Y. et al. Consensus statement on generalized anxiety disorder from the International Consensus Group on Depression and Anxiety. *J Clin Psychiatry.* 2001;62(11):53–58.

"I'm Having Problems with My Boyfriend"

CC/ID: 33-year-old single woman who works as a bartender in New York City and who presents for a psychiatric evaluation in the context of a failing relationship with her boyfriend of $1^1/_2$ years.

HPI: J.C. complains that she wishes to be able to get on with her life but feels "trapped into this dysfunctional relationship." When asked to clarify this dysfunction, she describes a long history of being attracted to "bad boys . . . I knew they weren't good for me, but I couldn't help myself." This insight has only emerged in the last few years. Regarding her current relationship, she reports that it went well at first; he frequently brought her flowers, told her he loved her, and spent most of his time with her. However, after a few months, when she began to become more enmeshed in his social world, she noticed his pulling back much of his affection and his becoming increasingly aggressive toward her. Now, she complains, when he goes out with his friends, she feels like she has only two options: (i) stay at home waiting for him to return, or (ii) accompany him and watch while he flirts with other women in the bar. Additionally, she has frequently been hit on by many of his friends, which he allows and laughs at. She describes feeling increasingly down on herself and hating how her life has turned. However, she does not feel able to break off the relationship, despite desiring to do so. Recently on football Sundays, he has been bringing his friends into the bar where she works, and inviting other women over to his table to flirt with while she serves them. She has thrice confronted him with her feelings of belittlement, and **each time he apologizes and is "good" for a week or so before reverting to his old routine**. She denies frank physical abuse.

She denies continuously depressed mood and any changes in sleep, appetite, psychomotor functioning, or suicidality. She further denies symptoms of panic attacks, nightmares, and excessive worry. She has been increasingly irritable in the last few months, but notes that she is irritable at her baseline.

PMHx: Experienced **multiple hospitalizations for asthma as a child;** never intubated.

PPHx: First contact at the age of 29 for psychotherapy for **excessive self-denigration** in the context of another relationship. She was in therapy for 2 years and left with greater insight into her dating experiences. She has never seen a psychiatrist and has never received psychiatric medications nor been hospitalized. She has no history of deliberate self-harm (including purging) or suicide attempts.

Substance Hx: Social alcohol use. Experimented a few times with hallucinogens in her early 20s.

Meds: None

FHx: Mother with depression

THOUGHT QUESTIONS

■ What do you imagine her mental status to reveal?
■ What facts are important to know in her social history?

CASE CONTINUED

MSE: *General:* well-groomed attractive woman, wearing excessive makeup. No obvious bruising. Well-related, calm, cooperative, and engaging, though with a very slightly seductive demeanor. Throughout the interview, she frequently enacts self-reproach, apologizing for crying, rambling, and feeling that she has not appropriately answered all the examiner's questions. When this is brought to her attention, she first apologizes for what she experiences as a criticism and then retreats into relative silence. *Speech:* normal in spontaneity, latency, rate, rhythm, and volume. *Mood:* described as frustrated. *Affect:* somewhat dysphoric, full range, appropriate, and congruent, with occasional crying episodes, though again it is noticed that she tries to hold back tears. *Thought process:* no formal thought disorder. *Thought content:* overwhelmingly apologetic and marked by frequent negative self-statements. She is clearly conflicted about her feelings toward her boyfriend, but frequently retreats into assuming she is the one who has done something wrong leading to his not liking her anymore. No delusions, obsessions, or phobias are evident. No SI/HI. No hallucinations. *Insight:* She has some insight intellectually in that she knows she should not stay with an abusive man, but emotionally she cannot bring herself to adjust her behavior. She knows she needs treatment. *Judgment:* generally intact, as are impulse control and cognition.

SHx: J.C. was born and raised in small town in upstate New York, the second of two girls. Her parents divorced when she was $1^1/_2$ years old, at which time she went to live with her grandmother in Virginia. She was visited by her mother many times but never saw her father. At the age of 6, she moved back in with her mother in New York. She describes her childhood as difficult, stating that she **frequently felt alone despite having many friends.** She relates multiple episodes of her father making plans with her only to leave her **stranded** when he did not show up. Her first sexual experience was in the middle of high school, when she **voluntarily had sex with three boys sequentially.** She says that she was interested in one of them and wanted to prove that she was cool. She has had a few long-term relationships in the past 13 years, with each of them having some component of **emotional abuse.** She denies a history of physical or forced sexual abuse. She completed 2 years of a local college, stating that it is **difficult for her to finish anything.** Currently, she lives with her mother and works as a bartender. Her current boyfriend is a salesman. She denies a legal history.

THOUGHT QUESTIONS

- What is the differential diagnosis?
- What part of the history is essential in making the diagnosis?
- Why does she stay with her boyfriend?

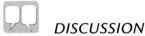

DISCUSSION

This patient has **dependent personality disorder.** In making this diagnosis, as in most personality disorder diagnoses, the **social history is paramount.** It is important to assess her lifelong pattern and level of functioning in relationships and interpersonal situations. While patients may experience depression and anxiety episodically, their personality usually remains constant with predictable responses to interpersonal experiences.

A core feature of patients with dependent PD is an **intense need for others to take care of them;** this leads to their being preoccupied with fears of abandonment. Unlike the borderline patient's fear of abandonment, that of the dependent patient is not associated with a contrasting and concurrent fear of being enmeshed and overwhelmed as well. They will go to **extraordinary measures to maintain relationships, frequently subjugating themselves in the process.**

Extending from these characteristics is their limiting their expression of their own desires, fearing that any assertion of their needs will be met with rejection. Thus, they tend not to express feelings of anger toward those who have abused them. In the MSE above, when the examiner commented on her frequent apologies for just being herself, she took it as a criticism, feeling discomfort at the prospect of asserting herself. Subjugating themselves at the expense of pleasing others is commonly found in patients with dependent PD. In its extreme form, dependent PD is manifest in patients' putting themselves in situations of abuse, and in its minor form in patients who continually look to others for reassurance and decision-making.

The psychology behind such self-denigration is that these patients tend to fear being alone more than anything else, such that they view (generally on an unconscious level) abuse as more tolerable than abandonment—in other words, the lesser of two evils. **Patients with dependent PD frequently have a history of childhood separations or childhood illnesses.** As children tend to experience separations from caregivers as their fault, this leads to an intense need to be loved and accepted at all costs and to limit self-assertion. Likewise, childhood illnesses are experiences of separation, but they also come with the parents' contextually offering more love and support to the child in the time of illness. Thus, the child is conditioned that with suffering comes love, and reciprocally, love comes with suffering.

Many patients with other axis II illnesses have dependent features but may be differentiated by the following: cluster A patients are less focused on issues of being cared for and intimacy; borderline patients express more rage and simultaneously fear abandonment and extreme closeness; histrionic patients bounce from relationship to relationship, while dependent patients maintain relationships for long periods; avoidant patients also fail to assert their own needs but tend to avoid contact rather than yearn for closeness; obsessive compulsive patients tend to subjugate themselves to rules at the expense of their affective desires, rather than to another person as in dependent patients (see Table 6-1 for a review of cluster C personality disorders).

TABLE **6-1**   Review of Cluster C—"Anxious/Fearful" Personality Disorders

Avoidant	Social inhibition, feeling inadequate, hypersensitive to criticism; avoiding people, occupational pursuits because of feeling inadequate	General population: 0.5–1% M:F = 1:1.	Intense desire for acceptance; overlap with social phobia
Dependent	Need to be taken care of, clingy, fear of separation, need for constant reassurance, helpless	2–3% of the population. Seen frequently in psych and medical settings because seeking help and support Possibly F > M	Intense need for relationships and social approval; treatment to help assertiveness Associated with depression and anxiety disorders
Obsessive-compulsive	Preoccupation with orderliness, perfectionism, inflexibility, control	1% in the general population M > F Not significantly associated with OCD	View their symptoms as positive; no intrusive obsessions or ego dystonic compulsions May be self-critical and lack social closeness and therefore may have increased depression

QUESTIONS

6-1. Which of the following are more likely to be found in the history of a patient with dependent PD?
   A. Closely knit family
   B. Childhood abuse
   C. Obsessive-compulsive personality
   D. Schizoid personality
   E. Healthy interpersonal relationships

6-2. The best treatment for dependent PD is
   A. Observation
   B. No treatment works for personality disorders
   C. SSRIs
   D. Low dose antipsychotics
   E. Psychotherapy

6-3. Which of the following are most commonly found with dependent PD?
   A. Comorbid bipolar disorder
   B. Comorbid borderline personality disorder
   C. Comorbid major depressive disorder
   D. Family history of somatoform disorders
   E. History of self-mutilation

6-4. The theorized reason behind a dependent patient's putting herself in situations in which she suffers is a
   A. Desire to feel pain
   B. Loss of control over her actions
   C. Focus on the negative
   D. Fear of abandonment
   E. Desire to get back at her parents

6-5. Patients with dependent PD will likely be most comfortable in a job in which they are
   A. In a supervising managerial position
   B. Factory or assembly line workers
   C. Commonly thought of for promotion
   D. Self-employed
   E. Under the direct supervision of a senior associate

ANSWERS

6-1. B. Dependent personality not infrequently develops in patients who have been exposed to childhood abuse. A way of looking at it is that they have been conditioned to experience love, attachment, and acceptance coincident with subjugation and suffering. Additionally, they tend to have a negative view of themselves and view interpersonal relationships as tenuous and requiring their profound effort to keep them going.

6-2. E. Dependent PD is by definition a character structure and a manner in which the patient interacts with the world. Further, it can be the cause of much suffering. Psychotherapy is the treatment of choice to address these issues. While SSRIs are effective for a superimposed depressive syndrome, they have little efficacy for core dependent traits. Low-dose antipsychotics may be useful for the affective instability and anger in borderline PD.

6-3. C. While theoretically any axis I syndrome can coincide with any personality disorder, for dependent PD, major depressive disorder tends to be the most comorbid. Patients with dependent

PD tend to view themselves negatively and minimize their interpersonal efficacy; it is not difficult to see how this can lead to a depressive syndrome. Depression is also very common in patients with borderline PD.

6-4. D. This is a case of the lesser of two evils, in which the prospect of being alone is much worse than is the pain sustained in an abusive relationship. It is not that patients with dependent PD seek pain or actually enjoy it; rather they are trying to minimize their experience of pain.

6-5. E. Patients with dependent PD are most comfortable in situations in which they are both accepted and can find secure interpersonal attachments. As they feel an overwhelming need to be liked by and please others (which is done at their expense), supervisory roles are difficult for them. Likewise, working on an assembly line would exacerbate their anxiety at needing to feel special; they would just be one of many. Dependent patients have much conflict over success and tend to associate promotion with abandonment and loneliness. They work well when under the direct and close supervision of a caring boss.

SUGGESTED READINGS

Gabbard GO. *Psychodynamic Psychiatry in Clinical Practice.* 3rd ed. Washington, DC: American Psychiatric Publishing, 2000.

Bornstein RF. Dependency in the personality disorders: intensity, insight, expression, and defense. *J Clin Psychol.* 1998;54(2): 175–189.

Hill EL, Gold SN, Bornstein RF. Interpersonal dependency among adult survivors of childhood sexual abuse in therapy. *J Child Sexual Abuse.* 2000;9:71–86.

Widiger TA, Mullins S. Personality disorders. In: Tasman A, Kay J, Lieberman JA, eds. *Psychiatry.* Vol. 2, 2nd ed. Philadelphia: W.B. Saunders; 2003:1603–1637.

"I Don't Know What's Wrong"

CC/ID: 26-year-old SWM, recent business school graduate presents ambulatory to the emergency department with the complaint of "What's wrong with me?"

HPI: He describes feeling well until 1 month ago, when he left work, and while in a taxi, he became short of breath, had palpitations, and felt his throat closing. He was **frightened and dizzy,** and asked to go to an ED where he had "lots of tests." The symptoms passed in about 30 minutes, and he was pronounced "fine." The next week he had two more episodes and saw his internist, who again reassured him. As he became afraid of the attacks, he stopped taking taxis, but he continued to have **attacks on the bus and then on the street.** He began to work from home and would only go out with his sister. He worries that he is gravely ill and his doctor has missed something.

THOUGHT QUESTIONS

- What physical illnesses could cause his symptoms?
- What would you look for on physical examination?
- What would you look for in laboratory tests?
- What would you look for in social history?

DISCUSSION

Numerous medical illnesses, medications, and substances can cause these symptoms (Table 7-1). It is important to do a careful history and physical examination, and to review all medications prescribed, including over-the-counter and herbal formulations, as well as illicit drugs. For example, herbal meds containing ma huang (Ephedra) can cause tachycardia and anxiety.

TABLE 7-1   Conditions that Mimic Panic

Thyroid dysfunction (primarily hyper- but also occasionally hypothyroidism)
Seizure disorders (especially those originating in the temporal lobe)
Neuroendocrine tumors (carcinoid, pheochromocytoma)
Hyperparathyroidism
Stimulants (e.g., cocaine, amphetamines, caffeine)
Vestibular dysfunction
Hypoglycemia
Cardiac conditions (ischemia, arrhythmias, possibly mitral valve prolapse)
Depressant withdrawal (e.g., alcohol)

Adapted from Kaplan HI, Sadock BJ. *Comprehensive textbook of psychiatry*, VI. Baltimore: Williams & Wilkins, 1995.

On physical examination, it is important to assess for vital sign abnormalities (high blood pressure and pulse), palpable thyroid (and possible lid lag, exopthalmos, hyperreflexia, heat intolerance, tremor), heart murmur, and other physical manifestations of the conditions enumerated in Table 7-1. Laboratory evaluations should also rule in or out these conditions, and should include glucose, electrolytes including calcium, thyroid function, ECG, and urine toxicology.

When panic attacks occur it is frequently in the context of increased psychosocial stressors. Specifically, the onset of increased responsibility is associated with the development of panic disorder. Other factors include divorced status, aloneness, caffeine excess, and the loss of a parent at a young age (including divorce).

CASE CONTINUED

Meds: None

SHx: No substance use or ETOH. Recent new high-stress job.

VS: BP 125/70, HR 68 (from ED: BP 125/70, HR 90, O_2 sat on RA 99%)

PE: *Gen:* WDWN in no acute distress. *CV:* RR&R, no murmurs or clicks. *Neuro:* nonfocal.

Labs: Electrolytes, glucose, calcium, TSH: all WNL; ECG: WNL; Utox negative

MSE: *General:* Well-related, cooperative but anxious and manifesting some mild psychomotor agitation. *Speech:* slightly rapid. *Mood:* "worried." *Affect:* reactive, full range, and nervous. *Thought process:* logical. *Thought content:* preoccupied with his symptoms; no delusions, no hallucinations, no suicidality. *Cognition:* intact.

 ### THOUGHT QUESTIONS

- What do you think about his fear of being mortally ill?
- What is your working diagnosis?

 ### DISCUSSION

His concerns about illness could reflect multiple different pathologies, including major depression, hypochondriasis, generalized anxiety disorder, phobia, panic disorder, somatoform disorder, non-specific distress, and appropriate concern secondary to a nonpsychiatric physical illness. Each of these must be explored. Normal calcium makes hyperparathyroidism unlikely. He was not hypoxic or hypertensive during the attack, and he remained cognitively intact and conscious, further limiting the differential. He is taking no herbal meds or illicit drugs. He denies depressed mood, anhedonia, or neurovegetative changes. His activities are restricted for fear of attacks. He worries about a "grave illness" but is not fixated (as would occur in hypochondriasis or another somatoform disorder).

Given his symptoms, their progression, and his negative medical work up, the probable diagnosis is panic disorder with agoraphobia. Panic disorder is defined by at least four symptoms (Table 7-2) that occur spontaneously, peak in approximately 10 minutes, and are associated with marked worry about further attacks, "losing control," or dying. Of people with panic disorder, 10% to 15% have agoraphobia, which is a fear of going out because of worry about not being able to get help in the event of an attack.

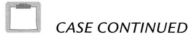 ### CASE CONTINUED

As are many patients who present with these frightening physiological sensations, he is relieved by the diagnosis of panic disorder: "I was grasping straws to explain what was happening to me."

TABLE 7-2   Signs and Symptoms of Panic

Palpitations	Chest pain/discomfort	Derealization or depersonalization
Sensation of choking	Nausea, abdominal distress	Fear of losing control or going crazy
Trembling	Dizziness, lightheaded	Paresthesias (numbness, tingling)
Fear of dying	Shortness of breath	Chills or hot flashes
Sweating		

Adapted from American Psychiatric Association. Task Force on DSM-IV. *Diagnostic and statistical manual of mental disorders: DSM-IV.* 4th ed. Washington, DC: American Psychiatric Association, 1994.

THOUGHT QUESTION

- What options are there for treatment of panic disorder?

DISCUSSION

Cognitive behavioral therapy (CBT) and medications are both effective. The goal of CBT is to help the patient see that the symptoms are self-limited and that fears are due to a misinterpretation of physical symptoms. Relaxation exercises help anxiety, and breathing techniques prevent hyperventilation which would usually lead to respiratory symptoms and paresthesias. A wide range of medications are effective, including tricyclic antidepressants (TCAs), serotonin reuptake inhibitors (SSRIs), benzodiazepines (BZDs), and monoamine oxidase inhibitors (MAOIs). The most commonly used medications are SSRIs. Agoraphobia tends to be the aspect of panic disorder that is the most impairing to one's functioning.

QUESTIONS

7-1. Which of the following is an important consideration in this patient's differential diagnosis?
- A. Social phobia
- B. Dysthymia
- C. Schizophrenia
- D. Mania
- E. Obsessive-compulsive disorder

7-2. Which of the following is correct concerning antidepressants?
  A. TCAs are not associated with weight gain.
  B. MAOIs do not cause orthostasis.
  C. SSRIs are safer in overdose than TCAs.
  D. TCAs are not associated with QT prolongation.
  E. MAOIs have fewer significant drug-drug interactions than SSRIs.

7-3. Which of the following is true in panic disorder?
  A. The prevalence is 20%.
  B. Identical twins have a 97% concordance.
  C. Panic attacks only occur as part of panic disorder.
  D. Family members have higher rates of panic disorder.
  E. Patients with panic disorder are no more likely to use emergency services than the general population.

7-4. Which of the following is correct concerning the biology of panic disorder?
  A. Clonidine (α_2 agonist) provokes panic.
  B. Lactate infusions prevent panic by stimulating the substantia nigra.
  C. CO_2 inhalation prevents panic.
  D. Yohimbine (α_2 antagonist) provokes panic by stimulating the locus coeruleus.
  E. Benzodiazepines directly open the chloride channel of the GABA receptor.

ANSWERS

7-1. A. The differential diagnosis for this patient with panic disorder with agoraphobia, including somatization disorder, also includes social phobia, which is a fear of embarrassment in public situations that the patient realizes is excessive. In panic disorder with agoraphobia, on the other hand, the fear concerns having an attack and being humiliated or unable to get away or get help. Major depressive disorder (MDD) may be complicated by occasional panic attacks, but these attacks do not lead to constant worry and fear and do not preoccupy the patient. However, panic disorder and MDD are not infrequently comorbid, usually with panic disorder coming first. This patient has no symptoms of mania or dysthymic mood.

7-2. C. SSRIs lack cardiovascular (e.g., QT prolongation) and clinically significant anticholinergic side effects, and therefore lack the toxicity associated with overdose that occurs with TCAs. However, SSRIs do carry a risk of sexual side effects (decreased libido, hyporgasmia and anorgasmia, and more rarely impotence). MAOIs cause orthostasis and require a tyramine-free diet to prevent malignant hypertension. It is important to give the patient realistic expectations about medications (e.g., it may take 3 to 6 weeks for a full effect). Start low and titrate slowly, as patients with panic may be very sensitive to the initial anxiety-inducing effects of these medications.

7-3. D. Approximately 2% to 4% of the population has panic disorder. First-degree relatives have a four- to eightfold increased risk. There is no psychiatric illness for which there is 97% twin concordance. In panic disorder, the concordance rate in monozygotic twins is 25% to 50%, depending on the specific criteria used; in dizygotic twins, the concordance is closer to 10%. Panic attacks are only one criterion for panic disorder, and they may be present in normal individuals as well as those with major depression, obsessive compulsive disorder, personality disorders, schizophrenia, somatoform disorders, or virtually any other psychiatric illness, including substance abuse. For a diagnosis of panic disorder, other conditions must be met; the attacks must be recurrent, unexpected, and associated with significant worry about future attacks or the implication of the attacks (e.g., dying). Patients with panic symptoms are highly frequent users of emergency medical services, and they frequently present to emergency departments many times before a diagnosis is reached.

7-4. D. In people with panic disorder, challenge with the α_2 antagonist yohimbine provokes panic attacks. The α_2 agonist clonidine does not cause panic symptoms. An infusion of lactate or exposure to CO_2 induces panic attacks in people with panic disorder as well as in those with a family history of the disorder. This may be because of increased firing of the locus coeruleus or hypersensitive brainstem CO_2 chemoreceptors. Benzodiazepines allosterically modulate the GABA receptor, making it more likely to be activated by endogenous GABA, but they do not directly open the channel.

📖 SUGGESTED READINGS

Otto MW, Tuby KS, Gould RA, et al. An effect-size analysis of the relative efficacy and tolerability of serotonin selective reuptake inhibitors for panic disorder. *Am J Psychiatry* 2001;158(12): 1989–1992.

Khan A, Leventhal RM, Khan S, et al. Suicide risk in patients with anxiety disorders: a meta-analysis of the FDA database. *J Affect Disord.* 2002;68(2–3):183–190.

Kumar S, Oakley-Browne M. Panic disorder. *Clin Evid.* 2004;(11): 1335–1342.

Roy-Byrne PP, Craske MG, Stein MB, et al. A randomized effectiveness trial of cognitive behavioral therapy and medication for primary care panic disorder. *Arch Gen Psychiatry.* 2005;62(3):290–298.

CASE 8

"I'm Having Trouble Sleeping"

CC/ID: 20-year-old female college junior without a psychiatric history, who presents to the student health center complaining of insomnia.

HPI: She describes having difficulty sleeping for the past 3 weeks, reporting minimal initial insomnia of 30 minutes a few times per week, but more constantly she finds herself **waking up very early in the morning,** unable to return to sleep. She always feels **tired,** has **difficulty concentrating,** and has fallen behind in her work. She spends all her time in her dorm "trying to work," but not getting anything done. She says, "It doesn't matter that I have no life, I don't enjoy anything, anyway . . . Everything and everyone bothers me." Her **appetite is poor,** and food has lost its taste. She describes feeling listless and unmotivated.

PMHx: None

Meds: None

PPHx: None

SHx/FHx: Born and raised in a small town, completed junior college, recently transferred to an out-of-state university. She used to be on the honor roll. The transition has been difficult, but she says, "I'm managing." She has a C average. One aunt is being treated with medications for "her moods."

VS: BP 120/70, HR 70, RR 12; weight 100 lbs, height 5'3"

PE: *Gen:* Thin, unremarkable. ROS: no hair or skin changes.

Labs: Recent routine labs WNL; TSH 1.2 (WNL)

MSE: *General:* Quiet, withdrawn but not guarded, mild PMR, eye contact fair. *Speech:* quiet, slow with some increased latency, mild psychomotor retardation. *Mood:* "Not great." *Affect:* constricted and dysphoric. *Thought process:* goal directed. *Thought content:* negativistic, no suicidality or psychotic symptoms.

THOUGHT QUESTIONS

- What was not asked that might be relevant?
- What is your differential diagnosis?
- What did you learn from her social and family history, and physical examination?

DISCUSSION

This patient presents with insomnia, but it is clear that this is not her only concern. She has associated anhedonia, irritability, and poor concentration, sleep, energy, and appetite, all of which seem to be impairing her ability to function at her previous level. Missing from the history are assessments of the following areas: **Weight loss, substance use, psychotic symptoms, and suicidality were missing from the presentation, as was a specific descriptor stating that there is no personal or family history of mania or hypomania** (as this would significantly widen one's differential and influence the manner of treatment). Additionally, a further evaluation of past relationships and interpersonal levels of functioning may be appropriate for an assessment for personality disorders which would further inform treatment. The differential diagnoses include the following:

- *Adjustment disorder with depressed mood:* She meets criteria for major depression, ruling this diagnosis out.
- *Bipolar disorder, mixed state:* She is somewhat irritable, distractible, and is not sleeping, but she feels she needs more sleep. She is not grandiose, nor is her speech pressured. Further, she does not describe other symptoms of mania (e.g., recklessness, increased goal-directed activity).
- *Substance-induced mood disorder:* We need to find out about her substance use history.
- *Depression due to a medical condition or medication:* We have no reason to suspect this, although routine screening of thyroid function is usually warranted. Her TSH was normal, as above.
- *Major depressive disorder (MDD):* Barring any new information, this is the most likely diagnosis. Her

family history of mood disorders is significant, but it is important to more specifically assess for a possible family history of bipolar disorder.

The rate of depression in families of unipolar depressed patients is 1.5 to 3 times higher than in the general population. The concordance rate for monozygotic twins is around 50%, while in dizygotic twins it is 10% to 25%. This patient may be having a difficult time with the transition to a university, and this may be important to address in therapy; other personality traits are also important and may have put her at risk for this episode of major depression, as well as predispose her to future suffering. Her physical exam did not show abnormalities which would suggest an endocrine or metabolic disturbance. Her weight is low, and it is important to discern whether she has a primary eating disorder as well as MDD, or if her weight loss is due to the depression.

 ## CASE CONTINUED

You further explore her history and note that she does not have a substance use problem, eating disorder, or personal/family history of bipolar disorder. You explain to her that she is experiencing a major depressive episode, and you invite her to participate in a research study including a PET scan, sleep study, and dexamethasone suppression test (DST).

 ## THOUGHT QUESTION

- What would you expect these tests to show?

DISCUSSION

In PET scans of depressed patients, parts of the **limbic system and prefrontal cortex** may show differing metabolic activity from healthy controls. Sleep studies in depression generally show **prolonged sleep latency (longer time to fall asleep), shortened REM latency (time from onset of sleep to the first REM period), early morning awakening, and decreased stage 3 and 4 sleep.** There are also abnormalities in the hypothalamic-pituitary-adrenal (HPA) axis, such as **increased plasma cortisol** and corticotrophin-releasing factor (CRF), as well as a blunted adrenocorticotropic hormone (ACTH) response to CRF. The DST further describes this **HPA axis abnormality,** in assessing the negative feedback sensitivity of the system. The patient is given dexamethasone (a synthetic cortisol-related steroid) at 11 pm, and plasma cortisol is drawn the next day at 8 am and 11 pm. Approximately 50% to 60% of depressed patients do not suppress further cortisol production. The DST alone is not a useful diagnostic tool because there are high levels of false-negatives and false-positives.

 ## CASE CONTINUED

You decide that she would benefit from the combination of psychotherapy and an antidepressant. Table 8-1 provides a more detailed description of antidepressant therapies. In formulating a treatment strategy, it is important to keep a number of things in mind. Can the patient function without immediate treatment? If not, this would clearly indicate more early use of medication. Did psychosocial stressors lead to the development of the current episode? What types of situations does the patient consider to be stressful, and how does she usually handle them? Such an evaluation would point the way to the prescription of psychotherapy and would influence its duration and focus (Table 8-1).

TABLE **8-1**   Review of Antidepressants

Class	Drug Example	Mechanism of Action	Side Effects	Comments
TCA	*Tertiary amines:* imipramine, amitriptyline *Secondary amines:* nortriptyline, desipramine	Block reuptake of serotonin (5-HT), norepinephrine (NE), and to a more limited extent, dopamine (DA)	Anticholinergic: dry mouth, impaired visual accommodation, constipation, urinary retention Cardiovascular: orthostasis, prolongation of the P-R interval, heart block, and increased width of T wave. Other: lowers the seizure threshold, weight gain	Need to check blood levels. Nortriptyline has a therapeutic window (50-150 ng/ml), while others have minimum therapeutic levels.

(Continued)

TABLE **8-1**   Review of Antidepressants (*continued*)

Class	Drug Example	Mechanism of Action	Side Effects	Comments
MAOI	Phenelzine, isocarboxazid, tranylcypromine	Block catabolism of NE, 5-HT, DA, tyramine	Orthostatic hypotension, insomnia, agitation, somnolence, impotence, delayed ejaculation, hypertensive crisis	Many drug/food interactions: *Vasoactive amines:* tyramine-containing foods (aged cheese, cured meat, red wine) may cause a potentially fatal hyperadrenergic crisis (diaphoresis, tachycardia, HTN, arrhythmias, etc.); meperidine is also a culprit. Serotonergic agents: "serotonin syndrome" (tachycardia, HTN, fever, myoclonus, hyperthermia, seizures, death)
SSRI	Citalopram (Celexa), escitalopram (Lexapro), fluoxetine (Prozac), fluvoxamine (Luvox) sertraline (Zoloft), paroxetine (Paxil)	Block the reuptake of 5-HT	Initial anxiety, headache, insomnia nausea, decreased appetite, delayed ejaculation, anorgasmia, decreased libido, weight gain, increased sweating, hyponatremia (rare SIADH). Use with care in children and adolescents; may rarely increase suicidal ideation or behavior during the first months of treatment.	Because of different effects on the cytochrome P450 system (particularly 2D6, 3A1), there are numerous different drug-drug interactions. Discontinuation syndromes are common (diaphoresis, flu-like symptoms, dysphoria).

(*Continued*)

TABLE **8-1**   Review of Antidepressants (*continued*)

Class	Drug Example	Mechanism of Action	Side Effects	Comments
SNRI	Venlafaxine (Effexor), duloxetine (Cymbalta)	Block the reuptake of 5-HT and NE	Same as for SSRIs. Duloxetine may increase serum trans-aminases, and may mildly increase BP. Increased BP is more common with venlafaxine.	Duloxetine is a moderate inhibitor of CYP2D6. Mydriasis has been reported with both, so they are contraindicated in narrow angle glaucoma. Discontinuation syndromes are common.
Other	Bupropion (Wellbutrin, Zyban)	Probably NE- and DA- enhancing properties	Agitation, dry mouth, insomnia, headache, migraine, nausea, tremor	May lower seizure threshold. Relative contraindications include seizure disorders, head trauma, and bulimia nervosa. Used in smoking cessation.
	Mirtazapine (Remeron)	Blocks pre-synaptic α_2 and post-synaptic 5-HT_2 and 5-HT_3 receptors Enhances activity at 5-HT_1	Antihistaminergic side effects, especially at lowerdoses (somnolence, dry mouth, increased appetite, weight gain)	Minimal cytochrome P450 inhibition, minimal orthostasis, sexual side effects uncommon.

QUESTIONS

8-1. Which of the following is a mechanism of action of antidepressant medications?

- A. Serotonin reuptake facilitation
- B. Norepinephrine reuptake inhibition
- C. Dopamine receptor blockade
- D. Cholinesterase inhibition
- E. GABA-A allosteric modulation

8-2. Which of the following statements about the treatment of depression is true?
    A. Antidepressant monotherapy is effective 95% of the time.
    B. Antidepressants usually show nearly full efficacy within 1 to 2 weeks.
    C. Cognitive behavioral therapy has been shown to be an effective treatment.
    D. Antidepressant medication is not lethal in overdose.
    E. The best studied short-term, time-limited therapy is psychoanalysis.

8-3. Match the antidepressant class with the BEST lettered answer:
SSRIs (e.g., fluoxetine, sertraline)
    A. Orthostatic hypotension
    B. Tyramine-free diet
    C. Anorgasmia
    D. Severe interaction with meperidine
    E. Priapism

8-4. Match the antidepressant class with the BEST lettered answer
Tricyclic antidepressants (e.g., imipramine, amitriptyline)
    A. Orthostatic hypotension
    B. Tyramine-free diet
    C. Anorgasmia
    D. Severe interaction with meperidine
    E. Priapism

ANSWER

8-1. B. Classes of antidepressant medications include tricyclics (TCAs, which block the reuptake of norepinephrine, serotonin, and, to a limited extent, dopamine), selective serotonin reuptake inhibitors (SSRIs), monoamine oxidase inhibitors (MAOIs, which block the breakdown of monoamines like dopamine and norepinephrine), and others (such as selective noradrenergic reuptake inhibitors and heterocyclic antidepressants). Dopamine receptor antagonists are used as antipsychotics, the most typical of which block the D_2 receptor. Benzodiazepines allosterically modulate the GABA-A receptor potentiating the effects of endogenous GABA. By contrast, barbiturates act as direct agonists to the GABA receptor. Cholinesterase inhibitors are used in the treatment of mild to moderate Alzheimer dementia.

8-2. C. Cognitive behavioral therapy is an effective treatment for depression and has been studied in a number of double-blind placebo-controlled trials. Antidepressant monotherapy is effective about 60% of the time. These medications do not work immediately, and though some effect is usually manifest in the first 2 weeks, it generally takes 3 to 12 weeks for a full response. Geriatric patients may require longer trials with slower titrations, but they generally require the same final doses. Some antidepressants are lethal in overdose (e.g., tricyclics cause cardiac conduction abnormalities). The SSRIs are the safest in overdose.

8-3. C./8-4. A. Common concerns for each class of antidepressants are as follows. TCAs: anticholinergic effects, sedation, orthostatic hypotension, weight gain, prolonged QT interval, lethality in overdose; SSRIs: nausea, diarrhea, headaches, delayed ejaculation, or anorgasmia; MAOIs: orthostasis, hypertensive crisis (need for tyramine-free diet and need to avoid certain meds (e.g., meperidine, serotonergic agents, sympathomimetic including decongestants), weight gain, and sedation; others: bupropion is contraindicated in seizure disorders and bulimia, and trazodone can result in sedation and rarely priapism.

SUGGESTED READINGS

Freemantle N, Anderson IM, Young P. Predictive value of pharmacological activity for the relative efficacy of antidepressant drugs. Meta-regression analysis. *Br J Psychiatry.* 2000;177:292–302.

Nemeroff CB. Neurobiological consequences of childhood trauma. *J Clin Psychiatry.* 2004;65(1):18–28.

Lieberman JA, Greenhouse J, Hamer RM, et al. Comparing the effects of anti-depressants: consensus guidelines for evaluating quantitative reviews of antidepressant efficacy. *Neuropsychopharmacology.* 2005;30(3):445–460.

"Is the Ozone Hole Affecting Me?"

CC/ID: 36-year-old single white woman who comes to your family medicine practice for a checkup.

HPI: R.T. is concerned about the ozone hole, radon, and pesticides, and wants a "complete check." Her only complaint is vague abdominal and neck pain that she attributes to food allergies. She also notes that at times she experiences tachycardia. She says she chose you because your phone number and the letters in your name "all come together favorably."

PMHx: None

Allergies: NKDA. Multiple "sensitivities" (e.g., wheat, corn, soy, dairy, eggs, latex, and many food additives). Her reactions range from fatigue to stomach or neck pain.

PPHx: None

SHx: Finished high school; worked as a waitress, a tarot reader, and at a few occult bookstores. She stopped reading tarot cards because "I saw much too much. . . ." She left two previous jobs because of vague paranoid concerns. She lives in an apartment, is not usually exposed to pesticides, and tends to stay indoors. Superficial friendships, usually around interest in the occult; no long-term relationships, uncomfortable around others; no use of illicit substances.

FHx: One brother with schizophrenia.

THOUGHT QUESTION

- What else would you want to know?

DISCUSSION

It is always important to inquire about medications, herbal preparations, and over-the-counter and illicit substances. Understanding more about her social relationships may be revealing. Additionally, one's understanding of her case would benefit from a more thorough exploration of possible abnormal perceptual experiences, delusional beliefs, anxiety, depression, history of suicidality, and to whom she has gone for help in the past. Finally, one should assess for any recent neurovegetative or affective symptoms.

CASE CONTINUED

Meds: Ma huang; shark cartilage; vitamins A, E, C, B_1, B_6, B_{12}; gingko biloba; valerian; melatonin

PE: WNL

MSE: *General:* Multicolored cape, dramatic make up, torn sneakers, fair eye contact, no psychomotor abnormalities. *Speech:* WNL. *Mood:* "Fine," though upon further questioning, she seems to have difficulty describing her emotional state. *Affect:* sometimes laughs at odd times, otherwise reactive. *Thought process:* some bizarre pauses, but otherwise no formal thought disorder. *Thought content:* overly metaphorical, overinclusive, and idiosyncratic ideas; no suicidal or homicidal ideation. No thought insertion or broadcasting, no frank delusions, but some paranoid ideas about people's motives. No auditory of visual hallucinations, but "In my work I have felt spirits of the dead." *Insight:* somewhat impaired.

THOUGHT QUESTION

■ What is this woman's most likely psychiatric diagnosis?

DISCUSSION

She likely does not have a current axis I disorder. She manifests **pervasive interpersonal deficits** (reduced capacity for and discomfort with close relationships), **cognitive and perceptual aberrations**, and **behavioral eccentricities** (Table 9-1). These characteristics seem to have been present for many years and have interrupted functioning in a variety of arenas. She meets the criteria for schizotypal personality disorder (PD).

Personality disorders are, by definition, a pervasive maladaptive pattern of behaviors that begin in early adulthood and affect functioning. **People with personality disorders generally experience their symptoms and behaviors as ego-syntonic,** that is, they do not necessarily see them as representative of an illness or as alien to their sense of themselves, and therefore often do not seek treatment. In contrast, **many patients with axis I disorders—primarily those with depressive or anxiety disorders—view their symptoms as ego-dystonic (or ego-alien)** and not in keeping with their sense of themselves. When patients with personality disorders present for treatment, the complaint is usually a superimposed axis I condition, or in the context of significant turmoil in an interpersonal, occupational, or romantic relationship.

DSM-IV defines three clusters of personality disorders. Cluster A ("odd") is comprised of paranoid, schizoid, and schizotypal personality disorders. This cluster is characterized by a disturbance of interpersonal relatedness and cognitive and perceptual functions. Cluster B ("dramatic") includes histrionic, narcissistic, borderline, and antisocial personality disorders. It is characterized by affective instability, impulsivity, and dramatic emotional expressiveness.

TABLE **9-1**   Criteria for Schizotypal Personality Disorder (5 required)

Ideas of reference (not delusions)
Unusual bodily experiences
Excessive social anxiety
Inappropriate or constricted affect
Lack of close friends or confidants
Magical thinking or odd beliefs (e.g., ESP, telepathy)
Behavior or appearance that is odd or eccentric
Odd speech (idiosyncratic, metaphorical)
Suspiciousness or paranoid thoughts

Adapted from American Psychiatric Association. Task Force on DSM-IV. *Diagnostic and statistical manual of mental disorders: DSM-IV.* 4th ed. Washington, DC: American Psychiatric Association, 1994.

Cluster C ("anxious") includes avoidant, dependent, and obsessive-compulsive personality disorders. It is characterized by the constriction of assertiveness and sociability in the service of avoiding anxiety.

There are many overlapping symptoms among personality disorders, thus the full criteria must be met to make a diagnosis. For example, in avoidant PD there is social anxiety and introversion, but unlike schizotypal PD, these symptoms diminish with familiarity, and unlike schizoid PD, avoidant patients desperately seek companionship and loving but are held back by their anxiety (schizoid patients generally do not desire interpersonal relationships). Unlike borderline PD, the cognitive-perceptual aberrations of schizotypal PD are more stable and enduring, whereas borderline patients may experience momentary and extremely brief agitation and so-called micropsychotic episodes. **People with schizotypal PD may resemble those with prodromal or residual schizophrenia.** Thus, the **diagnosis must be made longitudinally,** and in the absence of a history of schizophrenic symptoms. People with Asperger syndrome, a pervasive developmental disorder, have poor interpersonal interactions and emotional expressions, but they do not have the magical thinking and perceptual changes that are seen in schizotypal PD. Schizoid PD is a pervasive pattern of social detachment and restricted emotional expression, without the odd or eccentric behaviors or ideas in schizotypal PD (Table 9-2). Of note, some of R.T.'s physical complaints may be caused by her use of vitamins and herbal preparations. For example, ma huang is a sympathomimetic and could cause tachycardia.

 QUESTIONS

9-1. Which of the following is true about the relationship of schizotypal personality disorder to schizophrenia?
- A. A point mutation on chromosome 10 is strongly associated with schizotypal PD but not with schizophrenia.
- B. A three base-pair difference in the schizophrenia gene leads to schizotypal PD.
- C. There is no increased risk of schizotypal PD in first-degree relatives of schizophrenics.
- D. Similar neuropsychological abnormalities are seen in schizophrenia and schizotypal PD.
- E. There is no increased risk of schizophrenia in families of people with schizotypal PD.

TABLE 9-2 Review of Cluster A —"Odd Cluster" Personality Disorders

Schizotypal	Discomfort with and reduced capacity for close relationships; cognitive and perceptual aberrations; behavioral eccentricities	~3% prevalence, possibly M > F; increased in families of schizophrenics, and increased risk of schizophrenia in families with schizotypal PD	Correlates of CNS dysfunction in schizophrenia may be seen in schizotypal PD, including tests of visual and auditory attention and smooth pursuit eye movement.
Schizoid	Detached, restricted range of affect; disinterest in social relationships	0.5–7% prevalence, possibly M > F; possible family association with schizophrenia	Loners are rarely seen in clinical practice until their ego-syntonic isolationist traits and coping skills are threatened and acute symptoms arise.
Paranoid	Suspiciousness, over interpreting other's motivations or actions	0.5–2.5% prevalence, M > F	Suspicious individuals rarely present for treatment given their ego-syntonic paranoid traits.

9-2. Which of the following statements about the natural history of schizotypal PD is true?
  A. As children they are usually well integrated into their peer groups.
  B. They may exist more comfortably in fringe groups with odd beliefs.
  C. 30% go on to develop schizophrenic.
  D. The course most often waxes and wanes throughout life.
  E. 50% go on to develop schizophrenic.

9-3. Which of the following is correct about schizotypal PD?
  A. Low-dose antipsychotics may be useful for the perceptual disturbances.
  B. Most people with schizotypal PD worry they are "going crazy."
  C. Those with schizotypal PD are usually disturbed about their eccentricities.
  D. Rapport is usually easy to develop.
  E. Most seek treatment to become more "mainstream."

9-4. Which of the following is found in schizotypal PD?

A. It occurs in approximately 15% of the general population.

B. More than half will have major depressive episodes.

C. The M/F ratio is 1:10.

D. Comorbid bipolar disorder is common.

E. It is common in prison inmates.

ANSWERS

9-1. D. Correlates of CNS dysfunction seen in schizophrenia have been observed in schizotypal PD, including performance on tests of visual and auditory attention and smooth pursuit eye movement, and there is empirical support for a genetic association of schizotypal PD with schizophrenia. Such clinically apparent abnormalities linking different but possibly related conditions are termed "endophenotypes." However, there is no known "schizophrenia gene," and multiple genetic abnormalities have been found in schizophrenia. The prevalence of schizotypal PD is increased in the families of schizophrenics, and there is an increased risk of schizophrenia in families of people with schizotypal PD.

9-2. B. Although there is an increased risk of schizophrenia, only 10% to 15% of patients with schizotypal PD will go on to develop schizophrenia. As children they are likely to be isolated, teased, or ostracized, and they may withdraw into bizarre fantasies or have odd preoccupations. As adults, they may be drawn to fringe groups that support their odd beliefs. Depending on the group, this may provide companionship and structure or be deleterious. The course appears to be relatively stable throughout life.

9-3. A. People with schizotypal PD may seek treatment for anxiety, perceptual disturbances, or depression, especially if these symptoms become increasingly intrusive. These patients are often not fully aware of their oddness and isolation and consider themselves to be simply eccentric, creative, or nonconformist. Some are troubled by their perceptual experiences or by their inability to relate to or feel comfortable with others. The treatment should be cognitive, behavioral, supportive, and pharmacologic, as these patients often find the intimacy of exploratory psychotherapy to be too stressful. Rapport is difficult to develop, as increasing familiarity and intimacy may actually increase their discomfort. Practical advice is usually helpful, and individuals with schizotypal PD may benefit from social skills training directed at their odd behaviors, dress, and speech. Most empirical research on the treatment of schizotypal PD has evaluated the effects of medications, such as low doses of antipsychotics, to treat the perceptual aberrations and social anxiety.

9-4. B. Of patients with schizotypal personality disorder, more than half will experience a major depressive episode. Schizotypal PD occurs at a rate of approximately 3% of the general population, and is frequently codiagnosed with fragile X syndrome. Schizotypal PD may be slightly more common in men. There is no evidence showing an increased association with bipolar disorder. Antisocial PD is common in prison inmates.

SUGGESTED READINGS

Kendler KS, Gardner CO. The risk for psychiatric disorders in relatives of schizophrenic and control probands: a comparison of three independent studies. *Psychol Med.* 1997;27(2):411–419.

Koenigsberg HW, Reynolds D, et al. Risperidone in the treatment of schizotypal personality disorder. *J Clin Psychiatry.* 2003; 64(6):628–634.

Siever LJ, Davis KL. The pathophysiology of schizophrenia disorders: perspectives from the spectrum. *Am J Psychiatry.* 2004;161(3):398–413.

McGlashan TH, Grilo CM, et al. Two-year prevalence and stability of individual DSM-IV criteria for schizotypal, borderline, avoidant, and obsessive-compulsive personality disorders: toward a hybrid model of axis II disorders. *Am J Psychiatry.* 2005;162(5):883–889.

"My Wife's Lawyer Insisted I See You"

CC/ID: 32-year-old male, referred by his almost-ex-wife's lawyer, as part of a custody dispute.

HPI: At initial presentation, A.P. says nothing's wrong and gives you a letter from the lawyer. He states that the lawyer is a "shyster," and that his wife is "using the kids to get more money." He wants to have contact with them "because I'm their father" and "it looks good to women to be involved with your kids, right?" He denies psychotic, depressive, or manic symptoms, although he reports he can be quite impulsive. The letter from the lawyer requests that the wife have full custody. The patient doesn't actually contest this but "wants to give her a hard time."

PMHx: None

PPHx: Age 11 diagnosed with conduct disorder, treated with counseling.

SHx/FHx: His father was a "businessman" who moved frequently to avoid legal repercussions of shady dealings. Father abused alcohol, often beat his son, and abandoned the family when the patient was 9. His mother was depressed and passive. After the father left, she took A.P. to live with an aunt in a wealthy suburb. The **patient had trouble with fights, setting fires, truancy, lying, using marijuana and alcohol, and running away.** He said, "At 13 I began my fortune scalping tickets." He continued alcohol use in high school and college. In college he was charged with both **sexual assault and cheating** on exams, but the charges were dropped. He left college after 2 years to open an import business. He has worked in a number of ventures and implies he has interacted with organized crime. He had **three DWIs** in his 20s. He married at age 26: "It was fun at first," but he gloatingly admits to multiple episodes of infidelity. His wife instigated divorce proceedings when Bunny, his girlfriend of the moment, called his home. "If it wasn't for Bunny and her stupidity, I wouldn't be here."

THOUGHT QUESTION

- What else would be important to find out?

DISCUSSION

It is important to carefully evaluate his history of substance use as well as any episodes of impulsivity, especially those resulting in violent outcomes or other harm to others or himself. Additionally, a full assessment must include an evaluation of enduring personality traits, evident in his functioning in relationships and at work.

CASE CONTINUED

He uses cocaine "socially" about once a month. He drinks, "the usual amount": one drink at lunch, two to three in the evening, and beer with dinner. He denies morning withdrawal or escalation of use, although he does drive in the evenings: "I'm fine—I can hold my liquor." He describes his relationships as follows: "I'm the one in charge; these women just cozy up to me, and I go through them when I want"; in this vein, he denies that these relationships are turbulent. He also denies experiences of identity disturbance or parasuicidal behavior. His MSE is notable only for an overly ingratiating manner.

THOUGHT QUESTION

- What is the differential diagnosis in this case?

DISCUSSION

On axis I he may have a substance use disorder, but other illnesses are unlikely with this history. On axis II the **differential diagnosis includes borderline, histrionic, narcissistic, or antisocial PD.**

Table 10-1 presents a review of cluster B ("dramatic") personality disorders. He is grandiose and impulsive, symptoms also seen in narcissistic PD, but his symptoms are more about "getting one over on someone else" than about maintaining his own fragile self-esteem. Though this is a fine line, the difference is in the motivation behind the behaviors, and less about the behaviors themselves. For example, narcissistic patients may lack empathy

TABLE **10-1**   Review of Cluster B–Dramatic Personality Disorders

Antisocial	Disregard for and violation of rights of others; lying, illegal behavior, impulsivity, aggressiveness, remorselessness	Prevalence in prison: ~20%–50%; prevalence in population: ~3% of men, 1% of women Possible genetic predisposition	Childhood often characterized by physical or sexual abuse or neglect, with empathy and warmth discouraged or punished; associated with substance abuse and depression.
Histrionic	Excessive emotionality, attention seeking, seductive, shallow, theatrical, impressionistic or vague speech	Prevalence 2%–3%; much higher in psychiatric and medical populations Diagnosed in F >>> M	May have a higher rate of somatic complaints, depression, and substance abuse; so-called "global emotional thinking" describes impressionistic style
Narcissistic	Grandiosity, need for admiration, lack of empathy, exploitative, envious, arrogant, underlying very low self-esteem	Prevalence in population: <1-2% – 16% of psychiatric clinical populations M >> F	Sense of worth contingent upon accomplishment; associated with devaluing parenting; injury to self-image leads to depression, rage, or paranoia
Borderline	Instability of interpersonal relationships, self image, and affect; marked impulsivity	Prevalence in population: 2%–3%; much higher in clinical samples M:F = 1:3	Associated with childhood physical or sexual abuse; also associated with substance use, suicide (~9%), depression, eating disorders

TABLE **10-2**   Criteria for Antisocial Personality Disorder (3 of 7 required)

Failure to conform to social norms or laws
Deceitfulness, conning people
Impulsivity
Irritability or aggressiveness
Reckless disregard of safety of self or others
Consistent irresponsibility
Lack of remorse, rationalizing aversive behaviors

Adapted from American Psychiatric Association. Task Force on DSM-IV. *Diagnostic and statistical manual of mental disorders: DSM-IV.* 4th ed. Washington, DC: American Psychiatric Association, 1994.

for another's plight, but the organizing drive of their behavior is to protect their own fragile self-esteem rather than to see what they can get from hurting another, as would be manifest in antisocial PD. Additionally, he does not meet criteria for borderline PD (e.g., he does not have identity disturbance). He does not have histrionic PD symptoms (e.g., suggestibility or considering relationships more intimate than they are). He meets criteria for antisocial PD. He had a conduct disorder as a child, and has a pervasive pattern of disregard for and violation of the rights of others; he has been exploitative in his relationships and manipulates situations, as well as blaming others for his troubles and lacking empathy. He has more than three of the seven adult diagnostic criteria in Table 10-2.

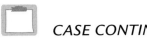 *CASE CONTINUED*

You ask him what goals he might have for treatment, and he offers to give you an "extra fee" to fill in the legal papers in his "favor". He does not express any interest in ongoing treatment or exploring his personality or behavior.

 QUESTIONS

   10-1. Which of the following statements about antisocial PD is true?
- A. It is found in 19% of men.
- B. It is found in 85% of prison inmates.
- C. It has not been associated with childhood sexual abuse.

    D. It has been associated with harsh discipline and physical abuse.

    E. The M:F ratio is approximately 25:1.

10-2. Which of the following may be helpful in diagnosing antisocial PD?

    A. EEGs, because they show an increase in theta activity in 80% of patients with antisocial PD.

    B. Neurological "soft signs" (e.g., low set ears), because they are seen in 30% of patients with antisocial PD.

    C. Criminality, because it is synonymous with antisocial PD.

    D. Presence of alcohol abuse and aggression.

    E. CT scans, because ventricular enlargement is pathognomonic for antisocial PD.

10-3. A psychological mechanism often seen in antisocial personality disorder is

    A. Externalization of blame

    B. Sublimation

    C. Internalization of blame

    D. Splitting

    E. Magical thinking

10-4. Which of the following is true about the treatment of antisocial PD?

    A. Behavioral therapy is an effective, validated treatment.

    B. Patients usually have poor insight into their illness.

    C. Atypical antipsychotics have been demonstrated to be useful.

    D. All of the above.

    E. None of the above.

ANSWERS

10-1. D. The rate of antisocial PD in prison and forensic settings has been estimated at 20% to 50%. The NIMH Epidemiological Catchment Area study indicated that approximately 3% of men and 1% of women have antisocial PD. Its etiology has been linked to a history of exposure to physical or sexual abuse or neglect, and growing up in an environment with excessively harsh, lenient, or erratic discipline in which feelings of empathy and warmth were discouraged or punished. Aggressiveness and exploitation are usually found to have been encouraged in families that give rise to patients with antisocial PD. Interestingly, however, there is also a clear genetic diathesis for this disorder.

10-2. D. Antisocial PD is often associated with substance use and aggression, but it is not synonymous with criminality. Although studies have found abnormal EEGs in this disorder and related conditions, there is no pattern that is useful in diagnosis, nor are specific neurological abnormalities commonly seen.

10-3. A. As was seen in this case, externalization of blame is commonly seen in antisocial personality disorder. Internalization is more often associated with depression. Sublimation is a mature healthy defense that allows people to channel their energies in constructive ways. Splitting is characteristic of borderline PD and is characterized by overvaluation and devaluation.

10-4. B. Patients with antisocial PD usually have very little insight into the fact they have a psychiatric problem. This represents a major barrier to treatment, and disinterest in treatment is commonly encountered. It is not clear which types of therapies are most useful in antisocial PD, and some evidence indicates that these patients respond very poorly to psychotherapy, much of which is based on empathic connection. Some medications have been used to address impulsivity, including SSRIs and anticonvulsants, but there is a lack of consistent evidence. Structured treatment settings may be helpful. These patients are at increased risk of suicide.

📖 SUGGESTED READINGS

Grant BF, Hasin DS, Stinson FS, et al. Prevalence, correlates, and disability of personality disorders in the United States: results from the national epidemiologic survey on alcohol and related conditions. *J Clin Psychiatry*. 2004;65(7):948–958.

Simonoff E, Elander J, Holmshaw J, et al. Predictors of antisocial personality. Continuities from childhood to adult life. *Br J Psychiatry*. 2004;184:118–127.

Verona E, Sachs-Ericsson N, and Joiner TE. Suicide attempts associated with externalizing psychopathology in an epidemiological sample. *Am J Psychiatry*. 2004;161(3):444–451.

CASE 11

"My Wife Left Me!"

CC/ID: 62-year-old businessman, self-referred with a complaint of, "I am furious and want to talk about this."

HPI: B.D. reports that his wife of 12 years has abruptly and inexplicably left; "I have no idea why." Upon exploration, it becomes clear that he has had a series of extramarital affairs, which his wife recently discovered. In describing his frustration over her leaving, he remarks, "She will never find anyone else. She's making a terrible mistake. We have a beautiful house, a boat, a membership in the best club." He later describes his **"magnetic" appeal to women,** and he oscillates between describing his ease at being able to move on to another woman and having trouble believing that his wife has left for good, stating that "she'll be back," despite the fact that the divorce papers arrived yesterday. He also talks a great deal about his successes in business and how much power he has in his company, far surpassing the **"little people I stepped on on my way to the top."** Similarly, in his initial phone call to you, he told you that his doctors include the chairmen of internal medicine and cardiology at the local academic medical center, and he queried as to your academic rank, your position in the local psychiatric society, and what schools you had attended. When asked directly about symptoms, he describes some difficulty falling asleep, but normal appetite, energy, and concentration. He remains able to work productively. He is offended when asked about suicidality, and states, "She's not worth it."

PMHx: Hypertension

PPHx: No history of conduct disorder. During second marriage went to couple's counseling once and tells a story about the therapist's incompetence.

SHx/FHx: Oldest and most successful of three boys raised by a strict father who gave literal and limited pats on the back for As and beatings for Cs. Mother left the family for a "famous actor . . .

79

you've seen him." B.D. has been successful in his education and business, currently working as an executive in sales. He was married 3 times, the first for 8 years, the second for 5 years to an intern at his company, and currently for 12 years to a former secretary. He has two children from his first marriage. He has no history of legal entanglements, nor history of substance abuse.

PE/Labs: Noncontributory

MSE: *General:* Well groomed, expensively dressed, fair eye contact, relatively denigrating though appeasing when he seems to want something; no PMA/A. *Mood:* "angry." *Affect:* appropriate though expansive. *Thought process:* goal directed. *Thought content:* grandiose themes, no delusions, and no abnormal perceptions. No suicidal or homicidal ideation. *Insight:* fair. *Judgment:* fair.

THOUGHT QUESTIONS

- Does this man have an axis I diagnosis?
- Does this man have an axis II diagnosis?

DISCUSSION

On axis I, this man does not meet criteria for major depression, dysthymia, or an adjustment disorder. To meet the criteria for an adjustment disorder, he would need to have symptoms that either cause marked distress in excess of what would be expected for the stressor, or significant impairment in social or occupational functioning. While frustrated over his wife's leaving him, he remains able to function at prior levels. On axis II, it is important to examine his enduring personality traits. **He displays a pervasive pattern of grandiosity, need for admiration, and lack of empathy, which is consistent with narcissistic personality disorder.** Narcissistic PD is indicated by the presence of five or more of the diagnostic criteria in Table 11-1. People with narcissistic PD are often vulnerable to threats to their self-esteem, and they may react defensively with rage, disdain, or indifference; however, at their core, they are actually struggling with feelings of insecurity and humiliation, though they consciously deny this. Narcissistic PD shares some traits with histrionic and antisocial PD. Both narcissistic and antisocial persons may lie and manipulate others, as well as having a lack of empathy or remorse for their actions; the narcissistic person is

TABLE 11-1   Criteria for Narcissistic Personality Disorder

Grandiose self-importance	Needs excessive admiration	Sense of entitlement
Preoccupied with fantasies of unlimited power, beauty, and success	Believes that he or she is special and can only be understood by other high-status people	Envious and believes others are envious of him or her
Interpersonally exploitative	Lacks empathy	Arrogant and haughty

Adapted from American Psychiatric Association. Task Force on DSM-IV. *Diagnostic and statistical manual of mental disorders: DSM-IV.* 4th ed. Washington, DC: American Psychiatric Association, 1994.

motivated by recognition and status, whereas the antisocial person may be motivated by the desire to subjugate others. Like histrionic persons, those with clinical narcissism may behave flamboyantly, often acting out their feelings, chronically seeking admiration from others.

CASE CONTINUED

It was clear that B.D. found it humiliating to ask for help, and he spent much of the session reporting on his successes and conquests. He seemed to want you to agree that his wife was a "fool" who was somehow at fault for the breakup or would end up returning to him. By being supportive but not colluding with these ideas, you are able to make a tenuous therapeutic alliance, and he makes another appointment.

QUESTIONS

11-1. In an interview, which scenario would suggest a diagnosis of histrionic PD?

    A. He was inappropriately laughing when talking of his breakup.

    B. He was speaking impressionistically and dramatically shifting between expressions of grief and happiness.

C. He was tearful and stated he couldn't eat, sleep, or work since his wife had left.

D. He was concerned that his wife had been taken over by an evil spirit.

F. He was talking about aliens having exchanged his wife for an imposter.

11-2. Which of the following best describes narcissistic PD?
A. The prevalence is 10% of the general population.
B. A belief that value is contingent upon emotional accessibility.
C. Feelings of insecurity are masked by arrogance.
D. It is more prevalent in women than men.
E. Frequent work with humanitarian aid groups.

11-3. Which of the following is correct concerning patients with narcissistic PD?
A. They are rarely very successful in their work.
B. They may have difficulty in work because of their significant paranoia about other's motivations.
C. They have an increased risk of depressive disorders.
D. In old age there is a 70% suicide rate.
E. They are known for their altruistic qualities.

11-4. Which of the following is correct about the treatment of narcissistic PD?
A. Therapists should never collude with the patient's self-importance.
B. Antipsychotics may be used to treat grandiosity.
C. Patients usually have good insight into their illness.
D. Role-play could be useful in couple's therapy.
E. Initial devaluation of the patient increases the likelihood of successful treatment.

ANSWERS

11-1. B. Histrionic PD is characterized by one's needing to be the center of attention, using appearance to draw attention, being inappropriately seductive, having rapidly shifting and shallow emotions, using an impressionistic style of speech and excessive theatricality, and considering relationships to be more intimate than they actually are. In the question, choice (A) could be suggestive of antisociality or a psychotic disorder; (C) is more consistent with a major depression or underlying dependent personality;

(D or E) could be either a manifestation of a schizotypal personality disorder or a brief psychotic disorder; (E) could also be a manifestation of a delusional misidentification syndrome (e.g., Capgras syndrome).

11-2. C. The prevalence of narcissistic PD is <1% of the general population and 2% to 16% of clinical psychiatric populations and is more prevalent in men than women. Narcissism may develop through devaluing parenting (as in this case), or from parents who are narcissistic themselves, leading them to view and value their children only according to and in keeping with the child's accomplishments. Narcissists may then grow to believe that a sense of worth or meaning is contingent upon accomplishment, and they must continually seek signs of recognition to compensate for feelings of inadequacy. Value is contingent on success, accomplishment, or status. Their feelings of insecurity may be masked by disdain, indifference, conceit, arrogance, or grandiosity.

11-3. C. People with narcissistic PD have an increased incidence of depression, as they are extremely sensitive to perceived blows to their self-esteem (i.e., the narcissistic injury), and they may be at increased risk for suicide. However, a 70% suicide rate does not exist at any age. Adolescents and young adults with narcissistic PD tend to be self-centered, dominant, and arrogant. As adults, they may display high levels of achievement, but their relationships with colleagues and their staff may be difficult due to their tendencies toward interpersonal exploitation rather than paranoid ideation. Success may also be impaired by their difficulty in acknowledging or applying negative feedback or constructive criticism. They tend to develop sexual relationships rather easily, but these are difficult to sustain because of their self-centeredness and lack of empathy. They are prone to mood disorders as well as substance-use disorders (especially cocaine).

11-4. D. As they tend to lack empathy, people with narcissistic PD usually have difficulty understanding that their behaviors may cause undue hardship to another. Thus role-play and role reversal may be useful in couple's therapy to help each member of the couple understand his or her role in the dyadic problems present in the relationship. Occurring as part of a personality disorder, narcissistic symptoms tend to be ego-syntonic (e.g., in keeping with the person's self-concept), and role-play may help patients become aware that their behaviors are maladaptive. It is difficult for these patients to admit that they have a psychological problem, thus they usually present for treatment of depression, substance abuse, or relationship problems. Regarding their narcissism, active confrontation is useful at times, but other times the patient may require more unconditional support. Cognitive-behavioral approaches emphasize increasing an awareness of these patients' impact on others and changing their attitudes toward themselves and others. There is no accepted pharmacologic approach to the treatment of narcissism, although pharmacotherapy may be used in the treatment of comorbid disorders. As the grandiose themes are not psychotic, antipsychotics are not indicated for this symptom. However, while not expressly indicated for this purpose, they do have clinical utility in helping to attenuate impulsivity and severe acting out.

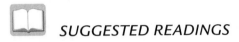 *SUGGESTED READINGS*

Zanarini MC, Skodol AE, Bender D, et al. The Collaborative Longitudinal Personality Disorders Study: reliability of axis I and II diagnoses. *J Personal Disord.* 2000;14(4):291–299.

Schiavone P Dorz S, Conforti D, et al. Comorbidity of DSM-IV personality disorders in unipolar and bipolar affective disorders: a comparative study. *Psychol Rep.* 2004;95(1):121–128.

Betan E, Heim AK, Zittel Conklin C, et al. Countertransference phenomena and personality pathology in clinical practice: an empirical investigation. *Am J Psychiatry.* 2005;162(5):890–898.

"My Boss Told Me to Come"

CC/ID: 39-year-old businessman presents stating: "My boss thinks I need help with my management style."

HPI: J.K. first confirms with you that the content of the sessions is confidential and will not "get back to" his boss. He somewhat tentatively admits that one of his subordinates, Bob, has recently transferred to another department, and he feels that this event has led him to be more **"testy" with his colleagues.** He describes running a department where three people report to him, and three report, in turn, to each of them. He is concerned that Bob may have taken some of the files when he left, and further, that one of the remaining two, Sam, is trying to undermine his authority in a possible bid for his job, or may be planning something similarly egregious with Bob. When the third person told him last week that she was pregnant, he accused her of "doing it on purpose" so that he would lose his department, leading to a merger with a larger division with Sam at the helm. He acknowledges that, reflecting on it, he may have "overdone it," but then reverses his position, stating, "Don't you think the timing is a bit **suspicious?** She *is* friends with Bob and Sam. . . ." He denies depressive, manic, and neurovegetative symptoms.

PMHx: None

PPHx: None

SHx/FHx: Mother was "extremely protective . . . She always said that you can't trust anyone better than yourself." He excelled in school, but had social difficulty throughout his childhood, which he explained as, "Other kids resented me. They were always trying to outmaneuver me, but I am very attuned to other people's motives." He had few friends and has never married. He describes being known as a "stickler" and "prickly" at work. His intelligence has helped him progress, despite a reputation for being hard to work with.

THOUGHT QUESTION

- ▪ What should be assessed in the physical and mental status examinations?

DISCUSSION

Given his symptoms and suspiciousness, it is important to carefully assess his thought process (for formal thought disorder), thought content (for systematized delusions or nonpsychotic overvalued ideas), and perception (for hallucinatory experiences). If he does manifest new onset psychotic symptoms, it would be important to perform thorough neurological and fundoscopic examinations, as well as considering neuroimaging (CT or MRI) and laboratory studies (RPR, TSH, basic metabolic profile) to rule out underlying organic causes.

CASE CONTINUED

PE/Labs: Noncontributory

MSE: *General:* Well groomed, anxious, guarded, fairly-related but distant. *Mood:* "angry." *Affect:* somewhat constricted; nervous and hypervigilant quality. *Thought process:* goal-directed. *Thought content:* preoccupied with suspicious themes, reaching the level of overvalued ideas, but no organized delusions, no perceptual abnormalities, no thought insertion or thought broadcasting. No suicidal or homicidal ideation. *Insight:* fair.

THOUGHT QUESTIONS

- ▪ Does this man have an axis I diagnosis?
- ▪ Does this man have an axis II diagnosis?

DISCUSSION

This man is suspicious of his co-workers, their actions, and their motives. On axis I, the most important considerations include schizophrenia and delusional disorder, both of the paranoid type. Paranoid schizophrenia is characterized by delusions (may be bizarre and may be highly systematized) and hallucinations (frequently well-formed audible voices that may provide a running commentary on the patient's actions or talk among themselves). A bizarre delusion might entail the FBI and newscasters' sending alien messages to him, leading him to insulate his hats with aluminum foil to prevent the transmissions; this delusion is bizarre in that it is not possible in the known physical world. Nonbizarre delusions may also occur, and include beliefs that are false but may be physically possible. For a diagnosis of schizophrenia, the patient must experience isolated bizarre delusions or a combination of delusions and hallucinations for at least 6 months. In delusional disorder, patients have nonbizarre delusions that do not interfere with other aspects of their functioning; that is, the patient might believe that the FBI is watching him, but his precautionary responses are limited to his making personal calls only on public phones. Importantly, these patients are generally able to function at work and in other spheres not affected by their delusional beliefs.

For axis II, we should examine his enduring personality traits. Throughout childhood, and continuing to the present, he has been socially isolated, somewhat rigid in his thinking, and has displayed a pervasive pattern of distrust and suspiciousness, feeling that people are out to manipulate him. A number of personality disorders can be included in this differential. People with narcissistic PD may be mistrustful; those with borderline PD may have micropsychotic episodes which may include and be manifest by paranoid thinking; people with avoidant PD are timid, socially withdrawn, anxious, and apprehensive; those with schizoid PD are socially isolated and choose solitary activities; and schizotypal persons may have paranoid ideation. The only disorder with predominantly and isolated paranoid symptoms is paranoid PD. Paranoid PD is indicated by the presence of four or more of the diagnostic criteria presented in Table 12-1.

TABLE **12-1**   Criteria for Paranoid Personality Disorder

Reading hidden messages into benign events	Bearing grudges
Unwarranted suspicion that people are exploiting or deceiving	Perceives attacks that others do not see and is quick to counterattack
Reluctance in confiding in others for fear of the information being used maliciously	Unwarranted suspicion about marital fidelity Preoccupation with doubts about friends' loyalties

Adapted from American Psychiatric Association. Task Force on DSM-IV. *Diagnostic and statistical manual of mental disorders: DSM-IV.* 4th ed. Washington, DC: American Psychiatric Association, 1994.

CASE CONTINUED

J.K. does not manifest and has not been experiencing any bizarre delusions, and his paranoia is not systematized or fixed, thus limiting it to the degree of an overvalued idea. Given his lifelong personality characteristics and functional impairment, he meets criteria for paranoid PD. Though he remains suspicious of your motives, he agrees to a trial of psychotherapy to help him improve his working relationships with his colleagues, but with the qualification that "I'm not going to let you change me."

QUESTIONS

12-1. Which of the following are possible theories for the etiology of paranoid PD?
- A. Modeling from the family.
- B. Cultural groupings have no effect.
- C. It may be a schizophrenia spectrum disorder.
- D. It has been definitively linked to childhood sexual abuse.
- E. A missense mutation on chromosome 6.

12-2. Which of the following epidemiological statistics is found in paranoid PD?
- A. The prevalence is approximately 10% of the general population.
- B. The prevalence is approximately 2% of the general population.
- C. It is more common in women than men.
- D. 40% of people with paranoid PD will have schizophrenic relatives.
- E. 60% of people with paranoid PD will have schizophrenic relatives.

12-3. Which of the following best describes factors related to the treatment of paranoid PD?
- A. They often seek treatment for their suspiciousness.
- B. They usually experience their paranoid traits as "alien" or "unlike me."
- C. They may seek treatment for anxiety.
- D. They do not have comorbid axis I disorders.
- E. Double blind placebo-controlled studies show profound effects from medication management.

12-4. Which of the following therapeutic techniques should be employed in paranoid PD?
   A. It is helpful to contradict the patient's paranoid beliefs.
   B. It is, at least initially, helpful to foster the patient's paranoid beliefs.
   C. It is helpful to encourage the patient to be more self-questioning.
   D. It is helpful to ignore the patient's paranoid beliefs.
   E. (A) and (C)

ANSWERS

12-1. A. Paranoid belief systems could develop through parental or group modeling. Paranoid beliefs do tend to be self-perpetuating; in refugee or minority groups, mistrust and suspicion may be normal and adaptive. Additionally, the paranoid person's behavior may cause reciprocal hostile responses in others, creating a "self-fulfilling prophecy." Though childhood sexual abuse has been linked to other disorders (e.g., borderline PD) and to various psychological problems, there is no known causal relationship with paranoid PD. There are no known gene mutations that cause paranoid personality disorder.

12-2. B. Although 13% of men and 6% of women may be characteristically mistrustful, only 0.5% to 2.5% of the population meets the diagnostic criteria for paranoid PD. Men are more often affected than women. Research suggests a genetic contribution to paranoid personality but, unlike that found in schizotypal PD, the findings are more equivocal about its relationship to the schizophrenia spectrum disorders.

12-3. C. People with paranoid PD usually experience their paranoid symptoms as ego-syntonic (i.e., part of who they are, and in keeping with their sense of self), rather than ego-dystonic (i.e, ego-alien). They therefore rarely seek treatment for their paranoid personality traits. In fact, their generalized suspiciousness and mistrust often preclude their presenting for treatment. However, they may come for treatment of a comorbid axis I disorder, such as anxiety, mood, or substance use, or for marital or occupational difficulties. Medications may be useful and are indicated in the treatment of comorbid axis I conditions; they have only marginal benefit in ameliorating symptoms inherent in the personality disorder. There is, however, limited evidence that low-dose antipsychotics may reduce some paranoid symptoms and that SSRIs may help with ruminative thoughts of suspiciousness.

12-4. C. Patients with paranoid PD frequently jump to conclusions that others have a malicious intent to harm the patient; this often results from their own fears and unrecognized aggressive impulses. The goal for the treatment of paranoid PD is to help the patient develop more self-reflecting and self-questioning capabilities. In time, this may facilitate an understanding of the contribution of paranoid traits to problems that are being experienced. This may be done by helping the patient to examine the reality of, and logic behind, the suspicions in a nonthreatening, nonjudgmental way. It is usually pointless to confront the paranoid beliefs; often this serves no other function than to alienate the patient. But fostering or supporting the paranoid beliefs is also counterproductive and may appear insincere or manipulative on the part of the therapist, especially when the patient is a prior looking for an underlying motive stop after therapist.

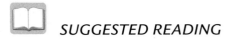 **SUGGESTED READING**

Bender DS. The therapeutic alliance in the treatment of personality disorders. *J Psychiatr Pract.* 2005;11(2):73–87.

"I Can't Stop Crying"

CC/ID: 43-year-old woman who presents for "depression," 6 weeks after her father's death.

HPI: T.C. describes feeling and functioning well until 8 months ago, when her father was diagnosed with pancreatic cancer. At that time she went into what she calls "hyper mode," researching treatments and endlessly talking to doctors. When her father's illness did not respond to traditional treatments, she insisted on experimental therapies, until finally she got a hospice involved. However, by this time, he was gravely ill and only survived for an additional 3 weeks. Since his death she has felt sad, tearful, lonely, and empty, and feels guilty that she did not do more. She has difficulty falling asleep, and she maintains a low to normal appetite, but her weight is unchanged. Her energy level is described as, "OK. I do what I have to, but I'm just going through the motions." She sometimes experiences a sensation as if her father is in the room, and occasionally has fleeting experiences of hearing his voice.

PMHx: None

PPHx: Major depression in college; took off one semester, no hospitalization, treated with psychotherapy and nortriptyline.

FHx: "They're all depressed on my mom's side, and they won't talk about it."

SHx: Eldest of three children, divorced 5 years ago, no children, successful management consultant.

THOUGHT QUESTIONS

- What would you like to clarify?
- What else is important to know?

DISCUSSION

It is important to clarify her experience of "hearing his voice." Phenomenological markers such as its origin (from where does it come?), localization (inside or outside her head?), clarity (as clear as the doctor's voice now?), content (mourning-based or bizarre?), precipitants (occurring in her father's room or in places not linked to him?), stability (does it disappear when she pays more attention to it?), and the explanation it is given (what does it mean to her?) are all important in the assessment of whether this experience is an illusion or an hallucination, and whether it is consistent with pathology or with grieving. This experience may be culturally congruent for this patient as a manifestation of grief. Understanding her relationship with her father may help shed additional light on the nature of her reactions. Paramount in an evaluation of symptoms following a loss is assessing whether this patient has been able to remain functional in interpersonal/social, occupational, and self-care realms.

As always, it is important to assess the risk for suicide. In their grief, people sometimes wish to "rejoin" their loved ones, and this may occasionally lead to a suicide attempt. Finally, one must rule out medical conditions or medication side effects that could be causing her symptoms.

CASE CONTINUED

Meds: None

SHx: Her mother died when she was 11, and she was very close to her father. After receiving her MBA, she joined him in the family business, which they sold when he became ill.

PE: WNL, no thyroid enlargement

Labs: unremarkable; TSH: WNL

MSE: *General:* Sad-appearing, well groomed, mild psychomotor retardation. *Speech:* slow but spontaneous and without increased latency. *Mood:* "Miserable." *Affect:* constricted and clearly dysphoric. *Thought process:* logical, goal-directed. *Thought content:* no delusions, no suicidal ideation. *Perception:* She explains she doesn't actually hear her father speaking to her, but sometimes "feels like he's there speaking in the next room."

THOUGHT QUESTION

- What is the differential diagnosis?

DISCUSSION

After experiencing a loss, such as death of a loved one, sadness and depressive symptoms are normal, and are typically seen as such by the individual. Specific symptoms may vary with one's culture, with the closeness of the relationship, and even with the type of death (sudden, violent, expected, etc.). Even if symptoms aggregate to that required for a major depressive episode, this diagnosis is reserved unless either symptom extends beyond 2 months (though this time marker is especially culturally sensitive), or if certain noncharacteristic reactions are present. As such, mood disorders can be diagnosed in the context of bereavement, especially when the following symptoms are present: functioning is severely impaired; suicidal thoughts exist beyond a feeling that one would be better off dead or should have died also; guilt extends beyond that related to what the survivor should or could have done at the time of death; morbid preoccupation with worthlessness; severe psychomotor retardation; and abnormal perceptual experiences beyond thinking that the survivor hears or transiently sees the deceased person.

In this case, the patient's father, with whom she had a close personal and business relationship, died of a rapid, severe, and painful illness less than 2 months ago. This is within the time expected for bereavement, and though she is sad and tearful, with decreased appetite and energy, it has not affected her functioning. She does not meet criteria for major depressive disorder (MDD). Adjustment disorder is diagnosed if the symptoms are greater than expected or are causing impaired functioning, but do not meet criteria for MDD. She does not meet criteria for this either, and thus has uncomplicated bereavement.

Atypical grief may include chronic grief with features of a depressive episode, inhibited or delayed grief, or even a mixed reaction with symptoms of neurosis or psychosis. Atypical grief may also be referred to as complicated, distorted, abnormal, or morbid bereavement.

CASE CONTINUED

You suggest she might benefit from counseling. She declines, stating she "just wanted to make sure she wasn't getting depressed again," and she promises to call if her symptoms worsen. She plans to spend the next 4 months visiting family across the country.

Six months later, she returns to your office saying, "I'm ill." She doesn't enjoy anything, has no appetite, has lost 15 pounds, has poor sleep, has no motivation to look for work, and cannot concentrate to file her tax return. She feels that she too has pancreatic cancer and that her recent comprehensive workup has "just missed it." On exam, her grooming is fair; she is psychomotorically agitated; she is preoccupied with the idea that she has cancer and talks much about the suffering that her father endured, saying that she'd "rather be dead than have to go through that." She denies wanting to die, but alludes to the fact that she will kill herself if she finds that she does have cancer.

QUESTIONS

13-1. Given the case scenario described above, what is her diagnosis now?
- A. Uncomplicated bereavement
- B. Adjustment disorder, with depressed mood
- C. Somatoform disorder
- D. MDD
- E. Hypochondriasis

13-2. Which of the following is appropriate management of a suicidal patient with psychotic depression?
- A. Prescribe a tricyclic antidepressant, and tell her to return in a month.
- B. Prescribe an SSRI, refer her for therapy, and follow up in 2 weeks.
- C. Prescribe an SSRI and an antipsychotic, and admit her to inpatient psychiatry.
- D. Prescribe an SSRI and an antipsychotic, refer her to therapy, and follow up in 2 weeks.
- E. Prescribe an antipsychotic and tell her to return in a month for followup.

13-3. Which of the following correctly describes the stages of grief as described by Kübler-Ross?

A. Denial, anger, guilt, bargaining, depression
B. Anger, guilt, sadness/depression
C. Denial, anger, bargaining, depression, acceptance
D. Denial, anger, guilt, depression, acceptance
E. Denial, anger, guilt, bargaining, depression, acceptance

13-4. What is considered a "normal" time course for symptoms of acute bereavement?

A. 2 weeks
B. 2 months
C. 12 months
D. 24 months
E. 36 months

ANSWERS

13-1. D. This woman currently meets criteria for a major depressive episode. She has anhedonia, poor sleep, energy, appetite, and concentration, and probably suicidal ideation. Given her feeling that she has pancreatic cancer, it would be important to assess whether this is actually a delusional belief, or if it exists primarily as a hypochondriacal or fear- or anxiety-induced response. As she is currently depressed in the context of her father's death, this new fear/belief may be an emotional mechanism of identifying with him, perhaps maintaining his presence after his death. If it is delusional, she is at much greater risk for suicide. Of note, pancreatic cancer may present as depression.

13-2. C. Given a diagnosis of major depressive disorder with psychotic features, it is important to assess for suicidality, homicidality, and one's ability to care for oneself. Assuming that the patient in the case does have a delusional belief of having pancreatic cancer, her suicidality takes on much greater weight. Although delusionality in and of itself does not mandate psychiatric hospitalization, this patient's suicidality is based on her delusion, and thus she requires an inpatient level of care; if she is not able to sign in voluntarily, then an involuntary commitment may be indicated. Additionally, delusionality would also lead to a different treatment from nonpsychotic depression, and would include both antipsychotic and antidepressant medications, as opposed to monopharmacy with antidepressants in a nonpsychotic depression. Electroconvulsive therapy is also an option. If she were to be treated as an outpatient (not recommended because of her impaired reality testing and suicide risk), a tricyclic antidepressant would be a poor choice because of its potential lethality in overdose.

13-3. C. Although people may experience guilt about various unresolved issues in their relationship to the deceased, or about what they could have done for the person around the time of death, guilt is not considered a usual stage of grief as defined by Elisabeth Kübler-Ross. According to her, the five stages of grief are (i) denial and isolation, (ii) anger, (iii) bargaining, (iv) depression, and (v) acceptance. These stages are useful in understanding the experience of grief, but they do not necessarily occur in order, and not everyone experiences all stages.

13-4. B. After a significant loss, symptoms similar to major depression may be present in an individual for up to 2 months, during which time they may still be categorized as "bereavement." If symptoms that meet criteria for major depression persist beyond 2 months, the person should be diagnosed with major depression (however, as stated in the case, this time marker is unique to DSM-IV and may not extend to all cultural groups). Certain symptoms are also suggestive of a major depression, and are enumerated in the presented case.

 SUGGESTED READINGS

Mulsant BH, Sweet RA, Rosen J, et al. A double-blind randomized comparison of nortriptyline plus perphenazine versus nortriptyline plus placebo in the treatment of psychotic depression in late life. *J Clin Psychiatry.* 2001;62(8):597–604.

Grande GE, Farquhar MC, Barclay SI, et al. Caregiver bereavement outcome: relationship with hospice at home, satisfaction with care, and home death. *J Palliat Care.* 2004;20(2):69–77.

Rothschild AJ, Williamson DJ, Tohen MF, et al. A double-blind, randomized study of olanzapine and olanzapine/fluoxetine combination for major depression with psychotic features. *J Clin Psychopharmacol.* 2004;24(4):365–373.

"Why is She Biting Herself?"

 CC/ID: 37-year-old female with Down syndrome who is brought in by her care workers for increased agitation.

HPI: Two months ago, soon after her mother's death from a CVA, D.G.'s 82-year-old father found that he was no longer able to care for her. Upon his moving to a senior assisted living facility, he arranged for her to live in a nearby residence for people with mental retardation (MR), where she has been for the past month. During this time, she has become increasingly upset, screaming at night, throwing food, and occasionally biting herself.

THOUGHT QUESTIONS

- What other elements in the history are important?
- What medical concerns might you have?

DISCUSSION

It is very important to **understand her baseline level of functioning** and to review her medications and medical history. Of people with Down syndrome, 33% to 50% have congenital heart defects, mainly endocardial cushion and ventricular septal defects; over 50% of patients have bilateral hearing loss; other associated abnormalities include gastroesophageal reflux, obstructive sleep apnea, and increased incidence of thyroid dysfunction, diabetes mellitus, cataracts, leukemia, and seizure disorders. Many of these comorbid conditions, if active, could increase discomfort and cause confusion and changes in mood or behavior, and hence a high level of suspicion is indicated. For example, if her blood glucose were poorly controlled, she might experience dramatic mood shifts.

Additionally, while stressors are significant in any evaluation of psychopathology, in patients with Down syndrome and in those with other cognitive developmental disabilities, seemingly minor disruptions in routine may precipitate severe symptoms and acting-out behaviors. In addition to the possibly depressogenic loss of her mother, this patient has experienced many additional disruptions in her daily life (e.g., mother not around, father not around, change in living environment, needing to rely on strangers to care for many of her needs). As such, it is vital to assess her understanding of the situation and look for signs and symptoms of depression, which may not be described in usual cognitive or emotional terms, but rather manifest as acting-out behaviors. Additionally, institutional or residential settings may be poorly staffed, and "acting out" may be a way of getting attention or gratification. Exploring the structure and quality of the residential placement may add clues to the cause of the behavioral change.

CASE CONTINUED

At baseline she is cooperative and affable, but she can be stubborn and manifest occasional outbursts. She is usually able to manage her own ADLs, including toileting, and has been able to help around the house, set the table, and so on. Until her mother's death, she participated in a daily sheltered workshop. Since moving, her appetite has been poor, she has developed enuresis, her participation in activities has been erratic, and she has frequently awoken during the night. The residential home in which she resides has only six residents, is well-staffed, and the environment seems quite supportive. Her father is in the process of selling his business, and he has been visiting only once a week.

PMHx: IDDM; no cardiac abnormalities

Meds: Insulin. Her glucose is monitored three times daily, as she adapts to the new eating routines at the residence, and now she is on a new stable regimen. *ROS:* negative.

PPHx: Once medicated with carbamazepine for behavioral outbursts as a teenager.

SHx: As above

FHx: Psychiatric, none

VS: WNL

PE: *General:* Small ears, flat nasal bridge, small mouth, slightly protruding tongue, single transverse palmar crease, upwards slanting palpebral fissures. Otherwise unremarkable.

Labs: Blood glucose 120

MSE: *Speech and behavior:* withdrawn, looking down, mildly psychomotorically retarded, speech slow. *Mood:* appears sad. *Affect:* somewhat labile though congruent and dysphoric. *Thought process:* two- to four-word sentences, though linear; some retardation in the rate of thought. *Thought content:* concrete. She appears to understand that her mother is gone and that she is living in a new place. She does not express suicidal ideation or the wish to harm anyone else. She has no evidence of psychotic symptoms.

THOUGHT QUESTIONS

- What do you think is contributing to this woman's behavior?
- What should be done?

DISCUSSION

As in most cases, the determinants of her symptoms and her behaviors are multifactorial. She has had multiple losses including her mother, home, sheltered workshop, and to some extent her father, who has been preoccupied with work. She is also transitioning to a new environment, with new people and routines. She may be yelling or biting herself because she is distraught and cannot express herself verbally. Things that may be helpful include restarting the sheltered workshop and arranging with her father to visit more regularly while she is getting adjusted. Her depressive symptoms should be monitored, and if they persist or worsen, an antidepressant should be considered. She may benefit from supportive therapy to help her during this difficult time of transition. For a review of the physical signs and comorbidities commonly found in individuals with Down's syndrome see Table 14-1.

QUESTIONS

14-1. Which of the following best describes the etiology or epidemiology of Down syndrome?

TABLE 14-1   Features of Down Syndrome/Trisomy 21

Physical signs	Low birth weight, small round head, high cheek bones, oblique palpebral fissures, epicanthal folds, Brushfield spots on iris, strabismus, small noses and ears, arched palate, protruding tongue, short limbs and neck, hypotonic muscles, single palmar crease with characteristic ulnar loops
Associated medical comorbidities	Umbilical hernias, duodenal atresia, deafness, Hirschsprung disease, congenital heart disease (atrial/ventral septal defects), respiratory infections, seizures and increased prevalence of dementia over 40 years

- A. The incidence is approximately 1 in 250 live births.
- B. It is usually caused by nondisjunction of chromosome 21.
- C. In most cases, the risk of having a second child with Down syndrome is 10%.
- D. In women over 40, the incidence is ~1 in 20 live births.
- E. Balanced translocations account for the majority of cases.

14-2. Which if the following statements is accurate concerning psychiatric symptoms in Down syndrome?
- A. Individuals are placid and pleasant and have no psychiatric illnesses.
- B. Aggression and impulsivity are not common.
- C. Children have fewer emotional problems than unaffected peers.
- D. Rates of depression are lower than in other populations of patients with mental retardation.
- E. Self-mutilatory behavior is common.

14-3. Which IQ level corresponds to moderate mental retardation?
- A. 20–34
- B. 35–49
- C. 50–69
- D. 70–90
- E. 90–110

14-4. Of the following conditions, which will this woman with Down syndrome almost certainly manifest as she ages over 40?
- A. Schizophrenia
- B. Vascular dementia
- C. Thyroid abnormalities
- D. Alzheimer disease
- E. Hemiballismus

ANSWERS

14-1. B. Most cases of Down syndrome are sporadic and are due to an extra copy of chromosome 21 caused by a nondisjunction during meiosis; the recurrence rate is <1%. In 4% of cases, one parent has a balanced translocation. The incidence is 1/800 to 1/1000 live births. If the mother is less than 35 years old the incidence rate is 1/2500; if the mother is over 40, it increases to more than 1/100.

14-2. D. In the DSM-IV, mental retardation is coded on axis II, along with personality disorders, as each significantly impacts the individual throughout his or her life in characteristic ways. While mental retardation may be thought of as an intellectual and cognitive retardation, personality disorders may be seen as a type of emotional retardation. These characteristics put the patient at risk for various superimposed illnesses, as intellectual and emotional flexibility, respectively, are compromised. As such, psychiatric symptoms tend to be more common in individuals with limited reserves (either cognitively or emotionally), than in their unaffected peers. However, in Down syndrome, there are lower rates of depression and of other psychiatric illnesses than found in other MR populations. However, common problems in Down syndrome do include hyperactivity, aggression, and impulsivity. Self-mutilation is characteristic of Lesch Nyhan and Cornelia de Lange syndromes. Self-injurious behaviors can also occur in individuals with autism, especially when they are stressed or acting out.

14-3. B. Though the precise cut-offs vary between classification systems, moderate mental retardation is defined as an IQ of 35 to 49. Most people with Down syndrome fall in this range, and with proper educational support, they may be able to attain a 2nd or 3rd grade level of education. An IQ of 49 to 69 is considered mild mental retardation and describes about 80% of people with MR. These individuals are usually able to function completely independently, although they may manifest concrete thinking and difficulty with environmental change or intellectual stresses. An IQ of 20 to 34 is considered severe, is associated with poor communication skills, and usually with organic abnormalities. These patients tend to require close supervision throughout their lives, but may be able to perform simple tasks and participate in their own care. An IQ of less than 20 is defined as "profound" MR, and most people with this level of intellectual functioning need total supervision throughout their lives. Though an IQ over 70 is normal, technically anything between 71 and 84 is considered borderline intellectual functioning.

14-4. D. The presence of plaques and tangles on autopsy is almost universal in persons with Down syndrome after the age of 40, and correlates with the presence of the Alzheimer phenotype. The Alzheimer precursor protein (APP) gene is located on chromosome 21, and it is hypothesized that the extra "dose" of this gene leads to the accumulation of A-Beta. Hemiballismus is a term describing intermittent gross movements on one side of the body, associated with a lesion in the contralateral subthalamic nucleus.

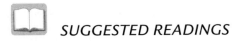 *SUGGESTED READINGS*

Nicham R, Weitzdorfer R, Hauser E, et al. Spectrum of cognitive, behavioural and emotional problems in children and young adults with Down syndrome. *J Neural Transm*. 2003;Suppl 67:173–191.

Roizen NJ and Patterson D. Down's syndrome. *Lancet*. 361: 1281–1289.

"I'm Fed Up with These Mood Swings"

CC/ID: 35-year-old married mother of two, who was referred by her gynecologist for complaints of mood swings and irritability before her menstrual periods.

HPI: I.R. noticed a change in her usual level of functioning about 1 year ago. Though she has always experienced **breast tenderness, a feeling of bloating, and the occasional tearful moment** in the week before her period, over the past year, these symptoms have steadily progressed to the point that both she and her husband have noticed that she has become **very irritable and angry.** Additionally, she complains of **hypersomnia and feeling very lethargic,** and she describes getting **very depressed** and finds it difficult to concentrate on her responsibilities. These symptoms are associated with a tendency to overeat with cakes and sweets. This constellation of symptoms begins about **2 weeks before her period is due** and resolves approximately 3 days into her cycle. She is extremely distressed by these symptoms and feels they are interfering with the quality of her relationships with her family. She denies the presence of suicidality.

PMHx: None

Meds: None

Allergies: NKDA

POb/GynHx: Menarche aged 13, always-regular menses.

PPHx: None

FHx: NIDDM, asthma, first cousin with schizophrenia.

SHx: I.R. is the second of four children. Her parents and siblings are all alive and well. She has been married for 8 years and has two children, a boy aged 6, and a girl aged 4. Both pregnancies and deliveries were normal. She is a homemaker.

PE/Labs: WNL

MSE: *General:* Well dressed, good eye contact and rapport. *Speech:* normal tone and volume. *Behavior:* some evidence of agitation, tearful at times, no abnormal movements. *Affect:* constricted and dysphoric, some lability. *Mood:* "awful." *Thought process:* logical and goal-directed. *Thought content:* preoccupied with concerns about performing poorly as a mother. Denies any suicidal or homicidal ideations. No evidence of perceptual abnormalities. *Cognitive function:* intact. *Insight:* good.

THOUGHT QUESTIONS

- What is your differential diagnosis?
- How can you help this woman?

DISCUSSION

Several differential diagnoses could be considered in this case:

Recurrent brief depressive disorder: In this disorder, the criteria are met for a major depressive disorder but the depressive episodes last from 2 days to 2 weeks and are not associated with the menstrual cycle. Not uncommonly found in patients with cluster B personality disorders.

Premenstrual syndrome (PMS): A large number of women experience some premenstrual symptoms including breast tenderness, bloating, carbohydrate cravings, weight gain, headaches, irritability, emotional lability, depressed mood, tearfulness, anxiety, or increased tension. These symptoms occur between ovulation and the onset of menses. However, in the majority of cases, these symptoms can be managed conservatively and do not cause drastic reductions in quality of life.

Borderline personality disorder (BPD): A personality disorder is characterized by pervasive patterns of behavior present since early adulthood. Although I.R. has episodes of impulsive overeating, affective instability, and anger, these symptoms are of relatively recent onset and she does not meet the criteria for this diagnosis.

Medical conditions: A substantial proportion of women presenting with premenstrual symptoms will actually meet criteria for other conditions such as anemia, chronic fatigue, endocrine abnormalities, endometriosis, fibrocystic breast disease, irritable bowel syndrome, migraine, or pelvic inflammatory disease. These should be ruled out and treated.

Premenstrual dysphoric disorder (PMDD): This disorder is also known as late luteal phase disorder. Premenstrual dysphoria is a severe form of premenstrual syndrome, which affects 3% to 10% of women. Because these women experience more severe symptoms that interfere with their quality of life, interventions should be considered. However, before definitively diagnosing I.R. with PMDD, premenstrual exacerbations of an underlying mood disorder such as bipolar disorder or major depression must also be considered and ruled out. Given the specificity of the timing and the severity of this patient's symptoms, she meets the criteria for this diagnosis. A personal past history of depression and a family history of PMS/PMDD are thought to increase the risk of developing this disorder. Changes in progesterone during the luteal phase are no longer thought to play a role, though hypoestrogenism may be implicated. Other endogenous substances that have been suggested to play a role include prolactin, prostaglandin, endorphins, testosterone, melatonin, cortisol, follicle stimulating hormone, and luteinizing hormone, but any definite causal links still need to be established. Psychological factors centering around menstruation and reproduction may also have an etiologic role, and these factors may be triggered by anything from life circumstances, age, or other idiosyncratic stressors. Conservative treatments include education, relaxation techniques, cognitive behavioral therapy, and increasing exercise. Alcohol and sodium intake should be decreased, and caffeine stopped. Antidepressant medications may be warranted.

CASE CONTINUED

I.R. is diagnosed with PMDD and is started on a combination of fluoxetine and supportive psychotherapy. Over several visits, her dose is titrated up to 40 mg daily with good effect. Six months later, both her physical and mental symptoms are much improved.

QUESTIONS

15-1. Which of the following best describes the symptoms of PMDD?

A. They rarely include insomnia or hypersomnia.
B. They usually occur during nonovulatory cycles.
C. They may be related to how an individual's brain reacts to normal variations in the serum levels of gonadotropins.
D. They may be caused by late luteal phase falls in the levels of progesterone and estradiol.
E. Symptoms usually begin before ovulation.

15-2. Which of the following is usually used in the treatment of PMDD?
A. Nortriptyline
B. Dantrolene
C. Fluvoxamine
D. Estrogen/progesterone contraceptive pill
E. Paroxetine

15-3. Which of the following statements best describes the treatment of PMDD?
A. Ovulation can be inhibited by gonadotropin-releasing hormone analogs or estradiol.
B. Progesterone therapy usually provides symptomatic relief.
C. Buspirone, a serotonin agonist, is ineffective in PMDD.
D. To be effective, SSRIs must only be given during the luteal phase.
E. Herbal and over-the-counter preparations should be avoided.

15-4. Which of the following agents is relatively safe to use in pregnancy?
A. Sympathomimetic agents such as methylphenidate
B. Methadone
C. Benzodiazepines
D. Barbiturates
E. Carbamazepine

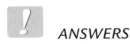

ANSWERS

15-1. C. The symptoms of PMDD are thought to be initiated by the mid-cycle peaks of progesterone or estradiol as opposed to late-luteal phase decreases in hormone levels. The criteria for this disorder include five or more of the following symptoms: depressed mood, anxiety or tension, labile affect, anger or irritability, a decreased interest in usual activities, impaired concentration, decreased energy, a change in appetite (either increased or decreased), and insomnia or hypersomnia. These symptoms should appear only after ovulation, should have diminished by days 4–5 of the menstrual period, and should be documented to occur in two or more consecutive cycles. Average age of onset is reported to be in the middle to late 20s, and sufferers have a strong family history of major depression. Remission has been reported during nonovulatory cycles, which may be spontaneous, suppressed, or due to menopause.

15-2. E. Estrogen/progesterone contraceptive pills are not used in the psychopharmacologic treatment of PMDD, as they are progesterone analogs and may actually increase symptoms. Although nortriptyline has been used as a treatment for postpartum depression, it is not usually used in PMDD. However, as a tricyclic antidepressant with primarily serotonergic properties, clomipramine may induce a remission of symptoms (and does so at doses less than those used for depression). Sertraline, fluoxetine, and paroxetine should be used as first line agents (citalopram as a second line option) at the doses used to treat depression. Fluvoxamine is not generally used to treat this disorder. Other agents under investigation include danazol (a synthetic partial androgen whose side effects may limit use to severe cases), gonadotropin-releasing hormone agonists (leuprolide), diuretics (spironolactone), bromocriptine, NSAIDs, and atenolol. Benzodiazepines have been used with limited success. Monophasic oral contraceptives may help bloating, tenderness, and breast pain. Dantrolene is a skeletal muscle relaxant used in psychiatry to treat neuroleptic malignant syndrome.

15-3. A. Treatment of PMDD may also include inhibition of ovulation with gonadotropin-releasing hormone analogs or estradiol. However, these may increase the risk of osteoporosis and cardiovascular disease and may not be suitable for long-term treatment. Buspirone, a serotonin agonist, may also be effective in PMDD. SSRIs have been reported to have response rates of over 60% in this disorder, and they may be given continuously (for those with more severe symptoms) or intermittently during the luteal phase (for those with milder symptoms); however this latter method may be associated with more side effects. They should be given at doses lower than or up to those used for depression. It has been reported that progesterone therapy does not provide symptomatic relief. Evening Primrose oil, *Ginkgo biloba*, and vitamin B_6 may give some relief, but their use remains controversial. Calcium and magnesium have been shown to reduce symptoms.

15-4. B. In patients with opioid dependency, methadone may improve obstetrical outcomes, by helping to increase nutrition and use of prenatal care, and low-dose methadone may actually decrease the rate of spontaneous abortions in opiate addicts. However, withdrawal effects may be experienced by the newborn. Although there is no evidence of teratogenic effects from sympathomimetics, their safety in pregnancy has not yet been established and is best avoided, even while breast-feeding. Benzodiazepine use in the first trimester has been associated with cleft lip and palate, and later use may cause withdrawal effects in the neonate; benzodiazepines are secreted in breast milk. Barbiturates are contraindicated in the first trimester due to possible teratogenic effects, and later use may cause a vitamin K–dependent coagulopathy in the infant. Carbamazepine should be avoided in both pregnancy and during lactation, as it is associated with several possible birth defects including spina bifida, craniofacial abnormalities, and developmental delay. Haloperidol is relatively safe in pregnancy, as is fluoxetine.

SUGGESTED READINGS

Freeman EW, Rickels K, Sondheimer SJ, et al.Continuous or intermittent dosing with sertraline for patients with severe premenstrual syndrome or premenstrual dysphoric disorder. *Am J Psychiatry*. 2004;161(2):343–351.

Halbreich U, O'Brien PM, Eriksson E, et al. Are there differential symptom profiles that improve in response to different pharmacological treatments of premenstrual syndrome/ premenstrual dysphoric disorder? *CNS Drugs*. 2006;20(7):523–547.

Altschuler LL, Cohen LS, Moline ML, et al. Treatment of depression in women: a summary of the expert consensus guidelines. *J Psychiatr Pract*. 2001;7(3):185–208.

Di Guilio G, Reissing ED. Premenstrual dysphoric disorder: Prevalence, diagnostic considerations, and controversies. *J Psychosom Obstet Gynaecol*. 2006;27(4):201–210.

Girman A, Lee R, Kligler B. An integrative medicine approach to premenstrual syndrome. *Am J Obstet Gynecol*. 2003;188(5).

Wyatt K, Dimmock P, Jones P, et al. Efficacy of progesterone and progestogens in management of premenstrual syndrome: A systematic review. *Br Med J*. 2001;323:776–780.

"I Know This Behavior Must Stop"

CC/ID: 35-year-old married male accountant who has come to your clinic seeking advice about decreasing his alcohol consumption.

HPI: K.Z. begins the interview by describing how he started drinking beer at the age of 16. Then, when he went away to college, he began to drink more often, getting drunk nearly each time. He states that, looking back, he had already lost control of his consumption. He experienced his first **blackout** at the age of 20. He was **arrested** one spring break for harassing a group of women, but the charges were dropped. Upon graduation from college, he attended business school where he continued to drink heavily 2 nights per week. After graduate school, he joined a firm of accountants and traveled often; he describes **going to bars alone and drinking until late.** Currently, on most nights, he drinks "a couple of beers" on the way home each evening, and has two or three more once home. He came seeking help following an episode when he **hit his wife** during a recent argument, and he is concerned about his behavior. He describes depressed mood, with poor appetite and difficulty sleeping. He was charged with **driving while intoxicated** 6 months ago. He **denies any altered tolerance, withdrawal symptoms, seizures, GI complaints, or changes in his pattern of drinking, other than unsuccessfully trying to cut back.**

PMHx: Childhood asthma. Never smoked.

Meds: None

Allergies: NKDA

PPHx: None. He denied any recent illicit substance abuse, though he smoked pot a few times at college.

FHx: His **grandfather was an alcoholic,** but his parents were strict teetotalers.

SHx: K.Z. has been married for 4 years and has a 2-year-old son. He has no siblings. He was passed over for promotion 6 months ago, and his last work review suggested that he was lagging behind his co-workers in productivity.

VS/PE: WNL

Labs: CBC, SMA 20 with LFTs WNL; tox. screen negative.

MSE: *General:* Appropriately dressed with good eye contact and rapport. *Speech:* normal rate and rhythm, though low volume at times. *Mood:* "terrible." *Affect:* constricted, and clearly dysphoric. *Thought content:* preoccupied with the toll drinking has had on his life. Denies suicidal or homicidal ideations. No perceptual abnormalities. *Thought processes:* no abnormalities. *Cognitive function:* intact. *Insight:* good insight into his problem and motivated to change. He becomes tearful describing the incident with his wife and is remorseful. He expresses guilt about this and his drinking in general.

 THOUGHT QUESTIONS

- What is your diagnosis?
- How can you best treat this man?
- What is his prognosis?

DISCUSSION

This patient meets the criteria for a diagnosis of **alcohol abuse** without evidence of dependence (Table 16-1). Substance abuse is described by a maladaptive pattern of use leading to clinically significant problems in at least one of four areas (e.g., job, personal health, legal, social/interpersonal). Though it is very important to obtain a good collateral history of the patient's drinking patterns, his drinking is clearly interfering with his functioning in several of these areas of his life, and his concern over its effects on his marriage has motivated him into treatment. Although his mood on interview is depressed, there is no evidence of symptoms consistent with a major depressive episode; of note, alcohol itself interferes with sleep patterns and appetite.

Nearly 10% of the U.S. population is affected by serious alcohol-related problems; men are affected more often and at an earlier age

TABLE 16-1 Criteria for Substance Dependence

A maladaptive pattern of substance use, leading to clinically significant impairment, manifested by 3 of 7 behaviors in any 12-month period

■ Tolerance: increased amounts of substance taken to reach effect

■ Withdrawal: substance is taken to avoid or to treat withdrawal symptoms

■ Substance is taken in larger amounts or over a longer period than intended

■ Persistent desire or unsuccessful effort to decrease or stop substance use

■ Much time is spent to obtain, use, or recover

■ Social, occupational, or recreational activities are given up

■ Substance use continues despite evidence of a physical or psychological problem

Adapted from American Psychiatric Association. *Task Force on DSM-IV. Diagnostic and statistical manual of mental disorders: DSM-IV.* 4th ed. Washington, DC: American Psychiatric Association, 1994.

than women. Genetics may contribute up to 60% of the risk of alcohol dependence. Those with antisocial personality disorder may be affected in early adolescence. Other common comorbid psychiatric conditions include bipolar disorder, depression, panic disorder, and social phobia. Abusers of alcohol generally do not develop tolerance, withdrawal, the craving to drink, or the pattern of compulsive use commonly seen in individuals with alcohol dependence; rather, abuse centers on the harmful consequences of repeated use. Conversely, in substance dependence, the criteria focus on the behavior of the individual as well as impairments caused by such behaviors and the development of tolerance or withdrawal symptoms. In other words, "abuse" describes continued use despite aversive consequences, and "dependence" describes these aversive consequences as well as a loss of personal control over use of the substance.

Though this patient's chief complaint concerns his distress over his alcohol use, patients commonly present for evaluation of medical complaints or symptoms of psychological distress rather than for substance problems outright. In order to effectively treat patients with substance problems, the physician must be forthright and nonjudgmental and should recognize her or his own views of drugs and drug use.

Good prognostic indicators include the presence of a stable job, family life, absence of comorbidities, and the ability to complete the full course (2-4 weeks) of an initial rehabilitation; this can lead to a 60% chance of abstinence for at least 1 year. Poor prognostic indicators include the presence of antisocial personality disorder, severe legal problems, and polysubstance dependence. Those who are homeless or have severe substance problems have only a 5% to 10% chance of 1 year of abstinence. Rehabilitation is based on helping patients achieve high levels of motivation to stop drinking and to adjust to a new alcohol-free life; preventing relapses is also crucial and nondrug-related support systems involving improved coping techniques need to be developed. Of note, in the treatment of dependence, brief interventions tend to only minimally change the environment or provide new skills, and do not generally alter drug-induced brain changes; therefore, a change in the patient's motivation (cognitive change) may be the best predictor of response.

CASE CONTINUED

K.Z. underwent a series of counseling sessions as an outpatient and attended AA meetings. His depressive symptoms improved about 2 weeks after stopping alcohol. His wife benefited from joint sessions, support, and attending AA meetings for family members. Six months later, K.Z. was promoted. He has remained abstinent from alcohol, and there were no further episodes of violence.

QUESTIONS

16-1. Which of the following is correct concerning treatment with disulfiram?
- A. A common side effect includes diarrhea.
- B. It can be started immediately after the last drink.
- C. It may be used safely in those with cardiovascular disease.
- D. Cough mixtures may provoke a severe reaction.
- E. It may be used safely in patients with schizophrenia.

16-2. Which of the following lab tests may indicate a pattern of heavy drinking?
- A. Decreased triglycerides
- B. Decreased carbohydrate-deficient transferrin
- C. Elevated γ-glutamyltransferase
- D. Decreased uric acid
- E. Equivalent elevations in both liver enzymes AST and ALT

16-3. Which of the following is accurate concerning psychiatric disorders comorbid with alcohol dependence?
  A. Such disorders may be present in 10% to 15% of patients.
  B. Depressive symptoms at presentation require immediate pharmacotherapy.
  C. Mood symptoms cannot be caused by alcohol.
  D. Suicide rates are increased.
  E. There is increased comorbidity of cluster A personality disorders.

16-4. Which of the following statements regarding the treatment of alcohol use disorders is correct?
  A. Bupropion is indicated.
  B. Naloxone is indicated.
  C. Acamprosate is indicated.
  D. Long-term treatment is less effective than brief counseling.
  E. Approximately 10% of alcoholic persons may achieve spontaneous permanent abstinence.

ANSWERS

16-1. D. Alcohol is metabolized by oxidation in the liver, via alcohol dehydrogenase to acetylaldehye, which is then converted via aldehyde dehydrogenase to acetate; then acetate is converted to CO_2 and water. A healthy liver oxidizes 0.75 oz. of 80-proof alcohol in 1 hour; in frequent drinkers, this rate is increased. Disulfiram (Antabuse) inhibits aldehyde dehydrogenase, and due to its toxic effects, should only be started at least 12 hours after the last drink. With even a small ingestion of alcohol, it produces an unpleasant reaction, including flushing, sweating, nausea, vomiting, headache, palpitations, and hypotension, even 2 weeks after the medication is last taken. Patients should be told to avoid all alcohol, including the minute quantities found in cough mixtures, aftershave, perfume, and vanilla extract. More extreme reactions with disulfiram include cardiovascular complications, unconsciousness, convulsions, and even death, depending on the amount of alcohol consumed. Disulfiram is contraindicated in psychosis, cardiac failure/ischemic heart disease, and pregnancy. Other side effects include constipation, liver toxicity, fatigue, metallic taste, decreased libido, hypothyroidism, and it may interfere with the metabolism of phenytoin and warfarin.

Given these risks, patients must be carefully selected for this treatment. It tends to function as a psychological deterrent to drinking and helps patients avoid acting on their cravings.

16-2. C. A level of γ-glutamyltransferase (GGT) over 30 U/L has 60% sensitivity and 80% specificity as a marker of recent heavy alcohol use (four or more drinks daily for several days or weeks). Other state markers useful for screening include the following: triglycerides >160 mg/dL; carbohydrate-deficient transferrin >20 mg/L (65% sensitivity and 80% specificity); mean corpuscular volume (MCV) >91 μm^3 (70% sensitivity and specificity); uric acid levels >6.4 mg/dL in men and >5.0 mg/dL in women; liver enzymes SGOT (AST) and SGPT (ALT) each above 45 IU/L, but not equally elevated (a 2:1 ratio of AST:ALT is classically described). Changes in normal levels after a period of abstinence may indicate a return to heavy drinking. Old rib fractures, cortical and cerebellar atrophy, and liver findings may describe chronic as opposed to acute alcohol use. (Adapted from *Kaplan & Saddock's Comprehensive Textbook of Psychiatry.* 7th ed. Philadelphia: Lippincott, Williams & Wilkins, 2000.)

16-3. D. 25% to 50% of suicides involve alcohol, and suicide may occur in up to 15% of those with alcohol dependence and risk may be additionally increased by the presence of comorbid psychiatric conditions, including anxiety disorders, depression, bipolar disorder, schizophrenia, and other substance dependence. Depressive symptoms may often be seen at initial presentation as well as during detoxification. However, one cannot diagnose a primary psychiatric illness if its onset has been within 4 weeks of stopping heavy drinking. Depressions, panic attacks, and psychotic thought processes occurring in the context of alcohol problems usually improve rapidly and then disappear, and do not usually carry the same prognostic implications as actual major depressive episodes, panic disorders, and schizophrenia. At the end of several weeks, most alcoholic patients are left with mood swings or intermittent symptoms of sadness that can resemble cyclothymic disorder or dysthymic disorder. Even those mild and intermittent depressive symptoms are likely to diminish and disappear with time. The presence of the dysthymic symptoms usually indicates the normal course of a withdrawal syndrome and not an independent mood disorder. As such, mood symptoms should be reassessed approximately 4 weeks after stopping alcohol. Of course, the presence of more serious symptoms such as suicidal or homicidal intent clearly warrants intervention, and there is some limited data that early treatment of a co-occurring depression with medications may assist in the patient's abstinence (however, whether one should still wait 4 weeks is debatable). Approximately 50% of those with alcohol dependence meet criteria for another psychiatric disorder and up to one-third of all psychiatric patients have an alcohol problem that may have caused or exacerbated their disorder. Bipolar I disorder, schizophrenia, and antisocial personality disorder reciprocally carry well-established heightened risks for subsequent alcohol-related disorders; individuals with panic disorder or generalized social phobia also carry a small but statistically significant risk for alcohol abuse or dependence. For those with independent axis I diagnoses, treatment must also be directed at these disorders.

16-4. C. Acamprosate is a relatively new compound approved for the treatment of alcohol dependence. Though its mechanism of action is unknown, as an analog of glutamate it is thought to affect the brain's GABA/glutamate system. As chronic alcohol consumption may lead to a compensatory long-lasting upregulation of excitatory and downregulation of inhibitory transmitters in the brain, acamprosate may mitigate this effect by restoring the excitatory glutamate system to normal. It is also thought that acamprosate reduces the "high" associated with alcohol, thus decreasing craving and relapse. Naloxone (Narcan) is an opioid receptor antagonist given intravenously to treat opiate overdose; it is not used in alcohol use disorders. However, its oral analog, Naltrexone (ReVia), is also an opioid antagonist and helps to diminish craving as well as alcohol's reinforcing effects. Treatment should also involve individual, group, couples, and or family therapy. Motivation can be increased by providing education about the effects of alcohol. Confrontation in a nonjudgmental and persistent manner, setting realistic goals, and providing support and reassurance that recovery is possible are also required. Support for the spouses and families may be needed. Alcoholics Anonymous is a mutual, self-help group with a well-known 12-step program that may be a useful resource. Although, approximately 20% of alcoholic persons may achieve spontaneous permanent abstinence, and a small number of people are able to control their social drinking, in alcohol dependence and some cases of abuse, total abstinence is the goal.

SUGGESTED READINGS

Pettinati HM, Rabinowitz AR. Recent advances in the treatment of alcoholism. *Clin Neurosci Res*. 2005;5(2–4):151–159.

Lovinger DM, Crabb, C. Laboratory models of alcoholism: treatment target identification and insight into mechanisms. *Nat Neurosci.* 2005;8(11):1471–80.

Rinck D, Frieling H, Freitag A, et al. Combinations of carbohydrate-deficient transferrin, mean corpuscular erythrocyte volume, gamma-glutamyltransferase, homocysteine and folate increase the significance of biological markers in alcohol dependent patients. *Drug Alcohol Depend.* 2007 Jun 15; 89(1):60–65.

CASE **17**

"I Feel Fantastic"

CC/ID: 35-year-old male artist whom you have been treating as an outpatient for relatively long-lasting depressive episodes. At his current presentation, he claims to feel "fantastic."

HPI: Though A.D. had been suffering from a consistent and moderately severe depression for the past 4 months, he has recently shown response to a combination of antidepressant medications and psychotherapy. At present, he is quite thankful for the treatment, and describes his **mood as elevated** and his thinking as clearer. About 3 days ago, he **rapidly developed increases in energy, creativity, and activity levels.** He is also quite pleased that he **no longer requires 10 hours of sleep to function each day, stating that now he works well on only 4 to 5 hours each night.** He has been busy catching up with friends and working on new paintings. In fact, he invites you to an extravagant party he is planning to celebrate his improved mood. His medication has not been altered recently, and he denies any illicit substance or alcohol abuse. He also denies suicidal and homicidal ideations.

PMHx: Pyloric stenosis as an infant, treated surgically.

Allergies: NKDA

PPHx: A.D. has never suffered from a manic episode in the past, nor has he tried to harm himself or others. This was his third episode of depression since his initial presentation at age 20. He has been hospitalized only once, during his second episode. He describes that his episodes of depression usually end like this, with his suddenly experiencing a **complete reversal of his symptoms,** usually lasting for about a week or two, after which he returns to his usual baseline. Although he admits to some past abuse of cocaine and alcohol, he denies any use over the past 10 years.

FHx: No psychiatric disorders; glaucoma and NIDDM.

SHx: Eldest of two sons, parents alive and well. Graduated from art school and has been supporting himself by bartending and through some successful sales of his artwork. He is engaged to be married.

MSE: Appropriately dressed, with good eye contact and rapport. *Speech:* normal, not pressured. *Mood:* "fantastic." *Affect:* mildly elevated. *Thought process:* logical and goal-directed, without evidence of any thought disorder. *Thought content:* he is more positive about his future and creative abilities. No delusional material, no suicidal or homicidal ideation, no evidence of perceptual abnormalities. *Cognitive function:* normal. *Insight:* intact.

THOUGHT QUESTIONS

- What is your differential diagnosis?
- Do you feel that he needs a mood stabilizer?

DISCUSSION

In determining a differential diagnosis for this patient, one should first describe the type of episode he is currently experiencing, and then proceed to detail his illness on a syndromal level. Essentially, this patient is currently experiencing a hypomanic episode, with a few days of inflated self-esteem, decreased need for sleep, excessive goal-directed activity, and engagement in pleasurable activities. Importantly, though his symptoms do not reach the severe level of a manic episode and impair his functioning, they do represent a discrete change from his usual baseline self. Given the presence of hypomania, the differential diagnosis includes the following disorders.

Cyclothymic disorder: In this chronic, recurrent, milder form of bipolar disorder, the episodes of hypomania alternate with periods of dysthymia or "mini-depressions." These are interspersed with infrequent phases of euthymia. The mood may be extremely labile, lacking adequate precipitants, and may cause significant interpersonal difficulties, such as marital failure. It has a lifetime prevalence of 0.4% to 1.0%, with no gender differences. Up to one-third of persons with this disorder may progress to a full-blown major mood disorder.

Substance-induced mood disorder: Hypomania may be provoked by use or withdrawal from psychoactive substances, medications, ECT, or even phototherapy. There is a high prevalence of alcohol and substance abuse in mood disorders, and self-medication for mood symptoms can be a considerable problem. If significant mood symptoms persist after detoxification (1–2 months), there may be an underlying mood disorder.

Bipolar II disorder: Criteria include the history of one or more depressive and at least one hypomanic (not manic) episode. There is no psychosis (hallucinations or delusions). It may present with episodes of major depression followed by a relatively short period of hypomania, which lasts a few days. Alternatively, hypomanic episodes can precede and follow depressive episodes, as when major depression is superimposed upon a cyclothymic disorder. The mood in hypomania may be described as elevated, jolly, and infectious. Self-esteem and self-confidence can be increased but irritability and even violence may also be seen. The depressive episodes in bipolar II disorder may also present with mixed symptoms with increased drive, impulsivity, or flight of ideas. A.D. meets the criteria for this disorder.

Though this patient may appear as wholly functional and having a joy-filled time, his hypomanic symptoms are inextricably linked to long periods of depressive suffering, and they are more likely a manifestation of an underlying bipolar II disorder than an appropriate or pathological response to antidepressant medications. Thus it is not surprising that his depressions have been so difficult to treat, as the type of illness he has may not be responsive to antidepressant therapy, and may instead require a mood stabilizer (Table 17-1).

TABLE **17-1**   Lithium

Uses	Acute mania, prophylaxis of recurrent bipolar, unipolar, and schizoaffective disorders. May be used to treat aggressive behavior.
Pharmacokinetics	Rapidly absorbed orally. Not protein bound. Excreted unchanged by the kidney. **Rates of clearance depend on renal function** and follow sodium reabsorption in the proximal tubules. Increased sodium intake causes decreased reabsorption, and a sodium-restricted diet causes increased lithium reabsorption leading to toxicity.
Side effects	Generally related to blood levels. *Early:* Nausea, vomiting, diarrhea, fine tremor, dry mouth, fatigue, drowsiness, nasal congestion, and metallic taste. *Long term:* Nephrogenic diabetes insipidus due to resistance to antidiuretic hormone; hypothyroidism (females > males); cardiac effects include ECG changes (sick sinus syndrome and other arrhythmias); neurological effects include choreoathetosis, ataxia, dysarthria, tardive dyskinesia, and memory impairment; acne and alopecia; increased risk of Ebstein's anomaly in fetuses.

CASE CONTINUED

A.D. agreed to a trial of a mood stabilizer, and lithium was started and titrated with good effect. After a week, he was euthymic and continued treatment as an outpatient. As he is not currently manic, his antidepressants were continued with the thought of possible tapering and discontinuation.

QUESTIONS

17-1. Which of the following is correct concerning bipolar II disorder?
- A. It may be less common in those with a hyperthymic or cyclothymic temperament.
- B. It is easily distinguishable from recurrent major depressive disorder.
- C. It can occur in a rapid cycling pattern.
- D. With mixed depressive episodes, it usually responds to antidepressant monotherapy.
- E. It is less prevalent than bipolar I disorder.

17-2. Which of the following agents is approved in the United States for maintenance treatment of bipolar disorder?
- A. Divalproex
- B. Lithium
- C. Carbamazepine
- D. Olanzapine/fluoxetine combination
- E. Risperidone

17-3. Which of the following is true of patients with bipolar II disorder?
- A. They suffer less from atypical depressions than those with unipolar depression.
- B. They are easily diagnosed.
- C. They have higher rates of suicidal ideation or attempts than those with bipolar type I disorder.
- D. They often convert to bipolar I.
- E. Bipolar I is more prevalent in the relatives of bipolar II probands than bipolar I probands.

17-4. Which of the following is found in bipolar II disorder?
- A. Insight is usually impaired.
- B. There may be a seasonal variation in this disorder.
- C. There is a lifetime prevalence of 2%.

D. It often progresses to a full-fledged manic psychosis.
E. Comorbid conditions include narcolepsy and paranoid personality disorder.

ANSWERS

17-1. C. Rapid cycling occurs more commonly in bipolar II than in bipolar I disorder. Possible risk factors for rapid cycling include female gender, borderline hypothyroidism, menopause, abuse of minor tranquilizers, alcohol, caffeine, or stimulants, long-term use of antidepressants, and temporal lobe dysrhythmias. At times it may be difficult to distinguish between those who are recovering from a major depressive episode and hypomania, as patients may feel great relief as their depression lifts. However, many discrete symptoms of hypomania are not usually present in a resolving major depressive episode. Recent data indicate that bipolar II is more prevalent than bipolar I disorder. It has been reported that 30% to 50% of outpatients diagnosed with major depressive disorder actually fit the bipolar II pattern. Those with hyperthymic temperaments may have hypomania as their baseline level of functioning; this temperament describes patients who are cheerful, have high levels of energy, extraversion, and humor, and rarely need more than 6 hours of sleep per night. It has been theorized that those hyperthymic patients who develop depression may actually have a family history of bipolar disorder and may develop mania spontaneously. (Adapted from *Kaplan & Sadduck's Comprehensive Textbook of Psychiatry*. 7th ed. Philadelphia: Lippincott, Williams & Wilkins. 2000.)

17-2. B. The only agents approved for maintenance treatment of bipolar disorder in the United States include lithium, lamotrigine, olanzapine, and aripiprazole. Divalproex and carbamazepine are approved for treatment of acute mania, as are lithium, chlorpromazine, ziprasidone, and aripiprazole. Olanzapine and risperidone may be used for monotherapy or as adjunctive agents in acute mania. The combination of olanzapine and fluoxetine is approved for the treatment of acute depression in bipolar disorder. Acute mania generally responds to the administration of an antipsychotic agent—possibly combined with a benzodiazepine—concurrent with the introduction of a mood stabilizer. Maintenance treatment of bipolar patients generally requires lower doses than that used in the hypermetabolic manic state; additionally, in maintenance, patients are more sensitive to side effects than they are when acutely manic.

17-3. C. When the results of several studies were combined, up to one-quarter of patients with bipolar II disorder were reported to have experienced suicidal ideation or attempts (compared to 17% of those with bipolar I disorder). Bipolar II disorder tends to be underdiagnosed or even misdiagnosed, and these patients are more likely to have atypical or mixed depressions. This is usually a stable diagnosis, and patients rarely "progress" to bipolar I disorder. Bipolar I is less prevalent in the relatives of bipolar II probands than in the relatives of bipolar I probands.

17-4. B. Bipolar II disorder may manifest a seasonal variation, with the onset of a depression in the autumn or early winter followed by a hypomanic episode in the spring. However, hypomanic episodes usually arise spontaneously or in relation to a depressive episode. Bipolar II rarely progresses to a full manic psychosis. Insight is usually well preserved. Mood may be elevated or irritable, and the symptom of pathological distractibility is uncommon in hypomania. The change in mood (hypomania) lasts at least 4 days, without marked impairment of functioning or need for hospitalization. Patients often do not report these episodes of hypomania. Bipolar II has a lifetime prevalence of less than 1%. Comorbid conditions include eating disorders, substance abuse or dependence, ADHD, social phobia, panic disorder, and borderline personality disorder. Use of antidepressants alone (monotherapy) in this disorder requires careful consideration, as these medications may provoke an episode of mania or hypomania. Lithium, carbamazepine, and divalproex sodium are the most commonly used, but lamotrigine may also be effective (particularly for those with depression). Women tend to experience depression, mixed episodes, and rapid cycling more often than men, and may require treatment with antidepressants more often. (Arnold LM. Gender differences in bipolar disorder. *Psychiatr Clin North Am.* 2003;26(3):595–620.)

SUGGESTED READINGS

Yatham LN. Diagnosis and management of patients with bipolar II disorder. *J Clin Psychiatry.* 2005;66(1):13–17.

Berk M, Dodd S. Bipolar II disorder: a review. *Bipolar Disord.* 2005; 7(1):11–21.

El-Mallakh R,Weisler RH, Townsend MH, et al. Bipolar II disorder: current and future treatment options. *Ann Clin Psychiatry.* 2006;18 (4):259–266.

Post RM, Altschuler LL, Leverich GS, et al. Mood switch in bipolar depression: comparison of adjunctive venlafaxine, bupropion and sertraline. *Br J Psychiatry.* 2006;189:124–131.

"I Cannot Sit Still"

CC/ID: 50-year-old woman with a 30-year history of paranoid schizophrenia. During a routine outpatient visit, she complains of **feeling restless** and says that it is **difficult for her to keep sitting still.**

HPI: Though B.T. has been treated with oral antipsychotic medications for many years, her dose of haloperidol was increased 6 weeks ago because she was complaining of hearing whispering in her apartment when no one was around. She describes these feelings of restlessness began approximately 2 to 3 weeks ago, and she feels like she wants **"to jump out of my skin."** She reports that pacing seems to help slightly, but that she feels very uncomfortable throughout the day. Associated symptoms include trouble sleeping from the discomfort, anxiety, and irritability. She denies change in chronic delusional beliefs, re-emergence of auditory hallucinations, suicidality, or homicidality.

PMHx: Mild COPD, psoriasis

Meds: Haloperidol, 5 mg PO BID; benztropine, 1 mg PO BID

Allergies: NKDA

PPHx: B.T. was first diagnosed with schizophrenia at 20 years old. Since that time, she has been hospitalized eight times, the longest for 6 months. She has been treated with both depot and oral antipsychotic medications. She has never been suicidal or violent.

FHx: Her mother died at age 80 of a stroke, and her father at age 76 from liver cancer. One sister has recurrent major depression. One brother is an alcoholic.

SHx: B.T. is the youngest of nine children. She had graduated from high school and was working as a shop assistant when she had her first psychotic episode. She lived with her parents until they died, and has been living with her older sister since then. She describes herself as religious. She does not drink alcohol, and denies ever using illicit substances. She has smoked 15 cigarettes a day for the past 32 years. She receives long-term disability payments.

PE: WNL. *Neuro:* no cog wheeling, rigidity, hemiballismus, or choreiform movements. No focal lesions.

MSE: *General:* Appears older than stated age, food-stained clothing. Eye contact and rapport fair; only minimally guarded. *Behavior:* unable to sit still in the chair; swinging her legs and fidgeting; pacing around the room during the interview; orobuccal chewing movements and rhythmic involuntary movements of her tongue. *Affect:* mildly blunted. *Mood:* "All right," though upon greater examination, she describes herself as suffering. *Thought process:* logical, goal-directed, but some retardation in rate. *Thought content:* somewhat impoverished. Delusional material as at baseline. No suicidal or homicidal ideations. No perceptual abnormalities. *Cognitive function:* intact. *Insight:* fair.

THOUGHT QUESTIONS

- What do you think this woman is experiencing?
- What concerns do you have?
- How can you help her?

DISCUSSION

It appears that this patient has two acute problems:

1. **Neuroleptic-induced akathisia:** Objective signs of restlessness and/or the subjective report of feeling restless (particularly in the legs) characterize this **extrapyramidal symptom.** Patients may describe feeling anxiety, **muscular restlessness,** or that they want to **jump out of their skin.** Lying down may produce some relief. Akathisia occurs after **subacute exposure to neuroleptic medications** (dopamine antagonists), generally within a few weeks to a month of starting or increasing the medication. Likewise, it may also occur if anticholinergic agents are decreased, disrupting the sensitive striatal dopaminergic-cholinergic balance. It has also been described as resulting from serotonin reuptake inhibitors and calcium channel antagonists. Akathisia is a highly uncomfortable experience and is an important **cause of nonadherence** to medication. It is

important to recognize that many patients may incompletely be able to describe their symptoms, and instead may manifest them behaviorally by becoming agitated. One must be able to differentiate akathisia from agitation from other sources, as the latter may require increasing the antipsychotic medication, while akathisia is treated by decreasing the dose of the involved agent, adding a **beta-blocker** or benzodiazepine, or adding or increasing an anticholinergic agent. Other options include changing the neuroleptic to a low-potency agent or using one of the newer atypical agents, which may be associated with a lower rate of akathisia.

2. **Tardive dyskinesia (TD):** This extrapyramidal movement disorder usually appears after at least 3 months of exposure to neuroleptic agents, but it may appear sooner in older persons. It has been reported in about 15% to 30% of those receiving chronic antipsychotic treatment, and is much more likely with one of the older "conventional" antipsychotics than the newer second-generation medications. It is characterized by **involuntary rhythmic movements** of the tongue, jaw, trunk, or extremities. Movements may be **choreiform** (rapid, jerky, dance-like) or **athetoid** (slow and snakelike). Most commonly, TD affects the muscles of the mouth and face, or the fingers and toes. If severe, it may affect the trunk, or cause difficulties swallowing or irregular breathing, which may cause belching or even grunting. Movements may increase with emotion and decrease with relaxation/sleep. Anticholinergic medications usually worsen the condition. Tardive dyskinesias may worsen after stopping or lowering the dose of antipsychotics (withdrawal dyskinesia) and can be severe. Treatment involves switching to one of the newer agents that may be less associated with this condition, though prevention is clearly best. Clozapine may improve, or even prevent, tardive dyskinesia. The use of vitamin E remains controversial. Neurological or medical causes should be ruled out.

CASE CONTINUED

B.T. was given a short course of a beta-blocker, propranolol 25 mg po TID, to help control her akathisia. In the interim, her neuroleptic was switched to the atypical agent risperidone, providing good control of her psychotic symptoms. Her chewing movements gradually disappeared over the next few months and she is more comfortable.

QUESTIONS

18-1. Which of the following statements is correct concerning antipsychotic-induced dystonia?
- A. It is not caused by any other medications.
- B. These symptoms characteristically appear after 72 hours of treatment with antipsychotics.
- C. Young men appear to be at increased risk.
- D. Older women appear to be at increased risk.
- E. It is a benign condition.

18-2. Which of the following best describes neuroleptic-induced akathisia?
- A. It may be misdiagnosed as psychotic agitation or anxiety.
- B. Middle-aged women appear to be at increased risk.
- C. Beta-blockers, benzodiazepines, or anticholinergic agents should be maintained indefinitely.
- D. It may occur in approximately 5% of patients taking antipsychotics.
- E. It is only caused by psychiatric medications.

18-3. Which of the following is correct concerning neuroleptic-induced tardive dyskinesia?
- A. It is always irreversible.
- B. Increased risk occurs in men.
- C. Increased risk occurs with a history of mood disorder.
- D. Increased risk occurs in young adults.
- E. Distracting tasks tend to minimize the movements.

18-4. Which of the following is found in neuroleptic-induced parkinsonism?
- A. It is characterized by the triad of akathisia, muscle rigidity, and tremor.
- B. It is caused by postsynaptic D_4 receptor blockade in the basal ganglia.
- C. The tremor is more often seen at rest.
- D. Tremor only affects the limbs.
- E. Significant autonomic instability is usually evident.

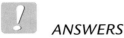

ANSWERS

18-1. C. Acute dystonia is caused by contractions of muscles resulting in abnormal movements or postures. Clinical symptoms depend on the muscle group involved. Laryngeal-pharyngeal spasm may cause impaired swallowing or breathing and necessitates urgent intervention (i.e., IV diphenhydramine 50 mg) and may require intubation. Other forms of acute dystonia include oculogyric crises affecting the extraocular muscles (eyes deviate and result in disconjugate gaze), spasms of the jaw causing trismus or grimacing, difficulties with speech, or abnormal positioning of the head (torticollis), trunk, or limbs. Onset is usually within 24 to 48 hours of starting a neuroleptic or after increases in the dosage of such agents. It may also be caused by other dopamine antagonists, such as metoclopramide (Reglan). Treatment of acute dystonic reactions includes immediate intramuscular (intravenous if laryngeal spasm) injections of antiparkinsonian/anticholinergic agents such as benztropine (Cogentin), trihexyphenidyl (Artane), or diphenhydramine HCl (Benadryl). Risk factors include being young, male, use of high-potency antipsychotics, and high doses of antipsychotics, especially IM. Of note, IV administration of haloperidol does not tend to cause dystonic reactions.

18-2. A. Akathisia may indeed be misdiagnosed as psychotic agitation or anxiety, especially in uncomfortable and distressed patients who cannot adequately describe their experiences. Treatment of akathisia with beta-blockers, benzodiazepines, or anticholinergic agents should be stopped after 2 to 3 weeks to see if the symptoms have subsided. Neuroleptic-induced akathisia is reported to have a prevalence of 20% to 75% and may be more likely to occur following the recent onset or increase of high potency antipsychotic treatments. Although it is generally caused by antipsychotics (both typicals and atypicals), SSRIs and calcium channel blockers are also implicated. Akathisia may be associated with poor treatment adherence and hence poor treatment outcome. There are recent reports of cyproheptadine (Periactin), a serotonin antagonist, being helpful in cases resistant to standard therapy. Neither gender nor age increases the risk of developing akathisia.

18-3. C. Possible risk factors for the development of tardive dyskinesias include increasing age, female sex, ethnicity (African American), a history of mood disorders, cognitive disorders, negative symptoms of schizophrenia, and long-term treatment with antipsychotics (more typical than atypical agents, though both are implicated). Other more controversial risk factors may include alcohol abuse, diabetes, and smoking. A history of extrapyramidal adverse effects, particularly those which develop early in treatment (e.g., acute dystonia, akathisia), or those more severe adverse effects such as anticholinergic-resistant akathisia may also be associated with the development of TD. It has been reported to be reversible in up to 90% of mild cases and 5% to 40% of all cases after stopping neuroleptic agents, with more than 50% remitting in 18 months. Reversibility is lower in the elderly. TD is associated with a poorer prognosis in schizophrenia. TD has been reported to occur in never medicated schizophrenics and healthy individuals. Distracting tasks such as finger tapping or mathematical challenges tend to exaggerate the movements.

18-4. C. Clinically, neuroleptic-induced parkinsonism is identical to idiopathic Parkinson disease, with a symptom triad comprising muscle rigidity, tremor, and bradykinesia or akinesia, which is a paucity or lack of spontaneous motor activity; akathisia is not part of this condition. The tremor of antipsychotic-induced parkinsonism is the least common symptom in the triad; it is 3 to 6 Hz, is most noticeable at rest, and may be intermittent and occasionally can be suppressed by the patient. With the exception of sialorrhea, the symptoms of autonomic dysfunction are not usually found in neuroleptic-induced parkinsonism. The muscle rigidity may be continuous (lead-pipe) or cogwheel (ratchet-like) in nature. The blockade of D_2 receptors in the nigrostriatal tract causes an imbalance between dopamine and acetylcholine. Prophylactic use of antiparkinsonian agents remains controversial but should probably be used in those at known risk and tapered as soon as possible. Otherwise, consider lowering the neuroleptic dose, changing the neuroleptic, or using low-dose antiparkinsonian agents.

SUGGESTED READINGS

Hansen L. A critical review of akathisia, and its possible association with suicidal behaviour. *Hum Psychopharmacol Clin Exp.* 2001;16:495–505.

Sachdev PS. Neuroleptic-induced movement disorders: An overview. *Psychiatr Clin North Am.* 2005;28(1):255–274.

Chou KL, Friedma, JH. Tardive syndromes in the elderly. *Clin Geriatr Med.* 2006;22:915–933.

"I'm Worried She Might Leave Me"

CC/ID: 42-year-old man referred to you by a colleague in the urology department for treatment of symptoms of **secondary impotence.**

HPI: D.Z. reports that this symptom started gradually about 6 months ago. Very distressed, he first went to see a urologist, who found **no evidence of any organic cause.** Though he was hoping for "an easy solution . . . I didn't know it was going to be psychiatric," he is hopeful, albeit embarrassed about this initial interview. He describes that his being unable to maintain an erection with his wife has made their arguing "even worse than before," and he has become more **anxious about his performance** and worries that his wife will leave him. He is, however, able to achieve an erection and **ejaculate while masturbating,** but with his wife he is unable to sustain an erection. He notes sincerely wanting to be able to please his wife, who is now under a great deal of stress upon her returning to the work force: "She's getting mad at me for this. First we argued about her going back to work; I'm not sure it's right for the kids. I saw that she was set on it, so I told her I'd try and support her however I can. Now this . . . if it's not one thing it's another between us." Additionally, he notes not being interested in "pills to help in that area." Though he describes mildly depressed mood and near-constant frustration, he denies neurovegetative symptoms of insomnia, appetite change, or other symptoms of major depression.

PMHx: None

Meds: None

PPHx: None

SHx: D.Z. is the middle of three sons. He has worked in the same firm since graduating from law school and is working toward partnership, putting in many late nights and weekends. He met his wife in college, and they dated for 2 years before they were engaged. They have been married for 15 years and have three children, aged 10, 8, and 4. He describes a "normal healthy sex life" until 6 months ago, when his wife returned to work full time. He admits to feeling that his wife should stay at home to raise the family as his own mother had done. He denies alcohol, nicotine, or substance abuse.

FHx: No relevant family history.

VS: Afebrile, BP 120/80, HR 65, RR 12

Labs: CBC and SMA 20, WNL; Utox negative

MSE: *General:* Well dressed, with good eye contact and rapport, occasionally embarrassed when discussing masturbation. *Speech and behavior:* normal. *Affect:* mildly anxious. *Mood:* "Fed up." He says he feels like a "failure as a husband and useless as a man." *Thought process:* logical, goal-directed. *Thought content:* no delusional material. No suicidal or homicidal ideation. No perceptual abnormalities. *Cognitive functions:* intact. *Insight:* good.

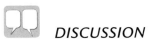

THOUGHT QUESTIONS

- What do you think is the diagnosis?
- What psychiatric conditions would you want to rule out?
- How can you treat this man?

DISCUSSION

A number of sexual desire, arousal, and orgasmic disorders are defined by current diagnostic criteria, and include the following. Each is listed under its associated phase in the sexual response cycle.

Sexual desire disorders (i.e., reduced fantasies about and desire to have sexual activity):

- Hypoactive sexual desire disorder
- Sexual aversion disorder

Sexual arousal disorders (i.e., inadequate vaginal lubrication, clitoral swelling, penile tumescence, or erection):

■ Female sexual arousal disorder

■ Male erectile disorder

Orgasmic disorders (i.e., lack of orgasm after normal sexual functioning and adequate stimulation, or ejaculation occurring with minimal stimulation):

■ Female orgasmic disorder

■ Male orgasmic disorder

■ Premature ejaculation

As this patient seems to have a normal sexual interest and drive, desire disorders are ruled out. Likewise, the orgasmic category does not fit, as D.Z. is unable to maintain an erection in order to orgasm (part of the diagnostic criteria include the presence of a normal sexual excitement phase); however, it would be important to inquire if he did have a history of an orgasmic disorder, which may have impaired his marital relations and secondarily led to the development of a disorder at an earlier point in the sexual response cycle (e.g., an erectile disorder). D.Z.'s symptoms are most consistent with **male erectile disorder,** also referred to as **erectile dysfunction (ED) or impotence.** ED is currently the preferred term. This disorder is characterized by a persistent or recurrent inability to maintain an adequate erection through completion of sexual activity. In lifelong cases, the man has never achieved an erection sufficient for intercourse; in acquired types, penetration has been previously achieved. As D.Z. is able to achieve an erection in some situations, this is referred to as situational erectile disorder. It has been reported that approximately 2% to 4% of men experience erectile dysfunction by age 35, but this increases to approximately 75% by age 80.

In order to arrive at the diagnosis of male erectile disorder, the dysfunction must cause **marked distress or interpersonal difficulties.** Additionally, one must rule out a psychiatric disorder, medication, alcohol, or substance use as etiologic. Important items in the differential diagnosis include low serum testosterone, diabetes, and medications such as psychotropics (e.g., tricyclic antidepressants, SSRIs, lithium, carbamazepine, antipsychotics), antihypertensives, diuretics, digoxin, statins, hypoglycemics, antiandrogens, estrogens, and substances (e.g., alcohol, heroin, methadone, cocaine, amphetamines, barbiturates). ED is reported to be strongly associated with the type of lower urinary tract symptoms commonly seen with prostatic hypertrophy. It is important to also consider that sexual desire may vary between individuals or in the same individual over time. However, desire is significantly affected by anxiety, depressed mood, stress, or **decreased levels of testosterone. Total (rather than situational) impotence is more likely to be associated with organic causes.** If the patient describes being unable to masturbate, a simple test to rule out total impotence is the nocturnal penile tumescence test which assesses whether the patient has nighttime erections. By and large, men who are unable to have an erection because of a psychological problem still have erections during deep sleep.

If the patient had a psychiatric disorder such as major depression, then appropriate treatment for the underlying psychiatric condition should be started. Remember, though, that many psychotropic medications themselves may cause sexual dysfunction. Though less likely to cause isolated erectile dysfunction, serotonergic agents (e.g., SSRIs) may inhibit orgasm or may decrease libido; for this reason they may be given to treat premature ejaculation or to patients with hyperactive sexual desires causing impairment.

In this case, D.Z.'s symptoms seem to be related to his marital problems, and these should be fully explored. He and his wife should be encouraged to attend couple's therapy. Selective phosphodiaesterase inhibitors such as sildenafil (Viagra) or vardenafil (Levitra) could be considered as part of the treatment. It is important to remember that both are contraindicated in patients who take nitrates and relatively contraindicated in those who take α-blockers.

CASE CONTINUED

While D.Z. was having difficulty dealing with the changes in his wife's role in the family, Mrs. Z. had been finding it increasingly difficult to manage her job as well as run the home and care for the children. She complained that her husband did not help out enough. The couple decided to obtain more professional housekeeping and childcare services, and in psychotherapy, D.Z. explored his concerns regarding his role in the home and the changes that were taking place. His symptoms of anxiety, frustration, and depressed mood diminished. The couple then began an integrated program of sexual therapy, using behavioral and insight-oriented techniques including initial nongenital mutual pleasure giving. Gradually this was increased to include sexual activity. D.Z. found occasional use of sildenafil citrate (Viagra) beneficial when he was particularly stressed. Both partners were pleased with the results of this combination of treatments.

QUESTIONS

19-1. Which of the following correctly describes sexual side effects encountered in patients with psychotic disorders?
A. Erectile dysfunction (ED) due to antipsychotics is irreversible in 25% of patients.
B. Antipsychotics can cause decreased libido only in males.
C. Yohimbine may be used safely to treat impotence in patients with psychosis.
D. Antipsychotics may cause priapism, painful orgasms, or retrograde ejaculations.
E. Antipsychotics may cause decreased prolactin levels, and therefore ED.

19-2. Which of the following is true concerning impotence?
A. In younger men, 50% of cases are secondary in nature.
B. Diabetes is the leading cause of impotence in the United States.
C. It is inevitable in old age.
D. It is not caused by Parkinson disease.
E. Erection is dependent on the sympathetic nervous system.

19-3. Female orgasmic disorder is
A. More common after 35 years of age.
B. An uncommon sexual disorder of women.
C. Also known as inhibited female orgasm or anorgasmia.
D. Never caused by psychiatric medications.
E. Caused by psychological factors that usually include anger toward maternal figures.

19-4. Which of the following is correct concerning the treatment of impotence in males?
A. Sildenafil (Viagra) is rarely contraindicated.
B. Sildenafil (Viagra) may be associated with mania.
C. Organic causes require specialized treatments.
D. About 25% of men have an organic cause for their impotence.
E. Surgical interventions are unnecessary.

ANSWERS

19-1. D. Erectile dysfunction caused by antipsychotic medications may be mediated by dopamine receptor blockade, elevations in prolactin, or adrenergic receptor antagonism. A number of medications have been found to help treat this distressing side effect. Bromocriptine, a dopamine agonist, has been reported to restore erections, but in some cases may exacerbate psychosis. Yohimbine, an α_2-antagonist, has been used to treat anorgasmia and impotence; it should be used with care, as it may induce dysphoria, anxiety, or worsen psychotic symptoms in some patients. Anticholinergic agents have also been reported to be helpful (also in priapism or painful orgasms). Priapism is a painful erection that lasts more than 6 hours and must be treated immediately to prevent penile damage and permanent loss of potency.

19-2. B. Erectile dysfunction may be secondary to various medical conditions: Parkinson disease, diabetes (the leading cause of impotence in the United States), cardiovascular disease, renal, hepatic, endocrine, urologic, or neurological disorders (e.g. multiple sclerosis, tumors, infarcts, spinal cord lesions, peripheral neuropathies and neurosyphillis), hypothalamic/pituitary dysfunction, medications, or trauma. Primary (e.g., psychogenic) ED usually occurs when an individual feels anxious or guilty; this may be followed by a vicious cycle of performance anxiety and performance difficulties. In younger men about 80% of cases are primary, but in older men about 50% are primary and 50% are secondary. Although approximately 75% of men may be impotent by 80 years of age, it is not inevitable. Good health and an available partner are important promoters of continued potency. The neural pathway involved in erection includes the limbic system and the parasympathetic nerves to and from the sacrum. The sympathetic system is involved in ejaculation.

19-3. C. The most common type of sexual disorder experienced by women, female orgasmic disorder is the persistent or recurrent inhibition of the female orgasm following a normal sexual excitement phase. Though no association has been found between specific patterns of personality traits or psychopathology and orgasmic dysfunction in women, many different and idiosyncratic psychological factors may be associated with this disorder, such as fears of pregnancy, rejection, or loss of control, or feelings of guilt about sexual activity or hostility toward men. Likewise, female orgasmic disorder may affect one's body image, self-esteem, or relationship satisfaction. Reciprocally, many women tend to experience an increase in their orgasmic capacity as they experience a wider variety of stimulation and acquire more knowledge about their own bodies. Not surprisingly, orgasmic capacity in women may increase with increasing sexual experience, leading the disorder to be more prevalent in younger women. Incidentally, sex therapy may use "sensate focus" techniques as well as individual or couples therapy. Once a woman learns how to reach orgasm, it is rare for her to lose that capacity, except in instances of poor sexual communication, relationship conflict, mood/anxiety or general medical disorders, or in the context of psychological distress such as after experiencing a traumatic experience (e.g., rape). Additionally, female orgasmic disorder may be associated with the use of some tricyclics, MAOIs, antipsychotics, and SSRIs.

19-4. C. Between 50% and 80% of men may have a medical (i.e., nonpsychological) cause of their erectile dysfunction. So-called organic causes need specialized assessment and treatment. Sildenafil citrate (Viagra) may be considered to treat ED from a variety of etiologies (e.g., psychogenic, diabetes, cardiovascular disease), but it is contraindicated in those who take nitrates as it may cause life-threatening hypotension. It is a nitric oxide enhancer that increases blood flow to the penis by inhibiting cGMP, causing smooth muscle relaxation in the corpus cavernosum and hence dilation of the penile vessels. It takes effect 1 hour after ingestion and may last up to 4 hours. Most common adverse effects include flushing, headache, or benign hypotension, but it may also be associated with serious cardiac events, depression, anxiety, and seizures. It is not associated with mania. Other treatments include oral prostaglandins, local injections of transurethral prostaglandin E1 (alprostadil), as well as a variety of surgically implanted devices. (Seftel AD et al. Erectile dysfunction: etiology, evaluation and treatment options. *Med Clin North Am,* 2004;88(2).)

SUGGESTED READINGS

Seftel AD, Mohammed MA, and Althof SE. Erectile dysfunction: etiology, evaluation, and treatment options. *Med Clin North Am.* 2004:88(2):387–416, xi.

Thomas DR. Medications and sexual function. *Clin Geriatric Med.* 2003:19:553–562.

Beutel ME, Weidner W, Brähler E. Epidemiology of sexual dysfunction in the male population. *Andrologia.* 2006;38: 115–121.

"Am I Addicted?"

CC: 32-year-old stockbroker who has come to your clinic with a cocaine habit.

HPI: Ms.C began using cocaine about 2 years ago, starting with occasional use, but over the last year, her **consumption has increased,** and she is concerned. She feels her **work is slipping,** often canceling appointments with clients. Though admitting to **driving under the influence** of cocaine, she denies any legal problems. **She denies symptoms of withdrawal.** She describes only using cocaine intranasally, and denies other methods such as freebasing or smoking crack cocaine. She denies use of any other illicit substances.

PMHx: Elective termination of pregnancy at age 19.

Meds: None

Allergies: NKDA

PPHx: None

FHx: No psychiatric history. Her father had a myocardial infarction at age 52.

SHx: She has one sister aged 28 and a brother aged 26. She did well at college and graduated from business school. She dates regularly. She never smoked and has three or four drinks (scotch) at least 3 nights a week.

Labs: Utox positive for cocaine

Mental status: *General:* well dressed with good hygiene, eye contact, and rapport. *Speech and behavior:* normal. *Affect:* full range. *Mood:* euthymic. *Thought process:* logical and goal-directed. *Thought content:* no delusional material elicited; denies perceptual abnormalities, suicidal, or homicidal ideations. *Cognitive function:* intact. *Insight:* good. Guilty and remorseful about her drug use, she feels that she is beginning to desire "a hit" more often, and this scares her. She is well-motivated to obtain treatment.

THOUGHT QUESTIONS

- Do you think she meets the criteria for cocaine abuse or dependence?
- What do you know about stimulant intoxication, effects, and withdrawal?
- What treatments are available?
- Are you concerned if she were to become pregnant?

DISCUSSION

Ms. C. meets the criteria for cocaine abuse, as it has interfered with her work obligations, and she has used cocaine even in hazardous situations, such as while driving. These problems have occurred over a period of a year, without evidence of withdrawal, altered tolerance, increasing amounts, persistent efforts to cut down or give up, or increasing the time given to procuring the drug. Therefore, she does not meet the criteria for dependence but she does manifest abuse.

Cocaine stimulates the central nervous system to increase activity. Stimulants that are often abused include amphetamine, cocaine, and designer stimulants such as methylenedioxymethamphetamine (MDMA), also known as "ecstasy" (see Table 20-1 for brief overview). Although these drugs may cause visual effects, they are not hallucinogens like lysergic acid (LSD, acid) or phencyclidine (PCP, angel dust). It has been reported that 10% to 15% of those who snort stimulants go on to become abusers. Stimulants may also be combined with each other or with other substances (e.g., heroin with cocaine, also known as a "speedball").

Intoxication and effects: Cocaine can induce feelings of euphoria, well-being, increased alertness, and decreased need for food or sleep. The rush and euphoria produced by cocaine reinforces its use. Associated cues may provoke a craving to use. **Cocaine's reinforcing effects are due to its ability to produce high levels of intrasynaptic dopamine in the nucleus accumbens.** It is not clear how long intermittent use can continue before progressing to dependence. **Cocaine also inhibits the reuptake of serotonin and noradrenaline; this may account for some of the toxic effects seen.** Heavier or binge use may cause anxiety, depression, fatigue, suspiciousness, hallucinations, or irritability. Intoxication may cause

TABLE 20-1   Review of Main Psychostimulants

Cocaine	Half-life approx. 4–6 hours for metabolites. May be detected in urine within 4 hours of use and up to 3 days or more in a regular user. False positive Utox may be caused by use of topical anesthetics containing cocaine. Due to this short half-life, **intoxication rarely needs treatment unless psychosis develops.** Propranolol may be used for severe withdrawal symptoms. Disulfiram has been reported to be useful in cocaine dependence.
Amphetamines	Half-life approx. 6–12 hours. May be detected in urine for 2–3 days after use. False positive Utox may be caused by ephedrine, antiparkinsonian medications (amantadine and selegiline), chlorpromazine, and some antidepressants (bupropion, desimpramine, and trazodone). Street names include "crank," "crystal," "ice," and "meth;" ice is the free-based form, which can be smoked, and its effects may last much longer. Intoxication effects include dizziness, tremors, mydriasis, elevated BP, hyperreflexia, hyperthermia, tachycardia, and tachypnea. **May become aggressive, agitated, grandiose, and paranoid, with impaired judgment.** Haloperidol and other antipsychotics may be used to treat psychosis, with benzodiazepines for seizures. Treat acute intoxication by acidifying the urine with ammonium chloride. Longer use may lead to depression, poor concentration, parkinsonian features, dyskinesias, and neurotoxicity. **Long-term effects may be seen in attention and motor skills; anatomical changes include limbic gray matter deficits and smaller hippocampi.** May develop tolerance and dependence and may keep using to avoid depression from withdrawal.
MDMA	Can cause acute severe toxicity with disseminated intravascular coagulation, hyperthermia, hepatotoxicity, rhabdomyolysis, seizures, and renal failure. May cause increases in heart rate, BP, and myocardial oxygen consumption. **Chronic use may lead to severe paranoia, which may slowly resolve. May cause cognitive and mood impairments.**

tachycardia, arrhythmias, BP abnormalities, pupillary dilatation, diaphoresis, chills, stereotypical behaviors, hyperactivity, grandiosity, respiratory depression, seizures, confusion, and chest pain, as well as those symptoms mentioned for binge use. Insight into the drug effects is usually retained. **Cocaine may induce mood, anxiety, and sleep disorders, delirium, or a persistent (or recurrent) psychosis with visual and tactile hallucinations ("cocaine bugs," formication), paranoia, and lost insight.** Initially cocaine may enhance sexual performance, but later it may have the opposite effect. Cocaine hydrochloride is used for snorting or injecting. When treated with alkali and organic solvents cocaine may be used to freebase; here, the effects of inhalation are more rapid. Crack is a variety of freebased cocaine formed by heating cocaine with sodium bicarbonate producing a hard white substance that is smoked. Both freebasing and intravenous use may be associated with a more rapid progression to dependence. Cocaine may be detected in the urine for up to 72 hours after short-term use, and up to 2 weeks in heavier users.

Pregnancy: Use of cocaine in pregnant women is associated with increased risk of spontaneous abortions, premature birth, placenta previa, and **abruptio placentae,** as well as increased fetal morbidity, mortality, and teratogenic effects (e.g., microcephaly, urinary tract abnormalities). Infants may experience a "withdrawal" syndrome with poor feeding and sleep, and irritability. Cessation of cocaine use in pregnancy is recommended. Long-term effects are not clear.

Withdrawal: Cocaine withdrawal may be associated with significant depressed mood. Withdrawal effects are usually the opposite of those seen in intoxication, and include hyperphagia, somnolence, dysphoria, and irritability.

Comorbid psychiatric illness: If depression is still evident a week or two after withdrawal, then an underlying depression should be considered, as use of cocaine may reflect patients' self-medicating; however, formally, withdrawal must have been over for 4 weeks for a diagnosis of major depression. Studies have shown that 12% to 30% of schizophrenic patients use cocaine. It has been suggested that this use may be to improve negative or depressive symptoms or to help with the adverse effects of antipsychotics. Cocaine users have increased lifetime rates of panic disorder, major depression, cyclothymia/hyperthymia, mania/hypomania, phobias, and attention-deficit disorder. The prevalence of antisocial personality disorder is reported in up to a third of users. Lifetime comorbidity for alcohol problems is also high (up to 50% of those seeking treatment).

CASE CONTINUED

Ms. C. was treated with a combination of individual and group therapies over the next 6 months. These included psychoeducation, and psychodynamic and supportive methods. She has abstained from cocaine use and cut down on her alcohol consumption.

QUESTIONS

20-1. Ms. C. asks you if there are any long-term problems associated with using stimulants. You tell her that

A. Pulmonary edema, myocardial infarctions, and hypothermia may occur.
B. The "crash" associated with stimulant use lasts only an hour or two.
C. Pulmonary edema, cardiomyopathy, and strokes may occur.
D. There are no known effects on pregnancy.
E. Classic bipolar disorder may occur.

20-2. Cocaine's cerebral effects may include which of the following?
A. Inhibition of dopamine reuptake in mesolimbic and mesocortical neurons
B. No effect on noradrenergic, serotonergic, and cholinergic neurons
C. Diminished effects with chronic use
D. Visual impairment
E. Protection from seizure activity

20-3. Which of the following is correct about cocaine?
A. Its plasma half-life is 30 to 90 minutes.
B. Its metabolite can be detected in urine for up to 2 weeks.
C. It is the most commonly used illicit drug in the United States.
D. There is no increased risk in combining cocaine with alcohol.
E. Withdrawal effects are usually short in duration.

20-4. Which of the following is *accurate* concerning the treatment of cocaine dependence?
A. There is a consensus as to the benefits of pharmacologic agents.
B. Amitriptyline and dantrolene have been reported to be helpful.
C. Propranolol is useful for long-term abstinence.
D. The prognosis is poor.
E. Cognitive behavioral therapy (CBT) may be more beneficial than interpersonal therapy (IPT).

ANSWERS

20-1. **C.** The possible long-term medical consequences of stimulant use include impaired alveolar diffusion, pulmonary edema, cardiomyopathy, arrhythmias, myocardial infarction, and ischemic strokes (the latter with cocaine in particular). Stimulants may also cause spontaneous abortions, abruptio placentae, preterm labor, fetal distress, developmental delays, and congenital malformations. Ischemia may also affect the intestines, the kidneys, or the testicles. Although acute intoxication may appear similar to mania in presentation, with agitation, pressured speech, and grandiose ideas, stimulant abuse is not significantly linked with the development of classic bipolar disorder. However, bipolar mania is a risk factor for stimulant use. Long-term psychiatric complications of stimulant abuse include aggressive behaviors, cognitive impairment, paranoia, and hallucinations. The "crash" associated with stimulant use begins within half an hour of use and is manifest by acute anxiety, depressed mood, and occasionally paranoia. This is usually followed by a hypersomnolent phase with vivid dreams, and it can last up to 4 days and may be accompanied by periods of binge eating. This is usually followed by an extended dysphoric/depressed phase; suicide may be considered.

20-2. A. Cocaine seems to exert its primary effects through actions on dopaminergic neurons in the mesolimbic and mesocortical areas. It may also affect noradrenergic, serotonergic, and cholinergic neurons. Increased sensitivity to a given dose may occur with chronic use, and seizures may be induced. Strokes (hemorrhagic or ischemic), vasculitis, and migraines may also occur. Hallucinations may occur as well and can be tactile in nature (e.g., formication). Visual impairment is not usually reported.

20-3. B. If cocaine is used briefly, its metabolites may be detected in the urine for up to 72 hours, but with chronic heavy use, this increases to up to 2 weeks. When used with alcohol, cocaine forms a long-lasting cardiotoxic metabolite called cocaethylene. Withdrawal symptoms include dysphoria, apathy, anhedonia, disturbed sleep, and drug craving. These symptoms may last for several weeks and have been reported to occur in approximately 50% of prolonged heavy users. Cocaine is the second most commonly used illicit substance used in the United States, after marijuana. It is mostly used by males between the ages of 18 and 25 years.

20-4. E. Treatment programs for cocaine dependence include a variety of cognitive-behavioral, supportive, and psychodynamic approaches, which may be used in an individual or group setting. CBT has been reported to be more successful in treating cocaine abuse than IPT. Twelve-step programs may be useful for those with concurrent alcohol problems. There is no formal consensus as to the benefits of pharmacological agents, and many different compounds are under investigation. Agents reported to be helpful include desipramine (not amitriptyline), bromocriptine, and amantadine. Dantrolene is a smooth muscle relaxant used to treat neuroleptic malignant syndrome. Other agents under further investigation include SSRIs, anticonvulsants, calcium channel blockers, and dopamine receptor antagonists. Propranolol may be useful in managing the symptoms of acute withdrawal, but not in maintaining abstinence. Pre-existing psychiatric conditions should be treated. The prognosis for cocaine dependence is better than that for opiate dependence (abstinence rates of over 50% at followup have been reported), but depends on the patient's incentive to abstain, available support systems, and use of alcohol or other substances. Those who freebase or use intravenously may do less well than those who snort.

SUGGESTED READINGS

Pozner CN, Levine M, Zane R. The cardiovascular effects of cocaine. *J Emergency Med*. 2005;29(2):173–178.
Rothman RB, Baumann MH. Balance between dopamine and serotonin release modulates behavioral effects of amphetamine-type drugs. *Ann NY Acad Sci*. 2006;1074:245–260.

CASE 21

My Orthopedist Told Me I Needed a Shrink

CC/ID: 55-year-old married woman who has been referred by orthopedics.

HPI: Mrs. P. has a 5-year history of low back pain which has been thoroughly investigated and for which **no organic cause has been found.** The pain develops suddenly and becomes worse over time, lasting several hours, during which time she has to go to bed. The **symptoms are not consistent with a known anatomical pathway.** This problem began after her youngest child went away to school. She is having difficulties taking care of the home, and sometimes her husband has to take time off from work to care for her.

PMHx: Hysterectomy aged 45

Meds: Ibuprofen, 800 mg po BID

Allergies: NKDA

PPHx: **Postpartam depression** after birth of last child, responded to a tricyclic antidepressant and psychotherapy. No history of suicide attempts.

FHx: Hypertension

SHx: Mrs. P. is the youngest of four children. She married at age 23 and has two children. She is a homemaker and describes her marriage as satisfactory. Her husband is an accountant and often works late and travels for business. She does not drink or smoke. She denies any history of substance abuse.

MSE: *General:* appears her stated age and is clearly in pain, wincing as she moves and grabbing her back. *Speech:* normal rate, rhythm, and volume, though spoken in a rather tense manner. *Behavior:* normal. *Affect:* constricted and anxious at times. *Mood:* "fed up." *Thought process:* logical and goal-directed. *Thought content:* preoccupied with her pain; no delusional material elicited;

denies perceptual abnormalities; denies suicidal or homicidal ideations. *Cognitive function:* intact. *Insight:* limited into the possible role of psychological components of her condition.

THOUGHT QUESTIONS

- What are the possible psychological and social issues involved?
- What is the differential diagnosis?

DISCUSSION

Attention must be paid to how the patient feels about this condition. How disabling is it? Are there any undisclosed concerns about her health, her marriage, or her family? How does she feel now that her youngest has left home? How does she cope with this pain? What does she see in her future? Some or all of these possible issues may be causing concern. It is important not to challenge her belief in the underlying organic cause of her pain. Several differential diagnoses for her condition should be considered.

Depression: This disorder can often present with pain. The patient may have had previous episodes of depression without pain or a family history of mood disorders.

Somatoform disorders: In conversion disorder, the pain has symbolic meaning for the patient. Often there is a family member with similar problems. Treatment includes developing a caring therapeutic relationship and a supportive environment. Behavioral and other psychotherapeutic techniques aimed at resolving the patient's psychosocial problems as well as the conversion symptoms themselves may be successful. Most conversion symptoms remit spontaneously or with treatment.

Psychosis: The pain may be delusional in nature, and treatment should be aimed at the underlying cause of the psychosis, such as schizophrenia or dementia.

Malingering: This is the intentional production of false or exaggerated physical or psychological symptoms motivated by external incentives.

Undiagnosed medical condition: The patient's symptoms may come from a condition such as fibromyalgia. It is important to investigate any significant worsening of the condition or the development of symptoms suggestive of an underlying organic lesion. However, fibromyalgia itself is highly correlated with psychological factors.

Pain disorder: Also known as psychogenic or somatoform pain disorder. The DSM-IV-TR criteria for this disorder include pain in one or more anatomical sites, not caused by another medical or neurological condition, which causes significant distress or impairment of functioning. The pain is the main focus of the presentation. **Psychological factors are judged to have an important role,** and the pain is not better accounted for by a psychiatric disorder or dyspareunia. The pain is not intentionally produced or feigned. This patient meets these criteria. Pain is a significant cause of morbidity and mortality in the United States. Acute pain is defined as lasting less than 6 months; thereafter it is deemed chronic. **Pain disorders** have an age of onset usually in the fourth and fifth decades. Genetics may play a role as first-degree relatives are at increased risk for developing this disorder. **Individuals who have difficulty expressing their emotions or feel that physiological concerns do not deserve attention may manifest these as physical symptoms.** Some individuals have guilt and feel they deserve to suffer. Attention and the caring behaviors of others may serve as a "reward," or perhaps unwanted chores or activities may be avoided (i.e., secondary gain). The primary gain is the avoidance of the inner emotional conflict and psychological anxiety. In pain disorder, the pain can affect any system in the body, but psychological factors must play a significant role. Patients may deny any other problems in their lives except for the pain, and they may have significant medical or surgical histories. There may be comorbid substance abuse or dependence as patients self-medicate. Other comorbid psychiatric conditions include depressive disorders. **Evaluation** of pain disorders includes taking a good history, obtaining collateral information, and ruling out any possible underlying medical or neurological condition that could explain the symptoms. Pain that does not improve with pain medications or other treatments may have psychological origins. Psychiatric history is important for ruling out anxiety, depression, hysteria (conversion), or hypochondriasis. Also consider psychosocial stressors and any pending litigation. Treatment of pain disorders involves a multidisciplinary team focusing on behavioral interventions designed to enhance functioning and treating any psychiatric disorders. The important contributing role of psychological factors should be acknowledged in providing the patient with psychoeducation as to how these feelings may affect the perception of pain. This disorder can become chronic, and those with poor premorbid functioning, litigation concerns, or substance abuse or dependence may have a worse prognosis.

CASE CONTINUED

The patient is reluctant to try psychotherapy. She states, "If you think this is all in my mind, you're nuts." She finally agrees to try relaxation therapy. During this therapy she begins to talk, and it becomes clear that she is depressed. She agrees to a course of tricyclics, in combination with psychotherapy, physiotherapy, and relaxation training. She is encouraged to find a part-time job, and 3 months later is doing well.

QUESTIONS

21-1. Which of the following is correct about pain disorder?
A. Physical factors may have an important role.
B. This disorder appears to be more common in men.
C. There may be a family history of pain, depression, or substance abuse.
D. The focus of treatment is to remove the pain.
E. Defense mechanisms involved include rationalization.

21-2. Which of the following factors does not contribute to differences in response to pain?
A. Different tolerance thresholds
B. Stoicism
C. Intellectual abilities
D. Cultural heritage
E. Physiological makeup

21-3. Which of the following *may be* a clue that a patient's pain might include a significant psychological component?
A. Pain that wakes the patient from sleep
B. Good insight into the role of psychological factors
C. Pain consistent with dermatomes
D. Exacerbations during periods of increased stress or conflict
E. Absence of any secondary gain

21-4. Which of the following statements is accurate concerning patients who are malingering?
A. Patients usually refuse to undergo painful procedures.
B. Malingering may occur in 10% to 15% of patients seen by psychiatrists.
C. Patients are afraid of having a serious disease.
D. Patients may obtain relief from hypnosis.
E. Patients with this disorder wish to assume the sick role.

ANSWERS

21-1. **C.** There may be a family history of pain, depression, or substance abuse in patients with pain disorder. If there is an associated psychiatric disorder such as depression or anxiety, the pain may improve or resolve with appropriate treatment of the primary condition. Suicidal ideation in those suffering from chronic pain must be evaluated. The focus of treatment should be to regain functioning, and programs should be tailored to the individual patient. The patient's pain and difficulties should be acknowledged at each visit. Treatments can include NSAIDs, tricyclics, physical therapy, TENS (Transcutaneous electrical nerve stimulation) units, ultrasound, and nerve blocks. Relaxation therapy, hypnosis, or psychotherapy may also be of benefit. Close collaboration with the patient's other physicians is important. Psychological factors may have an important role in the onset, severity, exacerbation, or maintenance of the pain. Defense mechanisms used in this disorder include repression, displacement, substitution, and even identification with important role models who also have pain. This disorder appears to be twice as common in women as in men.

21-2. **C.** An individual's experience may depend on a variety of personal and cultural influences, including pain thresholds, stoicism, and previous experiences of pain. Intellect has not been shown to influence the individual's response to pain. Certain individuals may also be biologically predisposed (anatomically or physiologically) to experience heightened pain.

21-3. **D.** Pain may increase during periods of increased stress or difficulty. The secondary gain of this experience may be an unconscious avoidance of unpleasant situations or the gain of other forms of compensation. Other features that suggest a role for psychological factors in the pain include the following characteristics: pain that responds better to psychotropics than analgesics; pain that does not conform to known anatomical presentations (e.g., dermatomes); pain that may stop an individual from falling asleep but rarely wakes them; and pain that lasts for long periods and does not improve with distraction tasks. Although insight into the psychological factors involved may be very limited, there may be a symbolic connection with someone close to them (e.g., a headache in someone who lost a parent to a brain tumor). Pain disorder is also associated with poor premorbid functioning and may include difficulties with employment, relationships, and alcohol or substance abuse.

21-4. **A.** Unlike those with Munchausen syndrome, patients who are malingering often refuse to undergo painful procedures. Patients with factitious disorder wish to assume the sick role, but those who malinger often have a more tangible gain in mind (e.g., avoiding criminal responsibility or military duty, obtaining financial gain, medications, or a bed for the night). The patient's records may reveal that he or she has frequently presented in other settings as well. Malingering is found in 1% to 5% of patients seen by psychiatrists. Those with conversion disorder are usually seeking an answer, are more likely to be cooperative and dependent, and often do not present with such detailed histories behind their symptoms, as does the malingerer. They are also more likely to obtain symptom relief from hypnosis or suggestion, unlike the malingerer. The main difference between the differential diagnoses in this case is the patient's motive.

SUGGESTED READINGS

Leiknes KA, Finset A, Moum T, et al. Course and predictors of medically unexplained pain symptoms in the general population. *J Psychosomatic Res.* 2007;62:119–128.

Allet JL, Allet RE. Somatoform disorders in neurological practice. *Curr Opin Psychiatry.* 2006;19:413–420.

"My Nose Is Deformed"

 CC/ID: 24-year-old woman who is referred to you by a plastic surgeon for evaluation. She wishes to have surgery on her nose, which she feels is deformed.

HPI: She feels ugly and believes that the surgery will improve her life. There is **no obvious abnormality of her nose.** She has been more concerned about this since she broke up with her boyfriend 3 months ago. She thinks they broke up because he no longer found her attractive. She acknowledges that this is causing her considerable distress and is hindering her social activities.

 ## THOUGHT QUESTIONS

- What would be important to look for in her history?
- What possible differential diagnoses should you consider?
- How would you advise both the patient and the plastic surgeon?

DISCUSSION

A complete history and evaluation should be performed. In particular, **look for any evidence of depressive symptoms** such as poor appetite, disturbed sleep, low self-esteem, and poor self-image, as a depressive episode may have been triggered by her recent breakup with her boyfriend. Inquire about possible suicidal ideation. Ask about any substance abuse. **Explore her ideas about her apparent disfigurement, looking for delusional beliefs or psychotic symptoms. Look for evidence of obsessive-compulsive disorder.** Also, obtain information about her personality, focusing on her prior social and work relationships and how she copes with stress. Collateral sources of information should be considered. Also consider the possibility of an underlying organic disorder, such as a seizure disorder or an intracranial neoplasm. Several differential diagnoses should be considered.

Depression: If there were evidence of a depressive disorder, then treatment would include antidepressants and psychotherapy (cognitive-behavioral or insight-oriented therapy). She would also need support and education about depression.

Schizophrenia: If there is evidence of delusional ideas, ideas of reference, or perceptual abnormalities such as auditory hallucinations, this may be the initial presentation of schizophrenia. Treatment would include antipsychotics, support, psychoeducation, and rehabilitation.

Obsessive-compulsive disorder: Here the patient may be bothered with persistent, recurrent thoughts or images about his or her appearance. Patients with OCD may recognize that these thoughts come from their own minds and may try to suppress them. In this disorder, there are other obsessions, not only concerned with appearance.

Body dysmorphic disorder (BDD): This is a somatoform disorder in which individuals believe that a part of their body is abnormal. They often feel ugly and even repulsive. The minority of such patients may indeed have a minor defect, but the level of concern is out of proportion. It is more common in women. Individuals with this disorder usually present to plastic surgeons or dermatologists. It causes significant distress or impairment of functioning, and they are not reassured by others who deny the perceived defect. **The idea is not held with delusional conviction, but they often have poor insight into the nature of the problem** and may refuse psychiatric treatment. In BDD the defense mechanisms at play may be displacement, dissociation, distortion, projection, repression, and symbolization (Table 22-1). There may be a family history of OCD or mood disorders. There may be symptoms of depression, anxiety, and difficulties dealing with social situations. Although facial features are the most common features implicated, other areas of the body may be involved.

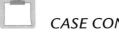

CASE CONTINUED

On further evaluation, you ascertain that she has no depressive symptoms. There is no evidence of OCD or psychosis. Her expectations of the surgery may be unrealistic, and the possible risks

TABLE **22-1** Overview of Defense Mechanisms

What is a defense mechanism?	Protects both patients and healthy people from being aware of intolerable, undesired, or feared thoughts, feelings, and impulses; allows the unconscious thought, feeling, or impulse to be indirectly expressed in a disguised form
Acting out	A direct behavioral expression of an unconscious impulse in order to avoid conscious awareness of the accompanying affect (e.g., the patient throwing furniture because the dinner cart is late)
Altruism	Using a constructive service to others to provide vicarious satisfaction (e.g., the unhappy divorcee volunteering in a soup kitchen)
Denial	A conscious refusal to accept external reality (e.g., the patient who has been diagnosed with cancer and leaves the hospital against medical advice)
Distortion	Grossly reshaping external reality to accommodate internal needs (e.g., the substance abuser who believes that amphetamines help clear his or her thinking)
Displacement	The shifting of feelings onto a less cared for object (e.g., the disgruntled employee who returns home and kicks the cat)
Dissociation	Temporary change of character or identity to avoid distress (e.g., the man who becomes bankrupt and develops amnesia)
Identification	Behavior patterns changed to emulate another (e.g., medical students wearing white coats on the wards)
Intellectualization	Excessively using reason to avoid affective experiences (e.g., the physician who has a terminal illness and discusses the details with colleagues constantly)
Isolation	An idea separated from its associated affect (e.g., an abused woman calmly plans to kill her husband)
Projection	Unacceptable feelings attributed to others; may become delusional (e.g., the person who wants to have an affair accuses his or her spouse of infidelity)
Projective identification	Unacceptable aspects of the personality dissociated and projected onto another, with whom the patient then identifies (e.g., the person who wishes to have an affair projects this onto a close friend whom he or she admires)
Rationalization	Reason used to justify unacceptable emotions and feelings (e.g., the individual who had an indiscretion blames it on a single martini)
Reaction formation	An unacceptable impulse is transformed into its opposite (e.g., the televangelist who rails against illicit sex caught on film with a prostitute)

(Continued)

TABLE 22-1   Overview of Defense Mechanisms (*continued*)

Regression	Attempts to return to earlier behaviors to avoid anxiety (e.g., the child who returns to wetting the bed when his parents separate)
Repression	Refusal to accept into consciousness a feeling or instinct; it is the basic defense mechanism (e.g., the angry wife of the traveling salesman forgets he will be out of town)
Splitting	Positive and negative aspects of relationships are separately and alternatively conscious; black and white thinking (e.g., the patient who thinks that his or her physician is wonderful until one day the physician is late for an appointment and is perceived as dreadful)
Sublimation	Unacceptable impulses directed in a socially acceptable manner (e.g., the male with aggressive impulses becomes a surgeon)
Suppression	Ideas or feelings consciously suppressed to minimize discomfort; the only conscious defense mechanism (e.g., the patient who has a life threatening illness decides to worry about it for only a limited time each day)
Turning against the self	Unacceptable aggression toward others expressed indirectly toward the self (e.g., the teenager who dislikes her stepfather superficially cuts herself after an argument)

and benefits are discussed. When you suggest that there may be a psychological component to this problem, she becomes very angry and storms out of your office. As you do not find any evidence of a formal psychiatric disorder, you convey this information to the surgeon. His decision may be helped by your assessment of her personality and expectations of the surgery.

QUESTIONS

22-1. Which of the following is true concerning body dysmorphic disorder?
- A. It is found in approximately 20% of those attending plastic surgery clinics.
- B. The disorder usually develops in middle childhood.
- C. There is a low rate of comorbid depressive disorders.
- D. SSRIs may be helpful.
- E. There is increased risk of psychotic disorders in families of probands with this disorder.

22-2. Which of the following is correct about those suffering from this disorder?
  A. The onset of symptoms is usually acute.
  B. They conceptualize the problem as only physical in nature.
  C. Surgery usually is successful.
  D. Surgery does not affect the development of psychiatric symptoms.
  E. Patients rarely retain bodily preoccupations even after treatment.

22-3. Which of the following is correct about the treatment of this disorder?
  A. Tricyclics or MAOIs usually are not useful.
  B. Pimozide may be helpful.
  C. Psychotherapy is not useful.
  D. Behavioral methods have no role
  E. Treatments should be short in duration.

22-4. Which of the following statements is accurate concerning the underlying psychological components of this disorder?
  A. Defense mechanisms used may include sublimation.
  B. Assessment of premorbid personality may reveal schizo-typal traits.
  C. Assessment of premorbid personality may reveal border-line traits.
  D. In psychodynamic terms, the disorder is viewed as resulting from the displacement of emotional or sexual conflicts onto an unrelated body part.
  E. It is associated with harsh punitive parental styles.

 ANSWERS

22-1. D. Studies have reported prevalence rates for BDD of 1% to 2% in the general population. Increased prevalence rates have been reported for certain patient populations: 12% among patients attending a dermatology clinic, and 2% to 7% of those attending plastic surgery clinics. This disorder usually develops in adolescence or early adulthood. There is a high rate of comorbid depressive and anxiety disorders, as well as an increased risk of suicide (particularly in women with reported facial defects). There is also an increased risk of having a comorbid psychotic disorder. SSRIs, which are both antidepressant and antiobsessional agents, may be helpful. There are increased rates of both OCD and depression in the families of the probands with this disorder.

22-2. B. The onset of symptoms in BDD is usually gradual in nature. Surgery is not usually successful in persons with this disorder; in fact, it may be followed by the development of more serious psychopathology (e.g., depression or worsening obsession over the perceived dysmorphology). Patients with BDD have limited, if any, insight into the possible psychological overlay to their symptoms. Even if there is no evidence of psychiatric symptomatology, there is still an increased risk of developing psychiatric disorders after surgery of this type.

22-3. B. Pimozide is a high potency typical antipsychotic agent that has been reported to be helpful, but care must be taken in view of the possible cardiotoxic effects of this medicine. It has a higher affinity for D2 than for D4 receptors and has a relative lack of noradrenergic antagonism. It does cause calcium channel antagonism and opioid receptor blockade. Trials of antidepressants such as tricyclics, MAOIs, or SSRIs may be helpful, particularly if there is a family history of mood disorder or OCD. SSRIs may be augmented with buspirone, antipsychotics, or carefully used in combination with other antidepressants. Unfortunately, relapse is common when medications are stopped. Psychotherapy (including cognitive-behavioral) and techniques such as desensitization, exposure therapy, social skills training, and assertiveness training may be beneficial in some cases. It is unclear how long treatment should be continued.

22-4. D. In psychodynamic terms, the disorder is viewed as resulting from the displacement of emotional or sexual conflicts onto an unrelated body part. Defense mechanisms may include dissociation, distortion, projection, repression, and symbolization. There is no significant evidence that the parenting styles of the patient's parents affect the development of this disorder. Assessment of premorbid personality may reveal shyness, sensitivity, self-absorption, narcissism, obsessional, or schizoid traits.

SUGGESTED READINGS

Phillips KA. The presentation of body dysmorphic disorder in medical settings. *Prim Psychiatry.* 2006;13(7):51–59.

Phillips KA, Pagano ME, Menard W. Pharmacotherapy for body dysmorphic disorder: treatment received and illness severity. *Ann Clin Psychiatry.* 2006;18(4):251–257.

Mackley CL. Body dysmorphic disorder. *Dermatol Surg.* 2005;31:552–558.

"My Wife Is Having an Affair"

CC/ID: 35-year-old married man who runs a microbrewery. His family doctor has referred him to your psychiatric clinic for assessment. His wife accompanies him.

HPI: The family doctor is concerned, as Mrs. P. reported that her husband has become increasingly suspicious of her over the previous 3 months, accusing her of having an affair. He apparently has been **searching for evidence** of this, and she believes that he has been following her. She has become quite frightened of him, although he has never actually threatened or hurt her in the past. Mr. P. tells you that he **knows his wife is having an affair,** although he is unsure exactly who her partner is. He has recently employed the services of a private detective and checks her phone bills, receipts, and clothing for evidence. He denies any history of violence.

PMHx: Appendectomy

Meds: None

Allergies: NKDA

PPHx: None. Denies abuse of or dependence on alcohol or illicit substances. Has never been a victim of violence. No legal problems.

FHx: Noncontributory

SHx: Mr. P. is the eldest of two boys. His parents are alive and well. He has been married for 10 years and claims that they were happy until recently. They have two children aged 8 and 6 years. He started the brewery after college and is very successful.

VS/PE: WNL

Labs: SMA with LFTs, CBC WNL, Utox negative

MSE: *General:* appears his stated age with good hygiene. Appropriate demeanor, with intermittent eye contact and fair rapport. *Affect:* guarded, suspicious. *Behavior:* no abnormal movements. He becomes agitated and somewhat hostile during the interview. *Mood:* "Fed up with all this carrying-on." *Thought process:* linear and without formal thought disorder. *Thought content:* systemized delusions of infidelity. Preoccupied with obtaining evidence. No delusions of control or persecution. Denies perceptual abnormalities. Denies suicidal ideation, but he admits to thinking about following his wife and murdering her with her lover (or murdering the man who he thinks is her lover). *Cognitive function:* intact. *Insight and judgment:* impaired.

THOUGHT QUESTIONS

- How should you proceed?
- What is important in his history?
- What is in your differential diagnosis?

DISCUSSION

Delusional or morbid jealousy is a symptom that can occur in a variety of conditions. **Underlying medical causes must be ruled out** and include intracranial neoplasm, stroke, seizure disorder, head injury, or dementia; this is particularly the case if this behavior represents a recent change from the patient's personality. Focal signs or symptoms may be evident on exam. Disinhibition and aggression may be seen with frontal lobe lesions. Several other differential diagnoses must be considered.

Substance abuse: Delusional jealousy has been described in alcoholics. Treatment is aimed at the substance abuse or dependence.

Paranoid schizophrenia: Marked feelings of jealousy may occur in schizophrenia and may be seen more commonly in females with this disorder. Other characteristic features of schizophrenia to aid diagnosis include thought disorder, blunted affect, and poor levels of psychosocial functioning.

Delusional disorder, jealous type (see Table 23-1): This is a rare disorder, which usually affects men. It may appear suddenly in those with no known past psychiatric history. Tactile or olfactory

TABLE 23-1   Overview of Delusional Disorders

Diagnostic criteria	1 month or more of nonbizarre delusions. Does not meet main criteria for schizophrenia (delusions/ hallucinations/disorganized speech, disorganized/catatonic behavior or negative symptoms). Level of functioning not severely impaired. If mood symptoms are present, they are brief. Symptoms are not caused by alcohol or illicit substances.
Subtypes	
Persecutory	This is the most common type of delusional theme: belief that the individual (or someone close to him or her) is being unfairly treated in some way.
Grandiose	Belief that an individual has special relationships with important people. May also believe that he or she has special knowledge, power, or worth.
Jealous	Belief that one's partner is unfaithful.
Erotomanic	Belief that another person is in love with the individual. This other person is usually someone of a higher position and may be unattainable (e.g., a rock star).
Somatic	Belief that the individual has a particular defect or medical illness.
Mixed	Mixture of above types of delusions, with none in particular as main theme.

Adapted from American Psychiatric Association. *Task Force on DSM-IV. Diagnostic and statistical manual of mental disorders: DSM-IV.* 4th ed. Washington, DC: American Psychiatric Association, 1994.

hallucinations may occur and are usually related to the delusional theme. Antipsychotics may be marginally helpful, but the disorder can be difficult to treat and may only be resolved by separation, divorce, or the death of a spouse. It is important to provide support for the wife. She may be taught ways of responding to the patient that can reduce levels of aggression.

CASE CONTINUED

His wife confirms that she has not been having an affair, and admits that given his behavior, she is concerned about the safety of herself and the children. A diagnosis of delusional disorder, jealous type is made. He refuses voluntary admission and is admitted involuntarily to inpatient psychiatry for further evaluation and a trial of antipsychotics.

QUESTIONS

23-1. What should you do about his homicidal ideation?
A. You have a duty to warn the wife and the relevant authorities.
B. This was told to you in a session and therefore is protected information.
C. You must call the police and have him immediately arrested.
D. You have to get his permission to warn his wife.
E. You do not have to be concerned about weapons; that is a police matter.

23-2. Which of the following is correct concerning delusional jealousy?
A. When concerned with spousal infidelity, it may be referred to as de Clerambault syndrome.
B. It may diminish on separation from the spouse.
C. It may diminish with reassurance or a confession from the spouse.
D. It is never associated with suicide and homicide.
E. Onset is usually very gradual.

23-3. His wife is most concerned about her husband and asks you if he can be treated and get "back to normal." What do you tell her about the management of such cases?
A. Management will involve an assessment of the risk of violence.
B. Patients rarely need to be hospitalized.
C. Psychoanalysis is usually effective.
D. Good prognosis may be indicated by a sensitive premorbid personality.
E. Good prognosis may be indicated by the lack of a clear underlying diagnosis.

23-4. Which of the following is relevant when assessing dangerousness?
A. A previous history of violence or harm to others
B. Harm or threats against specified individuals
C. Access to a weapon and knowledge of how to use it
D. Alcohol history
E. All of the above

ANSWERS

23-1. A. The Tarasoff Decision: In 1976, a Californian therapist was held responsible for the actions of a patient who murdered his girlfriend. The patient had repeatedly threatened to kill her. The Tarasoff "duty to protect" ruling states that the clinician must not only determine if the patient intends to do harm to others but must also take steps to prevent this, informing the relevant authorities and the intended victim as necessary. It is always important when evaluating the level of risk to determine the availability of weapons. States may have a prohibition of firearms policy, which states that after an individual has been placed on an involuntary hold for danger to self or others, he or she may not possess firearms for a period up to 5 years. An individual has the right to challenge this in court. A violation of this law may be a felony.

23-2. B. Delusional jealousy may diminish upon separation or death of the spouse. A confession of infidelity may only exacerbate the problem and may provoke an act of violence, so the wife should be warned against this. A delusion by definition is a fixed false belief, and reassurance does not help. Homicidal and suicidal ideation must be closely assessed. Othello syndrome is named after the Shakespearean character who murders his wife after he develops a delusion of her nonexistent infidelity. The onset of delusional jealousy is relatively acute in the majority of cases. De Clerambault syndrome is another name for erotomania.

23-3. A. Management will involve an assessment for the risk of violence. If the patient is deemed a danger to himself or others he may need to be hospitalized and appropriate precautions made to prevent the patient's absconding. If he is deemed not to be dangerous and a good therapeutic alliance may be reached, then outpatient treatment may be considered. Marital or sexual therapy may be necessary. Psychoanalysis is not reported to be the treatment of choice for this condition. Substance abuse treatment should be offered to those who may benefit from such interventions. Behavioral techniques to reduce aggression and anger management can be helpful. Separation from the spouse may be the only solution if there is clear risk of violence, a poor response to treatment, or if the prognosis is poor. Poor prognosis is indicated by an inadequate and sensitive premorbid personality, no clear underlying diagnosis, and long-standing duration of the problem.

23-4. E. The assessment of dangerousness can be very difficult to predict accurately, but the clinician must consider the following: Does the person have a history of previous violence or harm to others? Has he or she harmed or threatened a specific individual in particular? Has he or she ever been arrested, prosecuted, or even cautioned by the police? Did the patient use a weapon? Does he or she have access to a weapon and knowledge of how to use it? Does this person use alcohol or drugs that may affect his/her judgment or thinking? Does he or she have poor impulse control? Can the patient form a therapeutic alliance? Is he or she compliant with treatment? How does the clinician subjectively feel about the patient?

SUGGESTED READINGS

Charlton BG, McClelland HA. Theory of mind and the delusional disorders. *J New Ment Dis.* 1999;187(6):380–383.

Manschreck TC, Khan NL. Recent advances in the treatment of delusional disorder. *Can J Psychiatry.* 2006;51:114–119.

CASE 24

"I'm Always Miserable"

CC/ID: 25-year-old single woman who has reluctantly come to your office complaining of **having been depressed since she was a child.**

HPI: Ms. B. claims that this began when she was approximately 9 years of age, and has continued steadily since. She describes herself as a "gloomy" person who has continually struggled to maintain her job. Her mood is worse in the morning, and she has to force herself out of bed. Generally she **feels inadequate** and tends to brood about her lack of happiness. She has experienced periods when she has "not felt as bad" but without a frank change in her usual state or personality. She has never achieved the diagnostic criteria for a major depressive episode. Ms. B.'s life revolves around her job as an insurance assessor, and she has **few social activities, interests, or hobbies.** She **denies other vegetative symptoms,** symptoms of anxiety, or any recent stressors. Although she has felt hopeless at times, she denies any prior suicidal ideation.

PMHx: None

Meds: None

PPsychHx: None. No history of substance abuse.

FHx: One maternal aunt with recurrent major depression.

SHx: Middle of three daughters, parents alive and well. Graduated college with a B.A. Worked at the same insurance company since leaving college. Lives with roommate in a rented apartment.

PE: Unremarkable

Labs: CBC, SMA 20, TFTs, UA and Utox screen WNL

MSE: *General:* appropriately dressed, eye contact limited, hygiene good, demeanor is somewhat removed. *Speech:* monotonous, but normal rate and volume. *Mood:* "numb . . . empty." *Affect:* constricted and alternating between neutrality and sadness. *Thought* *process:* logical and goal-directed. *Thought content:* preoccupied with themes of inadequacy, suffering, and hopelessness. No evidence of suicidal or homicidal ideation. *Cognitive function:* intact. *Insight:* limited; she claims she is only here because her roommate "made me come."

THOUGHT QUESTIONS

- What is your differential diagnosis?
- Do you think she has an axis II disorder?
- How can you help this woman?

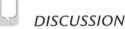

DISCUSSION

The differential diagnoses include the following:

Recurrent brief depressive disorder: This is not a differentiated entity in DSM-IV-TR, but research criteria are included in an appendix section. Criteria for a major depressive disorder are met and cause significant distress and impairment of functioning, but episodes last from 2 days to 2 weeks. These episodes can occur each month but are not associated with the menstrual cycle. May be associated with suicide attempts. Generally this is seen more often in primary care settings. Patients with this disorder tend to have more severe symptoms than those with dysthymia. This patient does not meet criteria for this disorder.

Cyclothymia: This disorder involves at least 2 years of mood instability, with both depression and hypomania, with or without normal mood in between episodes (see Figure 24-1). These episodes do not meet criteria for mania or moderate or severe depression, although such episodes may precede or follow this period of mood instability. Ms. B. does not meet these criteria.

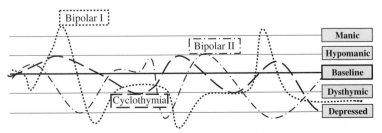

FIGURE 24-1. Graphic presentation of mood disorders

Dysthymia: This woman meets the criteria for this diagnosis with depressed mood most of the day, **for more days than not,** for a period **of at least 2 years.** During this time, she has had low energy, fatigue, low self-esteem, hopelessness, and some hypersomnia, though her appetite and concentration were normal. Other symptoms may include feelings of anger, irritability, inadequacy, or guilt. Patients with this disorder may become withdrawn from society and have significantly impaired functioning. During this 2-year period, she has never been without these symptoms for a period of over 2 months. She has not experienced an episode of superimposed major depression—so-called "double-depression"—but she may develop this pattern over time. Up to 40% of patients with depression may also meet criteria for dysthymia. **Patients with dysthymic disorder often tell you that they have always been depressed** and indeed they may have begun to

TABLE 24-1   Types of Psychotherapy

Psychodynamic	Usually several sessions per week; may use couch or be face to face with therapist. Therapy includes an analysis of transference reactions between the patient and the therapist or of defense mechanisms and interpersonal conflicts. In classical psychoanalysis, the therapist remains neutral. Patients have to be motivated for treatment and able to form a good "therapeutic alliance" (i.e., working relationship). This type of therapy may help those with character pathology or those who need adjunctive treatments such as medications. Also known as insight-oriented psychotherapy, it relates the development of symptoms to unresolved conflicts from an individual's childhood. In shorter forms there is less focus on free association and regression.
Supportive	The aim here is to strengthen the ego and to support reality testing. Good for acute crisis. Strengthens healthy defenses, reassures, and helps reframe thinking processes.
Cognitive behavioral	Tries to correct underlying distorted cognitive assumptions that an individual has about his orher world and that are causing distress. Therapy usually lasts 6 months. Sessions are structured and include homework tasks. Used in mood, anxiety, and eating disorders. The cognitive models of depression also apply to dysthymia.
Interpersonal	Focus is on current interpersonal skills. Usually time limited 12–16 weeks. Clarify emotions, reassure, and enhance interpersonal communication. Can work well in combination with medication.
Brief psychotherapy	Time limited up to 1 year. Research has shown these methods to be effective. Helps patients cope with current problems and crises as well as defined disorders such as depression.

have symptoms in childhood or adolescence. Comorbid disorders may include depression, anxiety, substance abuse, and borderline personality disorders. There are biological factors, as rates of dysthymia are increased in first-degree relatives, and there may be abnormalities of sleep as in depression ($\downarrow$ REM latency and $\uparrow$ REM density). Treatment can be difficult and includes a **combination of psychotherapy** (Table 24-1) **and antidepressants** (SSRIs, bupropion, or MAOIs). Augmentation of antidepressants with lithium or thyroid hormone may be helpful in some cases.

 CASE CONTINUED

Ms. B. is given a trial of treatment with a selective serotonin reuptake inhibitor (SSRI), but she is unable to tolerate any side effects. She begrudgingly agrees to return for psychotherapy, and you decide to embark upon a course of interpersonal therapy. Six months later, she is beginning to show some improvement in functioning.

 QUESTIONS

24-1. Which of the following is *not* correct concerning dysthymia?
  A. Patients with dysthymia may have symptoms that outnumber signs of depression.
  B. Brief hypomanic episodes may develop when patients are treated with antidepressants.
  C. Patients may have a family history of bipolar disorder.
  D. Dysthymic disorder and major depressive disorder are mutually exclusive.
  E. Patients may have a comorbid personality disorder.

24-2. Which of the following statements is *accurate* concerning dysthymia?
  A. It has a lifetime prevalence of approximately 15% in the general population.
  B. It is a sequel to well-defined major depressive episodes.
  C. It never presents in middle age and older.
  D. Most cases begin in childhood or early adolescence.
  E. There are different incidence rates for men and women.

24-3. Which of the following are *usually* found in patients with dysthymia?

A. Disturbed appetite and libido
B. Psychomotor agitation or retardation
C. Lethargy and anhedonia, which may be worse in the morning
D. Anxiety
E. Nihilistic psychotic features

24-4. Which of the following typically occurs during the course of dysthymia?
A. Children with this disorder frequently experience anxiety disorders later in life.
B. Children with this disorder frequently experience major depressive episodes later in life.
C. Those who present as adults tend to have more bipolar symptoms.
D. It is not helped by modified interpersonal therapies.
E. It usually responds well to medication.

ANSWERS

24-1. D. Patients with dysthymia often present with multiple subjective symptoms of depression that outnumber the actual, more objective signs of depression. Treatment with antidepressants may induce hypomanic symptoms in up to one third of those patients who present as adults, particularly if they have a family history of bipolar disorder. Those with dysthymia may have a family history of both depressive and bipolar disorders. Up to one third of psychiatric outpatients may suffer from dysthymia, which is frequently found in patients with personality disorders. A major depressive episode coexisting with dysthymia is colloquially termed "double-depression."

24-2. D. Its chronicity, subtlety, usual integration into the patient's personality and daily life, and the fact that it does not follow well-defined episodes allow dysthymia to be distinguished from major depressive disorder. Although most cases are of early onset (usually by the 20s), some studies have found that it may present in middle age or even in geriatric patients. The incidence rates do not vary between the sexes.

24-3. C. Patients with dysthymia do not usually exhibit marked disturbances in appetite or libido, but they may have more subtle features of psychomotor inertia, lethargy, and anhedonia, which can be worse in the morning. If these patients develop major depressive episodes, they may indeed present with the features characteristic of that disorder. Nihilistic delusions are associated with melancholic depression.

24-4. B. Children may experience frequent depressive episodes, which may become hypomanic, manic, or mixed in nature during adolescence. In fact those who develop this disorder early in life are at increased risk for developing major depression (20%) and bipolar disorder (5% develop type I and 15% develop type II). Adults who present tend to have a more unipolar (depressed) course. Patients with dysthymia are often unresponsive to traditional antidepressant therapies or they cannot tolerate the side effects of these medications. These long-standing symptoms lead to impaired relationships, social withdrawal, and impaired occupational functioning. Several specific types of psychotherapy may be beneficial in this disorder, including modified interpersonal therapy, insight-oriented psychodynamic psychotherapy, and the cognitive-behavioral analysis system of psychotherapy (C-BASP).

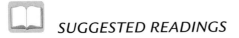 *SUGGESTED READINGS*

Klein DN, and Santiago NJ. Dysthymia and chronic depression: introduction, classification, risk factors, and course. *J Clin Psychol.* 2003;59(8):807–816.

Klein DN, Shankman SA, Rose S. Ten-year prospective follow-up study of the naturalistic course of dysthymic disorder and double depression. *Am J Psychiatry.* 2006;163(5):872–880.

De Lima MS, Hotopf M. Benefits and risks of pharmacotherapy for dysthymia: a systematic appraisal of the evidence. *Drug Safety.* 2003;26(1):55–64.

II

Adult Patients Who Present via Hospital Consultation

"Help Us With This Patient"

CC/ID: 29-year-old single white male for whom a consult has been requested by the medical unit for "behavior and depression."

HPI: The patient states that he has pancreatitis and is experiencing significant pain, which his team isn't treating. He denies depression or other mood or psychotic symptoms. He is "tired of the hospital and wants out" to get a job. You talk to the team and nurses. He has been admitted many times for complications of alcohol abuse, including pancreatitis. He was admitted yesterday with abdominal pain, lower extremity cellulitis, and fever. He has been told his amylase and lipase are normal and he does not have pancreatitis, but he disagrees. The cellulitis has focal purulent areas, and they suspect that he is causing the infection. Two nurses have been lobbying to increase his medications for abdominal pain. **He often asks the intern on the other team for tests or medications.** He told two nurses that he is depressed. **He causes discord among staff, is demanding, and at times is threatening. The team is angry, frustrated, and would like to transfer him to psychiatry.**

PMHx: Nine admissions in the previous 2 years for pancreatitis, gastritis, cellulitis.

Meds: From last discharge: fluoxetine, clonazepam, risperidone, gabapentin. Noncompliant. Now: IV antibiotics, thiamine, and folate.

PPHx: **Binge alcohol use since age 13,** two previous car accidents. No history of mania. Three inpatient psychiatric admissions: One overdose (OD) on alcohol, benzodiazepines (BZD), a tricyclic antidepressant, and acetaminophen with codeine, requiring an ICU admission. Two parasuicidal acts—small ODs with BZDs. Also three admissions for detoxification from alcohol. Last discharged the week before by the same team to a day program. He did not go. He went home, felt "empty," and began drinking "like I was outside

myself, watching me go to the bar." He carries a diagnosis of borderline personality disorder (BPD).

SHx/FHx: Patient states he has a Ph.D., was in the army, worked
as a medic, and was not in combat. His father abused alcohol, had
"rages," and left the family. His mother had depressions. He talks
about many jobs, but admits he has not had a full-time job in over
5 years.

VS: BP 120/80, HR 80

PE: WNL except *Abdomen:* diffuse tenderness, no guard-
ing or rebound. *Ext:* left leg red, indurated, covered in a bandage.

Labs: WBC slightly elevated, increased neutrophils

MSE: *General:* alert, appears older than 29, and is somewhat
ingratiating and overly familiar. *Speech:* normal rate and tone.
Mood: "I feel like crap." *Affect:* appropriately reactive though occasionally expansive. *Thought process:* goal-directed. *Thought content:* preoccupied with the "prejudiced" treatment he has received
by the medical team. No hallucinations, no suicidal or homicidal
ideation. *Cognition:* orientation intact.

THOUGHT QUESTIONS

- How do you understand his interactions with the treatment team?
- How would you recommend the inpatient medical
  team manage him?

DISCUSSION

The referring question may only hint at what the team wants or
needs. **The best strategy is to speak to the team prior to seeing
the patient to clarify what prompted the consultation.** Old charts
can be helpful in understanding previous presentations and treatments. In speaking to them, the points that you immediately notice
are (i) the anger that he engenders among the team, (ii) the splitting
that occurs among team members, and (iii) his noncompliance with
recommendations. He has alcohol dependence, BPD, a possible history of a mood disorder or substance-induced mood disorder, and
may have a factitious disorder or malingering. However, he currently denies depression. **Your role as a consultant is to facilitate**

his treatment; you should make sure that the team's anger is not causing them to overlook real symptoms like alcohol withdrawal. By helping staff acknowledge their reactions, including anger, loathing, and aversion, you can help improve his care.

People with BPD have characteristics that make them difficult to manage in a medical setting. They alternate between overvaluing and devaluing staff, and cause dissent and struggles as to how best to care for them. The medical staff needs to make unified decisions in order to avoid splitting by the patient. Consistent personnel or a designated person per shift can help allay a patient's worry about abandonment, which may in turn be manifested as anger or suicidality. Borderline patients often make conflicting demands and may manipulate staff in subtle and less subtle ways (e.g., threatening suicide). The patient needs to have clear limits set, which are agreed upon by all staff. The patient can also be presented with a behavioral contract that delineates what is expected of him during his hospital stay. When he is medically ready, you can assess his need for psychiatric admission.

 CASE CONTINUED

Using the above techniques, the staff is better able to manage the patient, his concerns, rages, and complaints. Staff discussions about his needs decrease their anger and dissent. They remain concerned about his possible self-inflicted cellulitis.

 QUESTIONS

25-1. Which of the following is *true* about this patient?
A. He has a high probability of abstaining from alcohol.
B. He is unlikely to kill himself.
C. He likely has stable long-term relationships.
D. He may be infecting himself to get access to care.
E. Psychoanalysis is the therapy of choice.

25-2. If he is causing his cellulitis to assume the sick role, his diagnosis is
A. Conversion disorder
B. Malingering
C. Factitious disorder
D. Munchausen by proxy
E. Somatization disorder

25-3. Which of the following is *correct* about Munchausen syndrome?

  A. Illness may serve to gratify the person's need for shelter.
  B. Because of a poorly defined sense of self, the sick role may offer a way to avoid legal obligations
  C. Abusive parenting may lead to associating nurturing and pain.
  D. It accounts for 20% of psychiatric consultations to inpatient medical units.
  E. It does not occur in children.

25-4. Which of the following is *true* about the treatment of factitious disorder?

  A. There is no proven treatment.
  B. Antipsychotics are effective in decreasing the service utilization of these patients.
  C. CBT is the treatment of choice.
  D. A team approach is not useful.
  E. Confrontation usually leads to resolution.

ANSWERS

25-1. D. He may be infecting himself to access care, unconsciously seeking psychological comfort. He is likely to relapse, and he may kill himself, either intentionally or inadvertently, or may have disabling sequelae of suicide attempts. Psychoanalysis may be upsetting to patients with identity diffusion and poor boundaries, and may cause borderlines to regress.

25-2. C. Factitious disorder involves intentionally producing symptoms for the sole purpose of assuming the sick role. If there is an incentive (e.g., financial), the diagnosis is malingering. Conversion disorder is marked by symptoms affecting motor or sensory function, not caused by a neurological or medical problem, and not created intentionally. Munchausen by proxy is characterized by someone creating symptoms in another (usually a parent creating illness in a child). Again, there is no financial gain or other incentive. These children have a high mortality rate.

25-3. C. Munchausen syndrome is an eponym for severe factitious disorder. Abusive, inadequate parenting may lead to associating nurturing with pain and feeling deserving of abuse. The prevalence is approximately 1% of psychiatric consultations and 4% of fevers of unknown origin. It is most prevalent in single, unemployed, estranged middle-aged men, and women in their 20s to 40s who have some medical experience (e.g., nursing). Comorbid personality disorders are common. Assuming the sick role has various psychological functions. An illness may get others to provide nurturance. A poorly defined sense of self may lead to feeling more in control in the well-defined role of a patient. Assuming the sick role to avoid legal issues or to obtain shelter would be consistent with malingering, rather than a factitious disorder.

25-4. A. There is no proven treatment for factitious disorder. Medications are not useful in factitious disorder itself. CBT has not been studied. Supportive therapy to address issues in day-to-day life, without colluding in the factitious disorder, may help. Confrontation may lead the patient to flee or act out. A team approach may decrease splitting and foster open discussion of the emotional, ethical, and legal issues associated with taking care of these complex patients.

SUGGESTED READING

Groves J. Taking care of the hateful patient. *N Engl J Med.* 1978 Apr 20;298(16):883–887.

CASE **26**

"This Patient Needs Chemo"

  CC/ID: 56-year-old single man who is refusing chemotherapy. You are called to assess his decision-making capacity.

HPI: This patient has a history of paranoid schizophrenia and was diagnosed with lung cancer 3 weeks ago. It is clear from imaging and bronchoscopic biopsy that he has stage IV adenocarcinoma with metastases to the liver. He is refusing chemotherapy. His oncologist says that he is "completely delusional" and that he frequently talks about the IRS and newscasters communicating with him through the "implants" in his brain.

THOUGHT QUESTIONS

- Does this man have the capacity to decide his treatment?
- What would be important to find out when examining him?

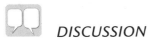 *DISCUSSION*

Capacity is based on the ability to
1. evidence a choice
2. understand the relevant information
3. comprehend risks and benefits
4. explain the rationale behind the decision.

To address the issue of this man's capacity to make this decision, we have to address these issues with him.

CASE CONTINUED

It is a difficult interview, because the patient is easily derailed and starts to talk about the implant the government put in his brain. He says he knows that he has lung cancer and that it has metastasized: "I guess all those cigarettes caught up with me." He says the doctors have told him about chemotherapy, and that there are treatments for the nausea and other side effects, but his chance of being alive in 5 years is almost none. He says, "I don't want to go through all that." His greatest concern is about pain, and he wants to be sure that he is comfortable: "My uncle had lung cancer, so I know what to expect."

PMHx: Noncontributory except lung cancer.

Meds: Risperidone, 3 mg BID; perphenazine, 12 mg BID; benztropine, 1 mg BID

PPHx: As above, over nine hospitalizations for psychosis.

FHx/SHx: Paternal uncle institutionalized; brother is an accountant, married with 2 children. Patient graduated from high school, has very few friends, started college but was hospitalized sophomore year; he returned for one semester but was unable to finish. 80+ pack/year smoking history. No illicit drugs.

VS: BP 140/80, HR 70, RR 12

PE: Noncontributory. *Neuro:* nonfocal.

MSE: *General:* unshaven, sitting in bed, withdrawn with fair eye contact, face slightly masked. *Speech:* normal rate and tone. *Mood:* "Not great." *Affect:* blunted and somewhat dysphoric. *Thought process:* thought blocking. *Thought content/perceptions:* ruminative about the implant. Auditory hallucinations—male voices commenting on his actions. Thought insertion from TV news. Delusions of reference, delusions of newscasters and the FBI channeling "government secrets" through his brain to be picked up by aliens. He denies a desire to hasten his death or commit suicide. *Insight:* into his psychiatric illness, poor.

You review his prognosis with his oncologist and his understanding about his life expectancy is correct. The oncologist believes that it is worth trying to induce some response in the tumor and that it may improve the patient's quality of life.

THOUGHT QUESTION

■ Do you think that this man has capacity to make this decision?

This patient can evidence a choice, and he is able explain the risks and benefits of treatment and why he does not want it. Although people with schizophrenia can have comorbid major depression, in this patient his refusal is not due to suicidality and depression. Though he is psychotic and has poor insight into his psychiatric illness, his psychosis is not impeding his ability to understand the treatment options and prognosis of his cancer. Thus, he has capacity to make this medical decision. The oncologist's opinion about quality of life is based on his own knowledge and beliefs. The patient does not have to agree with his physician to demonstrate capacity.

QUESTIONS

26-1. Which of the following is true about the legal aspects of capacity?
   A. Competence is decided by the court.
   B. Patients only need capacity to refuse treatment.
   C. Competence is decided by a psychiatrist.
   D. Primary care physicians cannot determine capacity.
   E. Competence is a variable function on a 5 point scale.

26-2. In which of the following scenarios could this patient possibly retain capacity?
   A. If he believed that the CIA had implanted and was manipulating the cancer.
   B. If the voices told him to refuse treatment.
   C. If the voices told him God would only accept a pure body with no chemicals.
   D. If he refused treatment because of his prognosis.
   E. If he denied that he had cancer.

26-3. Which of the following scenarios about decisional capacity is false?
   A. A patient with a stroke and aphasia definitely does not have capacity.
   B. Jehovah's Witnesses may refuse all transfusions.
   C. A Christian Scientist can refuse surgery or medication for appendicitis.

   D. A patient may have capacity to agree to a skin biopsy, but not to consent for a CT scan with contrast.
   E. A patient with Alzheimer disease may be able to appoint a healthcare proxy.

26-4. Which of the following patients probably has capacity?
   A. A patient with a severe major depression refuses treatment for a basal cell carcinoma because "it's all hopeless."
   B. A 40-year-old cancer patient who has hypercalcemia, hyponatremia, and a fluctuating mental status says, "No more."
   C. A patient with a 3-year history of bulimia with binging, vomiting, laxative abuse, and a potassium level of 2.1 says she can control her behaviors and doesn't need admission
   D. An 85-year-old woman with mild Alzheimer disease states that she doesn't want any extreme measures should she have a medical emergency.
   E. A 50-year-old woman with schizophrenia believes that the president gave her diabetes and therefore is refusing insulin because diabetes is a gift from the country.

ANSWERS

26-1. A. Competence is a legal determination. The decision is often made using information from a capacity assessment performed by a physician. Psychiatrists are most often called upon to make these determinations, but any physician can perform a capacity assessment. Patients require capacity to make any medical decision, although assessments of capacity are usually only called in the case of treatment refusal.

26-2. D. In all of the other scenarios presented, the psychotic symptoms were directly related to his understanding of his illness or treatment, and would therefore impair his ability to make an informed decision. While capacity assessments are usually called for when patients disagree with medical opinion, such disagreement does not in and of itself determine impaired decision-making capacity.

26-3. A. A patient with a stroke and aphasia may well have capacity to make certain decisions, if he or she can communicate a choice and understanding in some other way. Jehovah's Witnesses may refuse transfusions, and Christian Scientists may refuse surgery or medication if they are adults, despite the possible morbidity or mortality associated with these decisions. Capacity is decision specific. A patient may well have capacity to consent to a low-risk procedure, but not to consent for a CT scan with contrast, because the latter requires a more complex level of reasoning. To consent for the CT, the patients should understand why it was ordered, the risks of contrast, and the possible benefits of the test.

26-4. D. The woman with early Alzheimer disease probably has capacity to make these decisions. Alzheimer patients may not remember that they have filled in a healthcare proxy or signed a DNR, but especially in early disease their choices are usually reproducible and consistent with earlier wishes. The patient with cancer is delirious, and thus has impaired decisional capacity. In the other two cases, the psychiatric illnesses are directly interfering with the ability to make an informed choice.

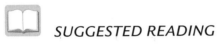 *SUGGESTED READING*

Miller SS, Marin DB. Assessing capacity. *Emerg Med Clin North Am*. 2000;18(2):233–342, viii.

"He Has AIDS. . . ."

CC/ID: 46-year-old homeless male who was admitted to medicine with PCP pneumonia and is beginning to recover. The team is concerned that he is cognitively impaired and depressed and has asked you to consult.

HPI: Mr. J. had been sick for about 2 weeks, thought he had the flu, and came to the ER only because he felt dreadful. He is mostly concerned that his friend Joe is taking good care of his shopping cart and all his belongings. During this admission, Mr. J. was diagnosed with AIDS and hepatitis C and started on medications. Upon inquiry he tells you that he is doing "just fine, thanks very much," though he also reports depressed mood "sometimes" but no anhedonia. He admitted that he has lost "quite a bit" of weight lately but cannot tell how much. His energy and appetite have "not been great . . . but what do you expect?" He denies any other neurovegetative signs or symptoms of depression or mania. He denies any psychotic symptoms or thoughts of harming himself or others. He says that he used to use methamphetamine, about 5 g per day intravenously, but says he gave it up about 2 years ago.

PMHx: He has been seen several times in the ER for dog bites, scabies, and several lacerations that required sutures.

Meds: Ritonavir (RTV) 600 mg bid, Zidovudine (AZT) 300 mg bid, and Lamivudine (3TC) 150 mg twice daily

Allergies: Says he is allergic to Haldol (haloperidol) but cannot tell you what happens to him.

FHx: Noncontributory

SHx: He grew up with six siblings on a farm in the Midwest. After high school, he moved out west wishing to be discovered for a career in the music business. His music career never took off and he was employed at the post office until he lost his job for being "unreliable." He never married and says that he does not have any children "that I know of." He usually panhandles and collects recycling cans and bottles.

Substance
Abuse Hx: He drinks "red liquor" when he has the funds. He denied any recent IVDA but admitted that he used methamphetamine for about 10 years. He tried crack cocaine and heroin but said that "meth" was his drug of choice. He smokes about 15 unfiltered "roll-ups" a day and does not want to give up.

MSE: *General:* Wearing hospital pajamas, appears much older than his stated age. Hair and nails are long and unkempt. There is no evidence of recent track marks on his arms. No abnormal movements are evident. *Speech:* low in volume and slow in rate. *Mood:* "all right." *Affect:* slightly constricted, alternating between dysphoric and neutral. *Thought process:* generally goal-directed, though circumstantial at times. *Thought content:* he expressed some vague paranoid ideations about this "fella who calls himself Gorgeous George" who he says has been threatening him lately, but this does not appear to be of delusional degree. Denied SI/HI hallucinations. *Insight and judgment:* fair. *Cognition:* MMSE scored 23/30, with scores of 3/5 for orientation to time, 1/3 for short-term memory at 5 minutes, and 2/5 for serial 7's.

THOUGHT QUESTIONS

- What do you think is going on with this man?
- What are the psychiatric complications of HIV/AIDS?
- How can you help him?

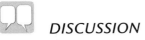

DISCUSSION

Psychiatric patients are at an **increased risk** of developing HIV, and there is reciprocally an increased psychiatric comorbidity in those infected with HIV. Comorbidities include the following:

1. **Depression:** Depressive symptoms may be undertreated in this condition, as they may be interpreted as a "normal reaction" to the illness. The differential diagnosis includes primary depression, grief, delirium, HIV dementia, or secondary to advanced HIV disease. **Antidepressants** have been shown to be safe in this population, but care must be taken with

interactions between them and the newer highly active antiretroviral therapies (HAART). SSRIs, SNRIs (e.g.,venlafaxine), and mirtazapine may be useful but may also be limited by side effects (Table 27-1). Noteworthy is mirtazapine which may stimulate a beneficial weight gain. Buproprion should not be used in those at increased risk of seizures (e.g., those with toxoplasmosis, CMV, or lymphoma). MAOIs and TCAs may have intolerable side effects (e.g., anticholinergic effects such as dry mouth, urinary retention, ileus, and cognitive impairment) and may also cause hypotension so should probably be avoided in advanced HIV disease in which hypotension often occurs. Other agents such as psychostimulants (methylphenidate) and testosterone replacement may improve depressive symptoms. Psychotherapy and bereavement counseling may also help. If depression is severe, then ECT may be considered. This population is at an **increased risk for suicide.**

2. **Mania:** A patient with HIV may have pre-existing bipolar disorder or develop it secondary to HIV, usually late in the course of AIDS. Pre-existing bipolar disorder is a risk factor for HIV, as manic patients often engage in unprotected sexual encounters. Care should be taken to **rule out an underlying infection/neoplasm or medication effect** (e.g., zidovudine) as a cause of manic symptoms in secondary mania. Lithium should probably be avoided in the treatment of secondary mania due to the increased risk of toxicity in this population. Valproic acid should be used cautiously, with frequent liver monitoring, as should carbamazepine, which can lead to agranulocytosis. Lamotrigine, gabapentin, and topiramate have been used off label. Secondary mania in HIV may require the use of high potency antipsychotics (e.g., haloperidol) or atypical antipsychotics.

3. **Anxiety:** Can be caused by various medications or be a symptom of other disorders, such as an adjustment disorder, delirium, or depression. Medications include buspirone (for generalized anxiety), benzodiazepines (use agents with short

TABLE **27-1**   Side Effects of Serotonergic Agents (agonists)

Receptor Subtype	Signs and Symptoms
5-HT$_{2a}$	Anxiety, agitation, insomnia, and sexual dysfunction
5-HT$_{2c}$	Decreased appetite and increased irritability
5-HT$_3$	Headache, nausea, and vomiting

half-lives and for short periods of time to avoid accumulation), low doses of the antidepressant trazodone, or antipsychotics if symptoms are severe.

4. **Psychosis:** First rule out any possible underlying medical or neurological cause. Use antipsychotics to treat but beware of possible drug interactions and increased risk of developing extrapyramidal side effects. Avoid low potency agents. HIV patients may be at increased risk of developing malignant neuroleptic syndrome.

5. **Cognitive disorders:** These include HIV delirium, dementia, and HIV-associated minor cognitive/motor disorder. Antiretroviral medications—zidovudine in particular as it easily crosses the blood-brain barrier—have been shown to improve cognition. Other agents being tried include nimodipine and memantine. Vitamins E, B_6, and B_{12}, antioxidants, and minerals (e.g., zinc) may also help. SSRIs and the MAOI-B selegiline are also under investigation. Delirium can occur at any stage but is more likely with advanced HIV; see list below for possible causes. Work-up may include neuroimaging, lumber puncture, labs, and EEG. Use a high potency antipsychotic (e.g., haloperidol) in low doses to control psychosis or agitation. Remember that patients with HIV are at increased risk of developing extrapyramidal side effects. If needed, short-acting benzodiazepines may be added if agitation is severe.

Differential Diagnosis for Causes of Altered Mental Status in Patients with HIV/AIDS

- Psychiatric disorders
- Substance intoxication or withdrawal
- Medication side effects
- HIV seroconversion
- CNS infection
- HIV dementia
- Opportunistic infections (e.g., bacteria, fungi, viruses, parasites, protozoa)
- Neoplasms (e.g., Burkett lymphoma, Kaposi sarcoma, CNS lymphoma)
- Endocrine (e.g., hypothyroidism, Addison disease)
- Seizures
- Anemia
- Vitamin deficiencies: A, B_6, B_{12}, E

CASE CONTINUED

You decide to try low-dose methylphenidate (Ritalin) in the morning. After a few days, the patient's mood has perked up, and his concentration is better. The social worker on the team has referred him to a shelter with supports for HIV patients and for a long-term specialized housing program. You refer him for outpatient medication management and psychotherapy.

QUESTIONS

27-1. Which of the following medication interactions is correct?
A. Ritonavir may decrease the levels of tricyclic antidepressants (TCAs).
B. Ritonavir may decrease the levels of SSRIs.
C. All protease inhibitors inhibit CYP3A4, thus increasing midazolam levels.
D. All protease inhibitors inhibit CYP3A4, thus decreasing pimozide levels.
E. Ritonavir may inhibit the metabolism of diazepam.

27-2. Which of the following statements accurately describes the interaction between CNS pathology and cognitive impairment in HIV?
A. Plasma HIV RNA levels may predict the development of dementia.
B. Characteristic neuropathology includes attenuation of the deep cerebral white matter.
C. HIV encephalitis is characterized by microglial nodules.
D. HIV leukoencephalopathy is characterized by diffuse myelin loss in the white matter.
E. All of the above are correct.

27-3. Which of the following is a risk factor for suicide in patients with HIV?
A. Loss of autonomy
B. Substance abuse
C. Personality disorders
D. Bereavement
E. All of the above

27-4. Which of the following is correct concerning methamphetamine use?

A. "Crank" is methamphetamine hydrochloride.
B. "Crystal" is methamphetamine sulfate.
C. Amphetamines block the metabolism of catecholamines.
D. Long-term use does not affect production of noradrenaline or dopamine
E. Tolerance does not develop.

ANSWERS

27-1. **C.** All protease inhibitors inhibit CYP3A4, causing decreased metabolism of both midazolam and triazolam. These ultra–short-acting benzodiazepines are contraindicated with protease inhibitors, as they may then accumulate and cause respiratory depression and sedation. Through this inhibition of CYP3A4, protease inhibitors are also contraindicated with pimozide, as the combination may cause increased levels of pimozide and thus an increased risk of arrthymias (QT prolongation). Ritonavir is a protease inhibitor that also inhibits the hepatic isoenzymes CYP2D6, causing an increase in both TCA and SSRI levels which may lead to toxicity. Ritonavir induces CYP2C9, causing a decrease in diazepam levels, possibly precipitating withdrawal symptoms.

27-2. **E.** All of the above are correct. HIV dementia may affect up to 30% of those with HIV. Gross pathology of the HIV dementia brain reveals atrophy, with ventricular enlargement, widened sulci, and attenuation of the deep cerebral white matter. HIV encephalitis is characterized by microglial nodules, which consist of inflammatory cells, macrophages, and microglia. HIV leukoencephalopathy is associated with white matter pallor and diffuse myelin loss.

27-3. **E.** All of the above are correct. Many people with HIV are at high risk for suicide. This may be due to pre-existing or comorbid psychiatric illnesses, substance abuse, and psychosocial difficulties. Other risk factors include bereavement, grief, feelings of guilt or hopelessness, poor social supports, isolation, fears about disease progression, becoming a burden, or a loss of independent functioning.

27-4. **C.** Both amphetamines and cocaine stimulate the release of catecholamines and block their reuptake. However, unlike cocaine, amphetamines also block the metabolism of catecholamines, thus prolonging the length of their intrasynaptic effects. "Crank" is methamphetamine sulfate, and "crystal" is methamphetamine hydrochloride. The initial effects of amphetamine use include elevations of pulse, BP, and respiration, as well as increased energy and decreased appetite. Long-term use of methamphetamine causes a decrease in the body's ability to manufacture catecholamines, leading to continued use of stimulants to achieve homeostatic normalcy. Tolerance develops quickly. Long-term effects include malnutrition, insomnia, hypertension, strokes, cardiac arrthymias, and poor dentition. Overdose leads to convulsions, hyperthermia, stroke, and cardiovascular collapse.

 SUGGESTED READINGS

Robinson MJ, Qaqish RB. Practical psychopharmacology in HIV-1 and acquired immunodeficiency syndrome. *Psychiatr Clin N Am.* 2002;25(1):149–175.

Colibazzi T, Hsu TT, Gilmer WS. Human immunodeficiency virus and depression in primary care: a clinical review. *Prim Care Companion J Clin Psychiatry.* 2006;8(4):201–211.

CASE **28**

"I Should Be Happy"

CC/ID: 29-year-old married woman whom obstetrics has asked you to see.

HPI: Mrs. S. had a normal delivery of a healthy baby 2 days ago. **Staff reports that she has not been sleeping and is irritable** when the team approaches her. She spends most of her time in bed crying and cannot be encouraged to attend to herself or her baby. This is her first child, and she claims that she is **not ready to be a mother.** Her husband was at the delivery and visits regularly, as do family and friends. Mr. S. says that she was a little "down" during the pregnancy, but she and others assumed this was normal. Although she is still experiencing some discomfort, she denies any serious pain or unusual physical symptoms.

PMHx: Appendectomy at age 19.

Meds: None

Allergies: NKDA

PPHx: None

FHx: A cousin has schizophrenia.

SHx: Mrs. S. is one of four children; both her parents are alive and well. She claims to have had a happy childhood and marriage. She works as a paralegal in a major law office downtown. The couple had recently moved into their own home in the suburbs. Prior to her marriage, she had a number of short-term relationships with professional men, two of whom were married at the time. She and her husband have been together for 3 years, and this was a planned pregnancy.

PE: Vitals were stable and WNL, some abdominal swelling and varicose veins.

Labs: CBC, SMA 20, TFTs, and UA all WNL

MSE: *General:* lying in bed, crying intermittently, with poor eye contact and low vocalizations. Poor hygiene. *Mood:* "terrible." *Affect:* constricted, dysphoric. *Thought process:* no formal thought disorder. *Thought content:* she feels a little guilty that she is not happier now that the baby has arrived and expresses concern about her ability to cope with the stresses of motherhood; no delusional material elicited, denies perceptual disturbances. She denies suicidal or homicidal ideations. *Cognitive function:* intact. *Insight:* some insight into her condition, wanting to feel better so she can go home with her new son.

 THOUGHT QUESTIONS

- Do you think Mrs. S. has a major depression?
- Does the history of depressive symptoms during pregnancy concern you?
- What else would you like to know from her family history?

 DISCUSSION

Mrs. S. has **postpartum blues** ("baby blues"), which may occur in 30% to 85% of women. **Crying, irritability, anxiety, rapidly shifting moods (from elation to sadness), and even euphoria at times** characterize the condition. This can be an exceptionally difficult time, as friends and family expect one to be happy. The blues generally appears after the third postpartum day and is a **self-limiting condition** that usually responds to reassurance, support, and some education about the condition. It usually peaks on day 5 and resolves by day 14. It has been associated with a more dramatic fall in serum free estriol levels than in those who do not get the blues. Neither prolactin nor progesterone has been causally implicated. Risk factors include a personal history of depression or PMDD, depressive symptoms during the pregnancy, and concerns about one's career, childcare, and relationships (Table 28-1). A family history of postpartum depression may also increase the risk. It has been estimated that **20% of women with postpartum blues go on to develop major depression within the first year after birth**. While up to 70% of women may experience depressive symptoms during pregnancy, only 10% to 16% meet diagnostic criteria for a major depressive episode during this time (similar to rates in

TABLE **28-1**   Risk Factors for Postpartum Depression
(may be cumulative in effect)

Factors in the mother's history	A personal history of depression (especially postpartum), depression during the pregnancy, family psychiatric history, poor relationship with own mother
Factors in the pregnancy	Unplanned, contemplated termination, previous miscarriage, recent previous stillbirth, illness during the pregnancy (medical or psychiatric), congenital malformations
Psychosocial/Interpersonal factors	Lack of social support from family and friends, mother's unemployment, stressful life events in the previous year (marriage, moving house, death, etc.), concerns about childcare, lack of partner, lifetime history of depression in the partner, marital difficulties

nonpregnant women). Allowing the mother to get sleep can help, as can allowing someone else to care for the baby at night. If insomnia is a significant problem, then careful short-term use of a low-dose benzodiazepine such as lorazepam or clonazepam may be needed. These women should be advised to avoid alcohol.

CASE CONTINUED

The patient and her family are reassured and discharged thereafter. You give her your card and advise them to call if any further problems arise. Six weeks later, you receive a phone call from Mr. S. requesting an appointment. Although she improved after leaving the hospital, it appears that his wife has begun to feel more depressed over the past few days. When you see Mrs. S. at your office, she is complaining of excessive fatigue, insomnia, poor appetite, and episodic feelings of anxiety bordering on panic. Her husband reports that she was initially agitated but now is more depressed. She is finding it difficult to cope and feels isolated.

THOUGHT QUESTIONS

- What is your diagnosis now?
- What treatment would you recommend if any?

Mrs. S. is now suffering from postpartum depression, which is classified in DSM-IV as a depressive disorder with a postpartum onset specifier. **Women often do not complain about their own mood at obstetric or pediatric checkups and physicians should proactively ask about these symptoms.** Postpartum depression is generally moderate to severe in nature, and begins insidiously after the second or third week postpartum (80% within 6 weeks). The prevalence in the community may reach 10% to 15%. Those with significant depression during pregnancy are particularly at risk. The disorder may continue for many months (average 6 to 9). Generally, neither length of pregnancy nor type of delivery has been shown to affect the rate of postpartum psychiatric disorders. No particular etiological causative agent has been identified, but various factors have been investigated, such as estrogen, progesterone, testosterone, corticotrophin-releasing hormone, cortisol, and thyroid hormone. It has been suggested that elevated levels of gonadal steroids in pregnancy may precipitate depression during pregnancy, which is then exacerbated after birth. Investigation of the possible etiological roles of other neurohormones and neurotransmitters is ongoing. Particular care must be taken to check the thyroid functioning of such patients, as they are at increased risk of hypothyroidism in this period. **Treatment is the same as for nonpuerperal depression, and the earlier it is initiated, the better the prognosis.** The Edinburgh Postnatal Depression Scale is a 10-item, self-rated questionnaire that can be used for screening.

QUESTIONS

28-1. Which of the following is correctly matched with its possible teratogenic effect?

A. Lithium	neural tube defects
B. Tricyclic antidepressants	neural tube defects
C. Carbamazepine	craniofacial abnormalities
D. Valproic acid	fetal goiters
E. Benzodiazepines	Ebstein anomaly

28-2. Which of the following is an accurate statement about the clinical manifestations of postpartum depression?
  A. The mother rarely experiences obsessional thoughts about harming herself or the baby.
  B. Irritability and anger are rare.
  C. Rapid weight loss is not a concern.

D. Lack of energy is easily distinguished from that due to normal aspects of caring for a baby.

E. Difficulties bonding with the baby may lead to feelings of guilt and shame which add to the suffering.

28-3. Which of the following psychiatric disorders has been reported to occur in children of mothers with postpartum depression?

A. Autism

B. Asperger syndrome

C. Childhood schizophrenia

D. Conduct disorders

E. Lowe syndrome

28-4. Which of the following is *correct* concerning the treatment of postpartum depression?

A. Antidepressants do not affect the infant in the long term.

B. Women should be encouraged to breast-feed.

C. Certain tricyclic antidepressants may be used.

D. Psychotherapy has no role to play.

E. Prophylactic antidepressants should be started as soon as the next pregnancy begins.

ANSWERS

28-1. C. The risk of neural tube defects (NTD) in those exposed to carbamazepine is 1%. Carbamazepine is also associated with increased risk of developmental delay, craniofacial abnormalities, and finger hypoplasia. Those exposed to valproic acid have a 1% to 2% risk of NTD, as well as an increased risk of intrauterine growth retardation. Neonates may experience withdrawal symptoms from tricyclic antidepressants (TCAs), which can include tachycardia, tachypnea, irritability, hypertonia, and cyanosis. Reviews of several studies of TCAs have reported malformation rates within the normal baseline rate of 2% to 4%. Lithium may cause cardiovascular malformations (Ebstein anomaly, a malformation of the tricuspid valve) if used in the first trimester in approximately 1 in 2000, which is less than previously reported. It is also associated with neonatal toxicity and goiter formation (can be assessed by ultrasound). Information about SSRIs is accumulating, and so far, no increased rates of malformation have been reported. However, higher rates of spontaneous abortion versus controls have been reported for women treated with both TCAs and SSRIs. Benzodiazepines are usually contraindicated during pregnancy except in the treatment of alcohol withdrawal or status epilepticus. The actual effects of benzodiazepines on the fetus remain controversial, with reports of increased risks of facial dysmorphism (cleft lip and palate), GI malformations (pyloric stenosis, inguinal hernias), cardiac and circulation defects, and hemangiomas in the CNS.

28-2. E. Difficulties bonding with the baby may lead to feelings of guilt and shame which add to the suffering. The mother may not talk about these feelings easily. Obsessional thoughts about harming themselves or the baby are common but again are not easily talked about. These thoughts are not usually associated with increased risk of infanticide or suicide, but should be explored to ascertain any delusional content or nature, indicating possible postpartum psychosis. Clinical features may be hard to distinguish from the adjustments to motherhood (e.g., poor sleep, decreased energy) but any significant changes in appetite, weight, insomnia, libido, and energy should cause concern. Rapid weight loss and an inability to taste or enjoy food may be early signs. Significant anxiety, anger, and irritability may complicate the syndrome.

28-3. D. Postpartum psychiatric disorders can interfere with the bonding between mother and infant. Attachment styles that are developed in this period of early life are critical for mood and affect regulation in adulthood, and disruptions can predispose to adult psychopathology. Even feelings of guilt may affect the later development of the child, adding to the mother's anxieties. This may occur even if the mother has recovered from postpartum depression. Conditions reported to be associated with maternal psychiatric illness include aggressive behaviors, conduct disorder, depression, and cognitive deficits. Autism, Asperger syndrome, and childhood schizophrenia were once believed to be caused by maternal parenting styles, but these theories have been debunked. Lowe syndrome is a genetically inherited cause of mental retardation.

28-4. C. Tricyclics are efficacious especially in those with insomnia. Studies have demonstrated the efficacy of standard doses of SSRIs such as fluoxetine (Prozac), sertraline (Zoloft), and SNRIs such as venlafaxine (Effexor). One's choice is guided by prior response and adverse effect profiles. Benzodiazepines, such as clonazepam (Klonopin) and lorazepam (Ativan), may help anxiety. No data suggest that one antidepressant is safer than another. Severe complications in the neonate appear to be rare but long-term effects are not known. If the patient wishes to continue nursing, antidepressants such as nortriptyline or desipramine can be used with careful monitoring. If severe, electroconvulsive therapy

(ECT) may be considered. Psychotherapy has an important role to play in helping the woman adjust to the demands of motherhood, her fears, and concerns about her own identity and perhaps career. Help integrating her into her new community should also be investigated; perhaps a local mother and baby group could help provide support. Risk of recurrence has been reported to be approximately 50%. Women with bipolar disorders have reported relapse risk of 25% to 40%. Women who have a previous history of depression have a 25% risk of developing postpartum depression. Studies have suggested that women with a history of bipolar disorder or puerperal psychosis benefit from prophylactic lithium therapy started at 36 weeks and no later than 48 hours postpartum. Other strategies include psychosocial interventions (education and support) or interpersonal therapy.

SUGGESTED READINGS

Beck CT. Predictors of postpartum depression: an update. *Nurs Res* 2001;50(5):275–285.

Larimore WL, Petrie KA. Drug use during pregnancy and lactation. *Prim Care* 2000;27(1):35–53.

Dennis CL, Stewart DE. Treatment of postpartum depression, part 1: a critical review of biological interventions. *J Clin Psychiatry*. 2004;65(9):1242–1251.

Bloch M, Rotenberg N, Koren D, et al. Risk factors associated with the development of postpartum mood disorders. *J Affective Disorders*. 2005;88:9–18.

"They Are Trying to Poison Me"

CC/ID: 24-year-old African-American woman admitted 2 days ago with an acute asthma attack. Her respiratory function is poor, and she may need ventilation. The patient is refusing this and wants to be discharged from the hospital.

HPI: Ms. J, has been treated with IV fluids, antibiotics, steroids, and nebulized bronchodilators. Today, **she detached herself from the IV** and is clearly quite agitated. These **symptoms started quite suddenly.** Her aunt, who is visiting, says that she has been feeling low for the previous month with poor appetite, low energy, bouts of crying, poor concentration, and disturbed sleep with early morning wakening. She said that she felt worthless and said her asthma is ruining her life.

PMHx: She has had asthma for 4 years. She has been hospitalized three times and has a history of agitation when treated with IV steroids.

Meds: IV methylprednisolone, antibiotics. Nebulized albuterol every 4 hours.

Allergies: NKDA

PPHx: None

FHx: Asthma, hypertension. Her mother had recurrent major depressions.

SHx: Ms. J. is the eldest child of four and was raised by both parents until the age of 10 when they died in a car accident. Living with a relatively irresponsible aunt and uncle, she was forced to care for her younger siblings. Nonetheless, she graduated high school and culinary college and works as a chef in a popular restaurant. She does not smoke or use illicit substances.

VS: Temp 39°C, BP 130/85, HR 90, RR 24

PE: *HEENT:* PERRLA, struggling to breathe and using accessory muscles. Cyanosis in her lips and mucous membranes. *Lungs:* Bilateral wheezes throughout lung fields. *CV:* tachycardia, no murmurs. *Abdomen:* soft, nontender, normal bowel sounds. *Neuro:* no focal abnormalities.

Labs: ABG: severe hypoxia and CO_2 retention; WBC 22,00; HgB 12, platelets normal; SMA7: elevated Glu; BUN/Cr WNL.

Mental status: *General:* restless and constantly fidgeting, fair eye contact but suspicious demeanor. *Speech:* low tone and volume, slow. *Affect:* agitated, anxious. *Mood:* "Fine," but when questioned more describes feelings of irritability. *Thought process:* illogical. *Thought content:* paranoid delusions, thinks the doctors are not real doctors and that they are trying to poison her; denies hallucinations. *Cognition:* oriented to person, but not time or place. *Insight and judgment:* impaired.

THOUGHT QUESTIONS

- What is your differential diagnosis?
- How will you treat her?

DISCUSSION

Differential diagnosis is as follows:

Delirium: Between **10% and 15% of general medical inpatients may be delirious at any given time** and may be missed or misdiagnosed. There are several possible causes for delirium in this patient (see Table 29-1 below for review). She is acutely hypoxic and may have an infective process in her lungs. Causes of delirium are manifold and include drug intoxication, withdrawal, infection, cardiovascular disease, neoplasms, trauma, or various metabolic or endocrine disorders. **Treatment includes attention to the underlying medical causes.** Patients should be nursed in a quiet, well-lit room, with careful attention to vital signs, fluid, and electrolyte imbalances. Agitation may require physical restraints. Low-dose haloperidol, up to several milligrams a day, is the agent of choice. Sedatives, antihistamines, and low potency agents should be avoided, as they may exacerbate symptoms.

TABLE 29-1   Causes of Delirium (nonexhaustive)

Medications	Psychotropics, anticholinergics, anticonvulsants, antiarrthymics, antihypertensives, analgesics (including opioids), and miscellaneous (aminoglycosides, cimetidine, NSAIDS, steroids, and salicylates)
Substance abuse	Intoxication: Hallucinogens (e.g., PCP) and alcohol Withdrawal: Alcohol, hypnotics, and sedatives
Cardiovascular	Arrthymias, congestive heart failure, and myocardial infarctions
Endocrine	Addison disease, Cushing syndrome, diabetes, hyper/hypothyroidism, hypo/hyperparathyroidism, and hypopituitarism
Hematological	Anemia, bleeding diathesis, and polycythemia
Infection	Intracranial: Encephalitis or meningitis (e.g., bacterial, fungal or viral) Systemic: AIDS, influenza, infectious mononucleosis, malaria, pneumonia, septicemia
Neurological	Head injury, Alzheimer disease, seizure disorders, cerebrovascular disease (strokes, arteritis, or hypertensive encephalopathy), MS, and space occupying lesions (abscess, aneurysms, hematomas, and tumors)
Toxins	Carbon monoxide, heavy metals, insecticides, and solvents
Traumatic	Burns, electric shock, and heat injuries

Steroid-induced psychosis: High-dose oral (e.g., prednisone 40 mg/day or its equivalent) or IV pulse therapy may cause confusion, hallucinations, psychosis, seizures, and hemiplegia. Symptoms usually develop within 2 weeks of receiving steroids but may occur at any time during treatment, even during withdrawal. Chronic use of steroids may cause irritability, euphoria, anxiety, or depression. The incidence of psychiatric symptoms ranges from 5% to 50%. Despite newer preparations this incidence does not appear to have changed. Symptoms are dose related.

Steroid-induced mood disorder: This tends to be **manic or hypomanic in presentation,** often with psychotic features, and may recur with steroid use (in particular with pulse therapy) and psychosocial stressors. Ms. J. does not have a history of previous mania or hypomania and does not meet these criteria.

Depression: Depressive symptoms preceded this admission. Her decision to reject treatment may reflect a suicide wish. This possible diagnosis will have to be confirmed with a careful history when the patient has medically improved.

CASE CONTINUED

She is treated with haloperidol and monitored for ill effects. Her respiratory function improved with appropriate medical treatment, and the steroids are tapered and then discontinued. On further questioning, she reveals that she has been very depressed for the past month to 6 weeks. She is started on a course of antidepressants and psychotherapy. She is followed in the outpatient clinic and 2 months later is doing well.

QUESTIONS

29-1. Which of the following is *correct* concerning delirium?
A. Patients are usually oriented to place.
B. It always develops slowly and tends to fluctuate.
C. It is mostly hypoactive in presentation.
D. There is a disturbance of consciousness, impaired attention, or ability to focus.
E. It is a rarely missed diagnosis.

29-2. In delirium, which of the following is *true?*
A. The EEG usually shows increased alpha activity.
B. There is evidence that it is caused by hyperfunctioning of the cholinergic neurons.
C. Impairment usually resolves in a few hours.
D. There may be increased mortality.
E. Thought disorder is rare.

29-3. Which of the following is *accurate* concerning steroid-induced psychosis?
A. It has been reported that men are at increased risk of developing this disorder.
B. Resolution usually occurs rapidly with discontinuation or reduction of the steroids.
C. A history of mood disorder appears to be a risk factor.
D. Lithium may be used prophylactically.
E. Tricyclics are the treatment of choice for depressive symptoms.

29-4. When informing patients about the possible side effects of steroids, which of the following would you warn them about?
A. Hypothyroidism
B. Acne and hirsutism

C. Hypotension
D. Weight loss
E. Diabetes insipidus

ANSWERS

29-1. D. Delirium, by definition, involves a disturbance of consciousness (with impaired attention or ability to focus) or cognitive impairment (orientation, memory, or language). It usually develops over a short period of time and tends to fluctuate during any 24-hour period. There is also evidence that it is caused by an underlying medical condition. Features of delirium include prodromal symptoms of anxiety, irritability, restlessness, and disturbed sleep. The course may fluctuate rapidly with poor attention, distractibility, altered states of arousal, psychomotor agitation or retardation (hyperactive, hypoactive, or mixed presentations), abnormal sleep, affective symptoms (lability with sadness, anger, or euphoria), disorganized thought processes, delusions, and abnormal perceptions. EEG may show diffuse slowing, but in those whose delirium is related to alcohol or benzodiazepine withdrawal, it may show low-voltage fast activity. Treatment is usually with antipsychotics, benzodiazepines, and most importantly, attending to the underlying medical condition.

29-2. D. Delirium is associated with increased mortality (particularly in the elderly) both in the short term and up to several months thereafter. It also may be the harbinger of a developing cognitive disorder in older persons. The EEG usually shows slowing with increased delta and theta activity. Theories about the pathophysiology of delirium include dysfunction of the reticular activating system, hypofunction of the cholinergic system (particularly in the basal forebrain and the pons), and increased GABAergic transmission. It usually resolves within days to a few weeks in most patients. Abnormalities of thinking (content and form) are common, and delusions of persecution may be prominent.

29-3. D. It has been reported that complete recovery from steroid-induced psychosis occurs within 2 weeks in 50% of patients and within 6 weeks in 90%. Women and those individuals with systemic lupus erythematosus appear to be at greater risk of developing steroid-induced psychosis. A history of mood disorder does not appear to be a major risk factor. Steroid-induced psychosis may occur without abnormalities in orientation. Treatment usually consists of tapering or stopping the steroid if possible. Antipsychotics may have to be used should steroids be medically imperative. Lithium prophylaxis has been used successfully in those who have required further treatment with steroids. Tricyclics should be avoided in this patient population as they may worsen symptoms

29-4. B. Steroid-associated complications include psychosis, pseudotumor cerebri, cataracts, glaucoma, hypertension, atherosclerosis, obesity, diabetes mellitus, adrenal-pituitary suppression, hyperlipidemia, delayed growth, loss of potassium, calcium, nitrogen, fluid retention, peptic ulcers, pancreatitis, fatty liver, leucocytosis, neutrophilia, lymphopenia, oral esophageal candidiasis, infection, muscle myopathy, osteoporosis, avascular necrosis, acne, alopecia, hirsutism, skin striae, atrophy, and purpura.

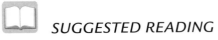 *SUGGESTED READING*

Cole MG. Delirium in elderly patients. *Am J Geriatr Psychiatry.* 2004 Jan-Feb;12(1):7–21.

CASE 30

"He's Uncontrollable"

CC/ID: 49-year-old, divorced white male 2 days post-op emergent appendectomy. You are consulted for help in treating his behavior—"extremely agitated . . . shouting at the staff . . . hallucinating."

HPI: On admission Mr. W, had been complaining of abdominal pain, nausea, vomiting, double vision, and a recent fall. He also reports some difficulties with his memory and is indeed a poor historian. The surgery was uncomplicated. Staff reported that the next day Mr. W. began to get quite anxious with a visible tremor and some dry retching. As the day progressed he became worse; by afternoon, he was picking at the bedclothes and openly responding to internal stimuli.

PMHx: Hx of fractured wrist, pre-op chest X-ray revealed several old rib fractures.

Meds: PRN oxycodone, using less than 20 mg per day.

Allergies: NKDA

PPHx: None known.

FHx: Father died of a stroke at 60, and elderly mother has IDDM.

SHx: Divorced, father of two. He lives alone in a small apartment and works as a welder at a local factory. He admits to taking a drink "now and then." No other details are available. He has smoked one pack per day for 30 years.

VS: Temp 101.5°F, BP 130/90, HR 110, RR 24

PE: *Gen:* thin, diaphoretic male with visible bilateral tremors, Dupuytren contractures, conjugate horizontal nystagmus, and a sixth nerve palsy. Spider nevi, mild gynecomastia, and abdominal distention. *Lungs:* mild expiratory wheezes throughout both lung fields. *CV:* tachycardia, no M/R/G. *Ext:* legs have bruises, decreased pinpoint sensation, and vibration sense. Otherwise, formal neurologic exam was impossible.

Labs: Elevated WBC, MCV 100 μm^3; SMA 20: elevated GGT 80 U/L, AST (SGOT) 50, and ALT (SGPT) 53.

MSE: *General:* appears older than his stated age, poor hygiene, disheveled, uncooperative with interview. *Speech:* mildly pressured with increased volume. *Behavior:* tremulous, agitated, and picking at the bedclothes. *Mood:* "I feel fine . . . it's these vermin that gotta go." *Affect:* fearful, but constricted. *Thought process:* tangential. *Thought content:* Preoccupied with the belief that there are rats in his bedding, suspicious of the medical staff. He says he can see and feel these rats as well as hear the staff say that they are going to "get" him. *Cognitive function:* exam limited, but attention and concentration are impaired. He is disoriented to time and place.

THOUGHT QUESTIONS

- What is your differential diagnosis?
- What other tests or investigations should be ordered?
- How should you treat this man?

DISCUSSION

The history, labs, and physical examination suggest acute **alcohol withdrawal delirium** (delirium tremens, DTs). This can be life threatening and may be seen in up to 5% of alcohol-dependent patients admitted to the hospital (see Figure 30-1). The DTs may present abruptly and unexpectedly during the hospitalization of an unsuspected alcoholic. **Patients may become very agitated, combative, confused, disoriented, and experience hallucinations** (micropsia, Lilliputian) and delusions (often persecutory in nature).

The differential diagnosis of a presentation consistent with the DTs includes intoxication with other substances (stimulants such as amphetamine, cocaine, or PCP), withdrawal from sedatives or hypnotics, overdose of anticholinergic agents, cerebral infections, hypoglycemia, and sepsis. He is also at increased risk of alcohol-induced seizures ("rum fits"). These are generalized tonic-clonic seizures and may be seen in up to one-third of alcoholics within 3 days of abstinence. They are likely to recur should the alcoholic relapse and then stop drinking again. **Focal seizures are uncommon and should raise concern about a focal lesion.** Status epilepticus is a medical emergency and occurs in less than 5% of cases.

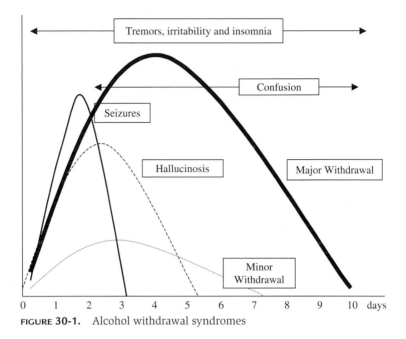

FIGURE 30-1. Alcohol withdrawal syndromes

Other substances that can produce withdrawal effects include narcotics and sedatives. Withdrawal is a symptom of dependence, features of which include three or more of the following in the same year: altered tolerance, evidence of withdrawal symptoms, increasing amounts consumed or used over increasing amounts of time, persistent desire or unsuccessful efforts to cut down or control substance use, large amounts of time spent procuring substance or recovering from its effects, continued use despite knowledge of the possible harm involved, and impairment of social, occupational, or recreational activities.

Wernicke encephalopathy: A triad of **ophthalmoplegia with nystagmus (cranial nerve VI), ataxia, and delirium** (encephalopathy) would suggest this diagnosis. Those with a genetic red cell transketolase deficiency are at higher risk. Intravenous glucose given to alcoholics can seriously deplete their already jeopardized reserve of vitamin B_1 (thiamine); thus thiamine is given prophylactically with glucose to many   patients in emergency settings. Untreated, Wernicke encephalopathy may lead to Korsakoff psychosis.

Delirium due to other medical conditions: Undetected head injury, hepatic encephalopathy, cardiovascular or cerebrovascular disease, seizure disorder, meningitis, or other infections may be present.

Investigations may include serum chemistries (including liver function), a complete blood count, a head CT, B_{12} and folate levels, thyroid function, serum toxicology, and perhaps blood cultures or a lumbar puncture. Alcoholics (in particular those who smoke) are at increased risk of head, neck, and GI cancers and may need a workup.

Screening for Alcohol use: Cage questionaire

- Have you ever considered **C**utting down on your drinking?
- Have you ever been **A**nnoyed by people commenting on your drinking?
- Have you ever felt **G**uilty about your drinking?
- Have you ever needed an **E**ye-opener (a drink first thing in the morning)?

Scores of 3 or more indicate possible alcohol dependence.

CASE CONTINUED

Mr. W. was started on chlordiazepoxide (Librium), 25 mg QID, and this was tapered every other day, stopping after 5 days without ill effect. On day 1, vitamin B_{12} and thiamine (100 mg) were given intramuscularly. Thiamine was then continued orally with folate supplementation when he resumed a normal diet. He was referred to an outpatient alcohol treatment program.

QUESTIONS

30-1. Which of the following is common in Korsakoff psychosis?
A. Retrograde amnesia
B. Impaired procedural memory
C. Patients do not confabulate
D. Reversibility
E. Clouding of consciousness

30-2. Which of the following statements concerning the effects of alcohol is correct?
A. Alcohol inhibits dopamine.
B. Alcohol potentiates NMDA receptor channels.
C. Alcohol inhibits GABA receptors.
D. Alcohol potentiates the effects of serotonin.
E. Alcohol inhibits nicotinic receptors.

30-3. Which of the following is *accurate* regarding alcohol use in the United States?
- A. The rates of alcohol abuse are approximately 15% for males and 3% for females.
- B. The lifetime risk of dependence is approximately 10% for men and 5% for women.
- C. The average American over age 14 consumes approximately 10 gallons of absolute alcohol per year.
- D. The age range of the greatest alcohol intake is the late 20s.
- E. Alcohol problems are encountered in less than 20% of hospitalized patients.

30-4. When treating the DTs, which of the following is a major consideration?
- A. DTs occur in about 50% of alcoholics.
- B. The associated mortality has been estimated to be about 35%.
- C. Complications may include infection or cardiovascular collapse.
- D. The danger period is passed after 2 days.
- E. Abnormal BP and pulse are the only manifestations of sympathetic hyperarousal.

ANSWERS

30-1. A. 50% to 70% of Korsakoff syndrome cases are irreversible. The alcohol-induced syndrome reflects both frontal lobe and diencephalic damage and may include confabulation, profound anterograde and retrograde amnesia, disorientation to time and place, personality changes, lack of insight, and a peripheral neuropathy. However, there is no clouding of consciousness (as seen in Wernicke encephalopathy) or impairment in procedural memory. Approximately 25% may recover fully, and 50% may show partial recovery with thiamine 50–100 mg daily for many months. Both Wernicke encephalopathy and Korsakoff syndrome are classified as alcohol-induced persisting amnestic disorders in DSM-IV-TR.

30-2. D. Alcohol affects a variety of neurotransmitters, neuropeptides, and receptors. Alcohol stimulates the release of dopamine in the nucleus accumbens, which may lead to craving effects. It also enhances the effects of serotonin at the 5-HT_3 receptors as well as nicotinic cholinergic and $GABA_A$ receptor complexes. Alcohol inhibits NMDA receptor channels, an effect which may play a role in the excitotoxic and hyperglutamatergic state of alcohol withdrawal.

30-3. B. The lifetime risk of dependence is approximately 10% for men and up to 5% for women. The rates of alcohol abuse are approximately 5% for males and 10% for females. Up to 30% of patients on general medical and surgical floors may have substance abuse problems, and nearly half of all trauma beds are occupied as a result of alcohol-related accidents. The DSM-IV-TR definition of alcohol abuse is a maladaptive pattern of use that leads to clinically significant impairment or distress as demonstrated by one or more of the following: failure to fulfill important obligations at home, work, or school; use in physically dangerous situations (such as driving); recurrent legal problems relating to alcohol use; and continued use in spite of continual or recurring social and interpersonal problems. These symptoms do not meet the criteria for alcohol dependence. Essentially, abuse refers to behavior and consequences while dependence refers to loss of control over use of the substance. The average American over 14 years old consumes approximately 2 to $2^1/_2$ gallons of absolute alcohol per year. The age range of the greatest alcohol intake is from the mid-teens to the mid-20s.

30-4. C. The DTs may begin within 8 hours after the last drink, peak in 2 to 3 days, and begin to diminish after 4 to 5 days, but they can persist in a mild form for several months. Treatment includes short-acting benzodiazepines such as lorazepam (Ativan) or longer acting agents such as diazepam (Valium) or chlordiazepoxide (Librium). Shorter acting agents should be used if there is any evidence of liver damage to avoid developing hepatic encephalopathy. Additionally, lorazepam, oxazepam (Serax), and temazepam (Restoril) are safest in patients with liver damage as these agents are metabolized solely by glucuronidation and metabolites do not accumulate. Due to the cross-tolerance between alcohol and benzodiazepines, large doses of these medications may have to be used to achieve any sedation. The dose can be tapered by approximately 20% per day until it can be safely stopped. Oral fluids should be encouraged and IV hydration may be needed. The DTs have a mortality rate of approximately 10% to 15%, and care must be taken to prevent dehydration, infection, hyperthermia, cardiovascular collapse, or respiratory depression. Take care to rule out any underlying trauma. The patients should be nursed in a well-lit, uncluttered room, with regular monitoring of vital signs, adequate hydration, and attention to fluid input and output. Signs of sympathetic hyperarousal include sweating, elevated temperature, tachycardia, hypertension, tremor, and mydriasis. Treatment also includes thiamine (initial dose 100 mg given IV or IM followed by daily oral supplementation), folate, and vitamin B_{12}. Seizures may precede the DTs in about 30% of cases and should be treated with IV benzodiazepines. Long-term treatment with anticonvulsants is not required. After recovery from the acute episode, the patient should be assessed for any residual neurological or cognitive deficits and offered appropriate rehabilitation.

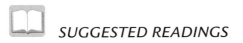

SUGGESTED READINGS

Daeppen JB, Gache P, Landry U, et al. Symptom triggered vs. fixed-schedule doses of benzodiazepine for alcohol withdrawal: a randomized treatment trial. 2002;162(190):1117–1121.

Wright T, Myrick H, Henderson S, et al. Risk factors for delirium tremens: a retrospective chart review. *Am J Addict.* 2006;15(3): 213–219.

Ferguson JA, Suelzer CJ, Eckert GJ, et al. Risk factors for delirium tremens development. *J Gen Intern Med.* 1996; 11(7):410–414.

III

Adult Patients Who Present in the Emergency Room

"I Am Special-God Is Sending Me Messages"

CC/ID: 23-year-old single white female brought to the ER by her worried parents.

HPI: Ms. W's parents report that she has **not slept for three nights.** She states she is too busy "securing world peace." She has spent the past **3 days cleaning her room** and surfing the Internet. Parcels are arriving, including a large telescope, which she says will help her monitor the night sky for "signals" from God. Her parents say she has been talking as if carrying on conversations with someone in her room. She has been **unable to work for 4 days.**

PMHx: None

Meds: None

Allergies: NKDA

PPHx: Depression at aged 19 which responded to psychotherapy.

SHx: She has one older brother. She graduated from art school with honors and was working in an advertising agency up until last week. No history of substance abuse, alcohol, or tobacco.

FHX: An aunt has bipolar disorder, and an uncle has recurrent major depression.

VS: Afebrile, HR 110, RR 20, BP 125/82

PE: Mild exophthalmus; otherwise normal exam.

MSE: *General:* difficult to interview, distractible, but funny with an infectious quality. Appears her stated age, hygiene good, eye contact limited, with psychomotor agitation. *Speech:* pressured, increased volume. *Mood:* "perfect." *Affect:* expansive. *Thought process:* thoughts racing, flight of ideas, intermittently making puns and rhyming words. *Thought content:* preoccupied with religion, feels she has been singled out for special messages. No suicidal or homicidal ideation. Auditory hallucinations + "God's voice in my head." No visual, or somatic hallucinations. *Cognitive function:* alert, but attention and concentration poor. *Insight and judgment:* impaired.

THOUGHT QUESTIONS

- How would you summarize this patient's presentation?
- What is the differential diagnosis?
- What would be important to consider in her history?

DISCUSSION

A combination of a careful history, collateral information, and mental state examination should guide your formulation. This patient's presentation clearly represents a **change from baseline functioning** for this young woman. Although she has had an episode of depression in the past, these current symptoms appear to be new for her. In addition to being markedly psychotic with auditory hallucinations and delusions of control, she has not been sleeping, has been purchasing expensive objects for bizarre reasons, and has been excessively goal directed. These symptoms, combined with functional impairment and telling findings on mental status examination, lead to the differential diagnoses presented below.

The differential diagnoses for this patient include several conditions:

Substance-induced mood disorder: This disorder could result from alcohol withdrawal, illicit drug use (stimulant or hallucinogen intoxication), and antidepressants (in a predisposed individual). While this patient denies abusing substances, it is still important to check a urine toxicology.

Mood disorder due to a general medical condition: Patients with thyrotoxicosis may present with dysphoria, insomnia, anxiety, pressured speech, and agitation. Look for sweating, palpitations, goiter, ophthalmic signs, or changes in weight, bowel habits, or menstrual cycle. Ms. W. is tachycardic with mild exophthalmus. A TSH should be checked. In temporal lobe epilepsy, partial complex seizures may present with disturbances of perception, mood, cognition, or behavior. Auditory or visual hallucinations, paranoia, and delusions have been reported. History and EEG usually confirm the diagnosis. Other medical conditions that may be associated with manic symptoms without evidence of previous bipolarity include systemic lupus erythematosus, rheumatic chorea, multiple sclerosis, Huntington disease, brain tumors, head injury, and infections such as AIDS or syphilis.

Major depression with agitation: These patients may present with insomnia, irritability, or agitation. The history differentiates this from mania. Ms. W. is not depressed.

Schizoaffective disorder: Concurrent affective (depression, mania, or mixed) and schizophrenic symptoms are present. There must be psychotic symptoms for at least 2 weeks without prominent mood symptoms. This patient does not meet these criteria.

Schizophrenia: Manic patients may be psychotic and disorganized. Patients may present with first rank symptoms (Table 31-1). However, an elevated, expansive affect is generally not seen in schizophrenia. Additionally, a period of functional decline precedes the development of frank psychosis. Ms. W. does not meet these criteria.

Mania: This patient presents with persistently elevated mood over the preceding week, insomnia, and increased goal-directed activity. She has inflated self-esteem, grandiosity, pressured speech, disordered thoughts, and has been shopping excessively. These symptoms are interfering with her ability to work and her relationships with others. This is a clear change from her previous behavior. These symptoms have not been caused by any substance, medication or underlying medical condition. Cognition is impaired. On the physical and labs, look for thyroid disease, recent seizure activity, or substance abuse. Inquire discretely about any possible recent sexual

TABLE **31-1**   Schneider's Ranked Symptoms[a]

First rank symptoms	Hearing one's own thoughts out loud, voices discussing or commenting on the patient in the third person, delusions of control (of patient's thoughts, actions, or impulses), thought insertion, and withdrawal, and delusional perceptions
Second rank symptoms	Perplexed affect, mood changes (may be depressed or euphoric), sudden onset of delusions

[a] Though once thought to be specific for schizophrenia, "first rank" psychotic symptoms may be present in different disorders. Up to 30% of patients with acute mania and 20% of those with depression with psychotic features may have first rank symptoms.

indiscretions or high-risk behaviors. It would be important to explore any family history of mood (and, if found, the treatment response) and other medical or psychiatric disorders, as well as previous episodes of depression or hypomania/mania. Look for any recent preceding stressors. Mania can occur as a single episode or may be recurrent. Its presence leads to a diagnosis of bipolar I disorder. Psychosis may be present and may or may not be mood congruent. Mania-congruent delusions include ideas of wealth and special powers. Individuals who are in a mixed episode meet the criteria for a manic episode and a major depressive episode on most days of a week. Specifiers include severity, psychosis, catatonia, and postpartum onset.

Hypomania, seen in bipolar II disorder, is a period of elevated or irritable mood that lasts 4 days but does not cause severe impairment in functioning or require hospitalization. Importantly, the symptoms of bipolar II must represent a clear change from baseline in a given individual. These symptoms must not be caused by any antidepressant treatments. The differential diagnosis for a manic episode includes bipolar disorder types I and II, cyclothymia, and mood disorders caused by either substances or a general medical condition (e.g., temporal lobe epilepsy).

Patients with bipolar disorder have a worse prognosis than those with major depression. As bipolar disorder progresses, the time between episodes may decrease, and the episodes themselves may last longer and sometimes become harder to treat. Additionally, periods of mania and hypomania wane while periods of depression increase. Only 50% to 60% of patients respond to lithium. Fewer and shorter manic episodes, late onset, few suicidal thoughts, and fewer comorbid conditions are associated with a better prognosis. Up to 15% of

TABLE 31-2   Treatments for Bipolar Disorder

Acute mania	Lithium, valproic acid, carbamazepine, chlorpromazine, haloperidol, aripiprazole, olanzapine, risperidone, quetiapine, zisprasidone
Maintenance	Lithium, lamotrigine, aripiprazole, olanzapine; valproic acid and carbamazepine are also used off-label
Depression in bipolar disorder	Fluoxetine-olanzapine combination, lithium, lamotrigine, olanzapine, quetiapine, ECT, transcranial magnetic stimulation (TMS), and light therapy; take care with conventional antidepressants which may cause a switch to mania/hypomania (buproprion is the least likely to do so)
Adjunctive agents	Benzodiazepines used for agitation, anxiety, and insomnia; topiramate used for obesity; gabapentin may be used for chronic pain, anxiety, and insomnia

TABLE 31-3   Side Effects of Mood Stabilizers

Lithium	Weight gain, acne, cognitive dulling
	Fine tremor at therapeutic levels; coarse when toxic
	Renal: pulyuria, polydipsia, nephrogenic diabetes insipidus
	Teratogenicity: Ebstein anomaly
Valproic acid	Weight gain
	Hepatotoxicity
	Pancreatitis
	Thrombocytopenia
	Polycystic ovary syndrome (controversial)
	Cytochrome p450 enzyme inhibition
	Teratogenicity: neural tube defects
Carbamazepine	Hepatotoxicity
	Granulocytopenia
	Cytochrome p450 enzyme induction (including its own metabolism)
	Teratogenicity: neural tube defects
	Hyponatremia
Antipsychotics	Weight gain (most with olanzapine; least with ziprasidone)
	Sedation (most with olanzapine and quetiapine)
	Diabetes mellitus (most likely with olanzapine)
	Long QTc (possibly most likely with ziprasidone)
	Tardive dyskinesia (most likely with typicals at rate of 5% per year)

patients will have four or more distinct episodes within 1 year and manifest rapid cycling bipolar disorder, a variant which may respond better to anticonvulsants than to lithium (Tables 31-2 and 31-3).

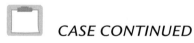

CASE CONTINUED

Labs: WNL; β-hCG negative

Ms. W. has no history of seizures, prior psychosis, or medical problems. She was started on divalproex sodium (Depakote), which was titrated to a blood level of 100 μg/mL. Support and psychoeducation were provided to the patient and her family. After 2 weeks, she was stable and was discharged with followup.

QUESTIONS

31-1. Which of the following is associated with bipolar I disorder?
A. Significantly earlier onset in males than females
B. Higher incidence in socioeconomic group 5

C. Increased risk of suicide
D. Higher incidence of depression in first-degree relatives than in unipolar depression
E. Easily diagnosed in adolescents.

31-2. Which of the following is correct concerning mania?
A. Lithium is the treatment of choice for mixed or dysphoric episodes.
B. If there is no response to a mood stabilizer in 2 days, treatment should be changed.
C. The manic episode may be followed by a moderate to severe depression.
D. It can easily be distinguished from schizophrenia
E. Patients are seldom violent or threatening.

31-3. Which of the following is correct concerning depression in bipolar disorder?
A. If severe with psychosis, preferred treatment strategy is monotherapy with an antipsychotic.
B. ECT is rarely indicated.
C. If severe without psychotic features, it should be treated with an antidepressant alone.
D. Of the antidepressants, buproprion is thought to be least likely to precipitate an episode of mania.
E. These episodes should be treated in the same way as traditional depressive episodes.

31-4. Which of the following is accurate concerning the treatment of bipolar disorders?
A. Untreated depressive episodes may last 3 months.
B. Untreated manic episodes may last 6 months.
C. Treatment of substance abuse is secondary to treatment of the primary bipolar disorder.
D. The main treatment for bipolar disorder is mood stabilizers.
E. Patients taking antipsychotics are not at increased risk of tardive dyskinesia.

ANSWERS

31-1. C. Suicide rates of up to 15% have been reported in both bipolar I and II. Bipolar I disorder has a lifetime prevalence of 0.4 to 0.6%, with equal prevalence among men and women. The mean age of onset is 30 years, but it can appear at any age. Females appear to have earlier age of onset, with predominantly depressive and mixed episodes, whereas mania appears to predominate in males. Mania in adolescents is often misdiagnosed as schizophrenia or even antisocial personality; younger children are frequently diagnosed with ADHD. Family history is an important risk factor; the morbid risk of bipolar disorder in first-degree relatives ranges from 3% to 8% as opposed to the 1% risk in the general population. Higher socioeconomic groups are reported to be at higher risk. Bipolar I patients with mixed episodes and those with the rapid cycling form of the disorder have a worse outcome than those with pure manic or manic and depressive episodes. The course of bipolar I tends to be manifest by an initial presentation of a depressive episode followed, perhaps years later, by a manic episode. However, an episode of either depression or mania may be followed immediately by the other. Overall, there is pattern of cyclic acceleration over time, with a trend toward shorter interepisode phases. There is a high likelihood of relapse in the bipolar disorders, with reported rates of 50% in the first 5 months after stopping lithium treatment, and up to 90% in the first 18 months.

31-2. C. After a manic episode, depression occurs in up to 50% of cases. Dysphoric mania or "mixed mania" is uncommon but is manifest by a combination of dysphoric symptoms and an excited mood. Other symptoms may include irritability, anger, agitation, grandiosity, pressured speech, insomnia, hypersexuality, confusion, and paranoid delusions of persecution. These states may be misdiagnosed as schizoaffective disorder. Mixed episodes occur in approximately 50% of bipolar sufferers during their lifetime, and tend to occur in females who have a dysthymic baseline or depressive temperament. Regarding treatment, mood stabilizers should be given for 1 to 2 weeks at adequate doses before switching. Divalproex is the treatment of choice for mixed episodes. Patients with severe mania may present with first rank symptoms as seen in schizophrenia. Patients with mania may be very labile, switching from euphoria to depression or irritability within a few hours. It has been reported that up to 75% of manic patients may be threatening or assaultive.

31-3. D. Depression in a bipolar patient requires special consideration, and few agents have been systematically tested in this group. An antidepressant may be added to a mood-stabilizing agent. If there is not a good response after an adequate trial, augmentation may be considered with thyroid hormone (25 µg QD) or lithium (target level 0.75 mg/L). Buproprion is the antidepressant thought to be least likely to precipitate mania. Alternatively, an SSRI or a SNRI agent may be tried, usually in conjunction with a mood stabilizer. Once the depression has been effectively treated, tapering and discontinuing the antidepressant should be considered. Psychosis should be treated with an antipsychotic agent—preferably an atypical, which may have antidepressant effects.

31-4. D. The main treatments for bipolar disorder are the mood stabilizers, though benzodiazepines (BZDs) and antipsychotics are usually employed in acute mania and occasionally for maintenance. Antipsychotics can be used in the treatment of nonpsychotic symptoms but are generally recommended for the more acute phase only, in view of possible long-term side effects; patients with a history of mood disorders may be at increased risk of developing tardive dyskinesia. Mood stabilizers include lithium (therapeutic range 0.6–1.2 mEq/L) and some anticonvulsants (e.g., valproic acid or divalproex sodium, carbamazepine, gabapentin, lamotrigine, and topiramate). Monitoring of blood levels helps to minimize toxicity and ensure adherence. In treatment-resistant cases, augmentation with BZDs such as clonazepam may help. ECT is used for highly resistant cases and those who cannot tolerate medication. Patients with bipolar I and II disorders have an increased risk of alcohol or substance abuse, and use even when in the euthymic state is not uncommon. The risks of impulsive behavior, HIV, and suicide become compounded. Psychotherapy has an important role in helping patients come to terms with the illness, increases adherence, and promotes a healthy lifestyle. A strong therapeutic alliance may improve treatment compliance and outcome. Untreated depressed episodes can last 6 to 9 months but when treated are reduced to 3 months. Untreated manic episodes may last 3 months.

SUGGESTED READINGS

Sachs GS, Printz DJ, Kahn DA, et al. The Expert Consensus Guideline Series: Medication Treatment of Bipolar Disorder 2000. *Postgrad Med*. 2000;Spec 1–104.

Culver JL, Arnow BA, Ketter TA. Bipolar disorder: improving diagnosis and optimizing integrated care. *J Clin Psychol.* 2007;63(1):73–92.

CASE 32

"I Feel Awful"

 CC/ID: 25-year-old single white heroin addict who comes to the ER feeling depressed and generally unwell.

HPI: Mr. T. has been using heroin for approximately 5 years, initially nasally, but injecting for the past 2 years. He is having **difficulty sleeping with early morning wakening, weight loss, and poor appetite.** He feels guilty about his drug habit, and wishes to stop. He is not sure if he wants to keep on living like this. He has never been in a drug treatment program. **He has tried to stop himself several times but has experienced intolerable withdrawal symptoms.** He has been using increasing amounts of heroin to achieve its usual effect. His life is focused on his drug use, and he is no longer working.

THOUGHT QUESTION

■ What would be important in his psychiatric or medical history?

There are extremely high lifetime rates of **psychiatric comorbidity in the substance abuse population, with reports of up to 25% of users having independent axis I disorders** and over 33% with axis II disorders. Each of these should be considered in his history. **Important to determine is whether his psychiatric symptoms predated or resulted from his drug use.** Also, dangerousness and psychotic behavior must be assessed. Medical illnesses are also highly prevalent: subcutaneous "skin popping" can lead to abscess and ulcer formation; sharing needles can lead to hepatitis (B and C) and HIV; infections and sclerosis can lead to edema of the extremities; contaminants may lead to pulmonary emboli and pulmonary hypertension; nonsterile procedures can cause septicemia or endocarditis; other serious possible complications include meningitis and brain abscesses.

PMHx: He **has never been tested for HIV;** he has not experienced jaundice, seizures, or neurologic problems.

Meds: None

Allergies: NKDA

PPHx: He denies any past psychiatric history, or suicidal or homicidal attempts.

Substance Abuse Hx: As in HPI. Binges on alcohol a few times per week; no history of DTs, seizures or withdrawal symptoms. Smokes cigarettes, 1½ packs per day. Tried cocaine a few times but never developed a habit.

FHx: His father is an alcoholic. One brother died from cystic fibrosis at age 15.

SHx: He is the oldest of four sons. He graduated high school but never completed junior college. He is currently using two bags of heroin a day. He also admits to drinking alcohol and having bought benzodiazepines on the street. He denied other illicit substance use. He has smoked 30 cigarettes a day since he was 15.

VS: Afebrile, BP 110/70, HR 68, RR 12

PE: *Gen:* thin, tattoo on arm. Track marks and few obvious veins. Otherwise relatively normal exam.

MSE: *General:* appears older than stated age, with poor personal hygiene. Eye contact and rapport fair. Slightly withdrawn. *Speech:* slow with low tone. *Behavior:* mild fidgeting during interview, no abnormal movements. *Affect:* anxious, dysphoric. *Mood:* "down." *Thought process:* logical and goal-directed. *Thought content:* guilty about drug habit and related activities. He admits to having suicidal ideation and has thought about jumping in front of a train. He denies perceptual abnormalities or homicidal ideation. *Cognitive function:* intact. *Insight:* fair.

THOUGHT QUESTIONS

- What investigations would you consider?
- How can he be treated?

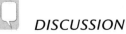

DISCUSSION

Investigations to consider are urinary/serum toxicology to confirm opiates or other substances. A false-positive Utox may be caused by quinine, poppy seeds, and rifampicin. His LFTs may be elevated, and a hepatitis screen may confirm infection. The VDRL may be false-positive (it is a specific but not sensitive test and may be falsely positive from a variety of nonsyphilitic causes). CBC may reveal infection or anemia. Chest X-ray may reveal pulmonary fibrosis. HIV counseling and testing should be offered.

Mr. T. meets the **criteria for opiate dependence.** He exhibits increasing **tolerance, withdrawal** symptoms, unsuccessful attempts to stop using, and reduced occupational activities due to his drug use. He is also dependent on nicotine, and abuses alcohol. Opiate abuse, as opposed to dependence, would imply that he has a maladaptive use of an opioid, which causes significant impairments over a 1-year period of time, but has not met the criteria for dependence.

There are a variety of opioid-induced disorders that may be considered in those who abuse opioids, including opioid-induced psychotic mood (usually mixed symptoms with irritability and depression), anxiety, sleep, and sexual disorders, as well as withdrawal and intoxication disorders.

Epidemiology: The lifetime prevalence is about 1% for heroin use with a 3:1 male to female ratio. Most patients manifest a genetic vulnerability toward substance abuse, perhaps mediated by abnormal opioid or dopaminergic receptors, which may be compounded by environmental psychosocial stressors.

Biology: Opioid dependence may be mediated by the dopaminergic reward system of the ventral tegmental area and its projections to the limbic system and other cortical areas, especially the nucleus accumbens. Opioids may actually decrease cerebral blood flow in certain areas. Opioids also affect other neurotransmitters, apart from dopamine, including acetylcholine, norepinephrine, and serotonin. As opioids depress noradrenergic activity, a compensatory hyperactivity develops, explaining some of the symptoms of opioid withdrawal (e.g., tachycardia, hypertension, tremors, anxiety); along these lines, α_2 agonists (e.g., clonidine) may be palliative. As opioids are analgesic agents, rebound pain is also a prominent component of withdrawal.

Comorbid disorders: Rates of psychiatric disorders are extremely high in opiate abusers, and include mood disorders, anxiety disorders including phobias, alcoholism (up to 30%), and antisocial PD. Lifetime rates of affective disorders are very high. Opiate addicts also have increased rates of physical morbidity and mortality, with overall death rates of approximately 1% per year in the United States. Suicide rates may be over 3 times higher than in the

TABLE 32-1 Review of Common Opioid Recpetors

μ (mu)	Analgesia, constipation, dependence, and respiratory depression
κ (kappa)	Analgesia, diuresis, and impaired consciousness
δ (delta)	Analgesia

general population. Other causes of death include infections and lethal combinations of alcohol and other psychoactive substances. Opioid use (especially intravenous) has been associated with increased rates of hepatitis and HIV/AIDS (from shared needles, unsafe sex, or prostitution), and remains a serious public health concern in cities with high numbers of intravenous drug abusers (Tables 32-1 and 32-2).

TABLE 32-2 Opioid Based Medication

Codeine	Tylenol #3; easily absorbed and converted into morphine. Used as analgesic in mild to moderate pain, and antitussive (for nonproductive coughs). Use with care in renal failure. Can cause seizure and nightmares. Inhibits cytochrome p450 enzyme 2D6.
Diacetylmorphine	Heroin; most commonly abused opioid, with rapid onset of action. Highly addictive. Derived from morphine. Can be injected, smoked, or snorted.
Fentanyl	Duragesic; used as adjunct for anathesia [SL1]or for severe pain (e.g., cancer patients). Transdermal patches (q72 hours) and lozenges available. Elderly may be very sensitive to its effects. May be abused by healthcare professionals. Contraindicated in raised intracranial pressure and severe respiratory disease.
Hydrocodone	Vicodin, Lortab; produced in combination with acetaminophen (e.g., Vicodin) or aspirin (e.g., Damason). May cause sedation. Inhibits cytochrome p450 enzyme 2D6. Preparations with aspirin should be avoided in those with known sensitivity to salicylates or NSAIDs, bleeding disorders, or in children with viral illness (concerns about Reye syndrome).
Meperidine	Demerol; do not give with MAOIs as may cause autonomic instability, seizures, coma, and death. Used for moderate to severe pain. May be abused by health care professionals.

(Continued)

TABLE 32-2   Opioid Based Medication (*continued*)

Methadone	Long half-life. May be used in severe pain and maintenance or detoxification from opioids. Avoid in severe liver disease and asthma. May cause arrhythmias, constipation, respiratory depression, and death (especially in opiate-naïve individuals). Tolerance does not develop to constipation. Inhibits cytochrome P450 enzymes 2D6 and 3A4.
Morphine	MS Contin (other brands available); used in moderate to severe and chronic pain. Use with care in renal failure. GI side effects include dry mouth, nausea, vomiting, and constipation. May cause anaphylactic reaction.
Oxycodone	Oxycontin, Percocet, Percodan; used for moderate to severe pain. May cause anaphylactic reaction. Abuse of extended release formulations is associated with fatal outcomes. Inhibits cytochrome P450 enzyme 2D6. Use with care in respiratory disease.
Pentazocine	Talwin; avoid in patients with liver disease. Used in moderate-severe pain and as an adjunctive in anesthesia. Use with care in those with seizures, head injury, and MIs. Pentazocine is a partial agonist, so will cause withdrawal symptoms in persons on methadone maintenance.

 CASE CONTINUED

In view of his depressive symptoms and suicidal ideations, Mr. T. is admitted to the psychiatric hospital. He is begun on methadone. After a week, his mood and physical symptoms have improved, and he is discharged to the care of a methadone maintenance program and outpatient followup.

 QUESTIONS

32-1. Which of the following is accurate concerning opiate intoxication?
    A. There is usually dysphoric mood.
    B. Cognition is rarely affected.
    C. If severe with anoxia, it may cause pinpoint pupils.
    D. It can be treated with intravenous naloxone.
    E. Hyperthermia is common.

32-2. Which of the following statements is accurate concerning withdrawal from heroin?

A. Symptoms usually develop within 4 hours after the last dose of the drug.
B. Severe withdrawal may include dilated pupils, irritability, and muscle and bone aches.
C. Generally, any severe symptoms will peak at 24 hours after the last dose of drug.
D. It may be followed by severe symptoms for many weeks.
E. It may include constipation.

32-3. Which of the following is ineffective in the treatment of opiate withdrawal?
A. Oral methadone
B. Oral naltrexone
C. Clonidine
D. Buprenorphine, a partial mu-agonist opioid
E. L-alpha-acetyl-methadol (LAAM), a longer acting alternative agent

32-4. Which of the following is true concerning the course and prognosis of opiate dependence?
A. Therapeutic communities have a low dropout rate.
B. Persons do not recover without formal treatment.
C. Methadone maintenance may decrease illicit opioid use and criminal acts.
D. Two out of three persons may relapse within 6 months.
E. It rarely affects neonates.

 ANSWERS

32-1. D. Naloxone is a short-acting opioid antagonist which, when given intravenously, may cause a rapid reversal of intoxication or overdose. Withdrawal symptoms may be precipitated when given at excessive doses or to a patient on chronic opioids. Importantly, as naloxone is short-acting, patients may slip back into a state of overdose as the naloxone wears off but the original opiate (heroin, morphine, methadone) is still present in the body. Opiate intoxification is marked by euphoria, apathy, agitation, retardation, or impaired thinking (e.g., impaired attention, concentration, and memory). Depending on the time course of presentation, opiate overdose is manifest by low blood pressure, cold, clammy skin, and hypothermia. Overdose may cause coma, respiratory depression, pulmonary edema, pinpoint pupils, and cardiac arrhythmias. If a severe overdose with anoxia develops, the blood pressure may fall dramatically, and the pupils may actually dilate. Medical complications of regular use include neurological disorders such as peripheral neuropathies, transverse myelitis, amblyopia, parkinsonian syndromes, and intellectual impairment. Contaminants may cause pulmonary emboli. Infection may lead to septic emboli, staphylococcal pneumonia, bacterial endocarditis, meningitis, or brain abscesses. Other infections may include viral hepatitis, tetanus, or HIV.

32-2. B. Withdrawal symptoms from opiates include diaphoresis, lacrimation, yawning, rhinorrhea, piloerection (going "cold turkey"), muscle cramps, bone aches, dilated pupils, hot and cold flashes, irritability, anxiety, disturbed sleep and nightmares, and drug craving. Other symptoms include abdominal cramps, nausea, vomiting, diarrhea, weight loss, muscle twitches, low-grade fever, hypertension, and tachycardia. With short-acting drugs like heroin or morphine, symptoms may begin within 6 to 8 hours after the last dose. If severe, symptoms generally peak around 48 hours after the last dose but may continue up to 10 days later. Cravings to use may last months or longer. Other abnormalities that may persist for some time include bradycardia, temperature dysregulation, and sleep problems. A protracted abstinence syndrome with poor sleep, bodily concerns, and poor stress tolerance may continue for many weeks.

32-3. B. As maintenance treatment, methadone is the gold standard for treating opioid dependence, and when given in low doses it is perhaps the most effective agent in treating opioid withdrawal. It rarely causes euphoria, depression, or sedation and has a long half-life (>24 hours). It is used most often in starting doses of 10–20 mg orally and up to approximately 40 mg maximum in 24 hours. There may be exceptions to this rule, but care should be taken to avoid toxicity (respiratory depression and death). Should a patient on methadone maintenance present to the hospital, efforts should be made to contact the clinic or outpatient provider to confirm the patient's regular dosage of methadone. L-α-acetyl-methadol (LAAM) is a longer acting alternative agent, given 3 times per week, but there have been recent concerns about possible serious cardiac effects. The α_2-antagonist clonidine may be used (TID or QID) to suppress opioid withdrawal symptoms produced by noradrenergic hyperactivity. Its main side effects include hypotension and sedation. Studies have shown that buprenorphine, a partial μ-agonist opioid, can suppress withdrawal symptoms with retention rates similar to methadone. It can also be used 3 times a week like LAAM. Naltrexone is an opiate antagonist used for preventing the high received with abusing opiates, for treatment of cravings in alcohol dependence, and for treatment of self-mutilatory behaviors in borderline personality disorder. It can precipitate opiate withdrawal.

32-4. C. Methadone may improve the functioning and productivity of opioid-dependent persons. As it significantly reduces the physiological craving for opioids, illicit behaviors are curtailed. It is suitable for once daily dosing, usually in doses of 20–70 mg. Most programs aim for eventual gradual withdrawal from methadone, and studies have reported abstinence rates of up to 40% in previous methadone users 6 years after methadone treatment. Blood levels of methadone may be decreased by barbiturates, rifampicin, phenytoin, carbamazepine, and alcohol. Other agents such as cimetidine may decrease its metabolism. Addicts may stay in therapeutic communities for up to 18 months and may gain benefits from such support, but dropout rates are high, with 50% leaving within 6 months. Persons may indeed recover from opioid dependence without formal treatment. Self-help groups include Narcotics Anonymous (NA), which follows the traditional 12-step model. Pregnant women who abuse opiates have a higher rate of miscarriage and stillbirth, and low-dose methadone may be used during pregnancy. The effects of opiates on neonates are significant: dependence is common, and withdrawal occurs after birth. Further, there are increased rates of maternal-fetal transmission of hepatitis and HIV. Public health interventions include education about the risks of opiate abuse or dependence, free condoms, needle exchanges, and education about the benefits of safe sex.

SUGGESTED READINGS

Sporer KA, Kral AH. Prescription Naloxone: a novel approach to heroin overdose prevention. *Ann Emergency Med.* 2007;49(2):172–177.

Van den Brink W, Haasen C. Evidence-based treatment of opioid-dependent patients. *Can J Psychiatry.* 2006;51(10):635–646.

Warner LA, Kessler RC, Hughes M, et al. Prevalence and correlates of drug abuse and dependence in the United States. Results from the National Comorbidity Study. *Arch Gen Psychiatry.* 1995;52(3):219–229.

"They Are Sucking My Thoughts Out"

CC/ID: 20-year-old student brought to the emergency room by his parents. His parents say he has been acting very strangely over the past few months, and this evening he told them that people are trying to kill him.

HPI: Over the past 6 months Mr. M. has become more withdrawn. Three months ago he stopped attending college classes and has been staying in his room. He has become **verbally aggressive** with his family and has refused to talk about his activities. He has been increasingly irritable, and when his parents have shown concern for his well-being, he has accused them of being "their agents." His personal **grooming has deteriorated,** and he has covered the mirror in his room. He **sleeps 9 hours a night,** and eats full meals, albeit alone in his room.

PMHx: None

PPHx: None

FHx: His mother has hypothyroidism.

SHx: He is the youngest of three sons; the older two are married. His father is a lawyer, and his mother is a kindergarten teacher. He has never had a serious relationship and was a "shy" child who did not have many close friends. He does not smoke or consume alcohol. He has always been religious and has never been in serious trouble.

Labs: Utox negative. TSH WNL. Other labs unremarkable.

MSE: *General:* thin and appears his stated age, with scraggly facial hair. He is wearing several layers of **unmatched clothing.** Eye contact and rapport are poor. Demeanor is both **suspicious** and occasionally **hostile.** *Speech:* almost pressured. *Affect:* irritable, though constricted. *Thought process:* tangential, idiosyncratic and vague thinking patterns, occasionally illogical. *Thought content:* says his thoughts are being "sucked out" of his head **(thought withdrawal).** He has delusions of reference, and admits to hearing the voices of two of his professors talking about him in the third person. He feels these men are trying to harm him with "physics machines" and that they are jealous of him. He denies other perceptual abnormalities, suicidal, or homicidal ideations. *Cognitive function:* intact. *Insight:* none into his condition. *Judgment:* fair regarding voluntarily accompanying his parents to the ER and allowing the interview.

THOUGHT QUESTIONS

- What is your differential diagnosis?
- How may these disorders present?
- How would you treat this young man?

DISCUSSION

There are several differential diagnoses.

Schizoaffective disorder: Depressive, manic, or mixed episodes occur concurrently with active symptoms of schizophrenia. Additionally, delusions or hallucinations must be present for at least 2 weeks without prominent mood symptoms. This patient has not met criteria for major depression or mania, so this is ruled out.

Schizophreniform disorder: The symptoms of schizophrenia (including prodromal ones) are present for at least 1 month but less than 6 months. Patients may eventually develop full-blown schizophrenia or mood disorders. This could be the diagnosis, although he is nearing the 6-month boundary and would then be diagnosed with schizophrenia.

Schizophrenia: The criteria for schizophrenia mandate that two or more of the following are present for a significant portion of the preceding month (or less, if treated):
- Delusions
- Hallucinations
- Disorganized speech
- Negative symptoms (flat affect, alogia [inability to speak], or avolition)
- Grossly disorganized behavior or catatonia

If the delusions are bizarre (i.e., clearly implausible, not understandable, and do not derive from ordinary life experiences; the government's putting crystals into one's blood for surveillance is bizarre, as opposed to one's being targeted by the mafia which is nonbizarre), or if the hallucinations are in the form of a voice making a running commentary on the person's thoughts or actions or two or more voices conversing with each other, then only one of the above symptoms is needed for the diagnosis. There must also be a significant social or occupational disturbance. The overall disturbance should have lasted 6 months, with at least a 1-month period of the symptoms above. Schizoaffective disorder and mood disorder with psychotic features must also be ruled out. As with other psychiatric disorders, substance use or an underlying medical condition should not be the cause of the symptoms. Mr. M. has the paranoid type with delusions and prominent auditory hallucinations. The prognostic and treatment implication of each subtype of schizophrenia remains unclear. See Table 33-1 below for an outline.

TABLE 33-1   Subtypes of Schizophrenia

Paranoid	Tends to be the least severe subtype; personality, affect, and cognition are usually well preserved. Onset may be later than in other subtypes, and the prognosis may be better. There is a preoccupation with delusions, or there are prominent auditory hallucinations. Delusions are usually persecutory or grandiose, but other types may also be expressed. Hallucinations with persecutory or grandiose content may be associated with increased risk of suicide or violence. If multiple delusions are manifest, a theme is usually present. No prominent disorganized behavior, speech, catatonia, or flat or inappropriate affects.
Disorganized	Tends to be the most severe subtype, with a continuous course and few significant periods of remission. Used to be called hebephrenic schizophrenia. Onset is often early and is associated with impaired premorbid personality. Diagnosed when disorganized behavior, speech, and flat or inappropriate affect (often described as silly) are evident. Disorganized behaviors may interfere with the individual's ability to perform activities of daily living. If delusions or hallucinations are present, they tend to be simple and without a clear theme.
Catatonic	Diagnosed whenever prominent catatonic symptoms are evident. ■ Immobility, which may be catalepsy, waxy flexibility ■ Purposeless and excessive motor activity

(Continued)

TABLE 33-1   Subtypes of Schizophrenia (*continued*)

	■ Negativism (motiveless resistance to attempts to be moved or to follow instructions) or mutism ■ Echolalia (repeating words or phrases spoken by another) or echopraxia (repeating actions of another) ■ Posturing, may be bizarre or involve stereotyped or manneristic movements, grimaces, or even automatic obedience
Undifferentiated	Although the main criteria for schizophrenia are met, they do not meet any of the distinct subtypes above.
Residual	To be diagnosed with this subtype there was at least one episode of acute schizophrenic symptoms, but now there are no significant positive symptoms or they exist in attenuated form. If delusions or hallucinations are present they are not prominent nor is there much affect. Negative symptoms are evident and are primary. May progress into complete remission or follow a more chronic course for many years.

The **treatment** of schizophrenia involves a combination of medications and psychosocial interventions. Typical antipsychotics refer to those that decrease or arrest the positive symptoms of psychosis more than the negative ones, and are more likely to cause extrapyramidal symptoms (parkinsonism, dystonia, or akathisia). Atypical agents have actions at both serotonin and dopamine receptors and produce fewer (or no) extrapyramidal symptoms. Animal models are used to distinguish atypicals from typicals, the latter of which cause catalepsy and stereotypical behaviors.

CASE CONTINUED

Management of this patient's schizophrenia consisted of a combination of antipsychotic agents and supportive, educational, and psychosocial interventions. The family was included in the work, which allowed for a more favorable prognosis. Mr. M. was admitted and started on olanzapine, which was titrated to 20 mg QHS. He responded well to medication without any adverse effects, and was discharged home after 6 weeks. He attends outpatient followup, but remains withdrawn and unable to return to school. He was referred for occupational therapy and vocational rehabilitation, and is currently working in a sheltered workshop. His parents benefited from education and support.

QUESTIONS

33-1. Which of the following statements is true about schizophrenia?
   A. It affects approximately 3% of the population.
   B. There are no geographical differences in distribution across the globe.
   C. Women may have an earlier onset than men.
   D. It may involve hypoactivity of limbic dopaminergic systems.
   E. Acute stressful life events may provoke acute episodes or relapses in vulnerable individuals.

33-2. Which of the following is accurate concerning schizophrenia?
   A. The causes are well understood.
   B. Brain imaging may reveal enlarged ventricles and cortical atrophy.
   C. Brain imaging may reveal decreased basal ganglia size.
   D. Monozygotic twins have a 90% concordance rate for this disorder.
   E. There is an increased rate of summer births in people with schizophrenia.

33-3. Which of the following statements is true concerning the prognosis of schizophrenia?
   A. Approximately 55% may achieve moderately good outcomes.
   B. Those who develop symptoms insidiously have a better prognosis.
   C. Suicide attempts may occur in approximately 30%, and about 10% succeed.
   D. Those who are single fare better.
   E. The earlier medication is begun in the initial episode, the more benign the course may be.

33-4. Which of the following is true concerning the treatment of schizophrenia?
   A. Rehabilitation programs are not useful.
   B. Family interventions may reduce rates of relapse.
   C. Clozapine is associated with agranulocytosis in 20% of cases.
   D. Clozapine is associated with seizures in 0.5% of cases.
   E. Augmentation strategies do not include mood stabilizers and antianxiety agents.

ANSWERS

33-1. E. Although the lifetime risk of developing schizophrenia is approximately equal in males and females, the peak age of onset for men is between 15 and 25 years, whereas in women the peak is between 25 and 35 years. Women also have another later peak of onset in their 60s. The incidence and prevalence rates are different across the globe, although the overall prevalence is 1% of the population. Increased rates have been reported in the west of Ireland and the northwestern parts of Sweden. Drugs that increase dopaminergic activity such as amphetamines and levodopa may induce positive symptoms of psychosis very similar to schizophrenia, whereas dopamine antagonists reduce the positive symptoms of schizophrenia. It is theorized that in psychosis, there is too much dopaminergic activity in the mesolimbic projections and too little activity in mesocortical projections. Impaired frontal lobe and executive function has been reported to result from this latter reduction in dopaminergic tone; in fact early descriptions of schizophrenia used the nomenclature "dementia praecox," meaning early dementia. Other neurotransmitter systems which may be involved include serotonergic, noradrenergic, GABAergic, and the glutamatergic NMDA receptors. Medication may help protect against the effects of both acute and chronic stressors. Stressors include life events (losses from the social field) and being in high expressed emotion environments (negative or judgmental comments being made about the patient).

33-2. B. Brain imaging in schizophrenia may reveal enlarged ventricles, cortical atrophy, decreased thalamic volumes, and enlarged basal ganglia, adding evidence to the theory that schizophrenia is a progressive developmental disorder of the brain. However, the actual causes of schizophrenia are not well understood. Although genetics play a role in some cases, other theories include neuroimmunovirologic mechanisms (theories include retroviruses, slow viruses, or maternal influenza) as well as hypoxic damage during gestation or birth (particularly for males). An excess of winter births has been found among patients with schizophrenia. Monozygotic twins have a concordance rate of 40% to 50%. There is a five- to tenfold increased risk of developing schizophrenia in first-degree relatives, even in those who have been adopted away. The risk if both parents are schizophrenic is 40%; one parent leads to an increased risk of 12%; and an aunt or uncle leads to a 3% increased risk compared to the risk of 1% in the general population.

33-3. E. Those who develop symptoms acutely rather than insidiously seem to have a better prognosis. The course of schizophrenia is variable; while some patients have one or more episodes but return to normal functioning, most others follow a more gradually deteriorating course. About 10% to 20% have a "good" outcome, and 50% have a poor prognosis with a chronic relapsing/remitting or deteriorating course. Many of those who are chronically ill may gradually improve in middle age; many also transform from the paranoid type to the residual type. Suicide occurs in approximately 15% of schizophrenic patients; risk factors include educated and previously successful young men, current depression, retaining insight into the illness, and following discharge from the hospital. Better prognosis is associated with the following: being married, having good psychosocial supports, later onset, acute onset with obvious precipitants or stressors, positive symptoms (as opposed to predominantly negative ones), higher premorbid levels of functioning, mood symptoms (particularly depression), and a family history of mood disorders.

33-4. B. Rehabilitation includes social skills training, vocational training, and supervised living arrangements, and is an important focus of treatment. Several studies have reported reduced relapse rates after family interventions (education, support, and advice) on how to deal with difficulties caused by the illness. Agranulocytosis may occur in about 1% to 2% of those treated with clozapine and may be life threatening. Seizures may occur in 3% and are dose related. Other side effects include drooling (sialorrhea), weight gain, constipation, dizziness, tremor, vertigo, visual problems, agitation, nightmares, sedation, diabetes mellitus, and myocarditis. While classic typical antipsychotics primarily block dopamine receptors, newer atypical agents have broader effects antagonizing both dopamine and serotonin. These include olanzapine (Zyprexa), risperidone (Risperdal), quetiapine (Seroquel), and ziprasidone (Geodon). Traditional dopamine antagonists include low potency (e.g., chlorpromazine) and high potency agents (e.g., haloperidol). Low potency agents are less likely to cause extrapyramidal symptoms (EPS), but are more likely to cause hypotension, sedation, and anticholinergic side effects. Depot preparations may be considered for long-term maintenance therapy for those with poor medication compliance or those at high risk of relapse. These agents consist of esterified decanoate preparations of haloperidol (Haldol) or fluphenazine (Prolixin). Those who do not respond to antipsychotics may require augmentation with mood stabilizers, antianxiety agents, or even ECT. Aripirazole is the newest antipsychotic agent. It acts as a partial dopamine agonist, such that if there is excessive dopamine, it binds the receptor preventing dopamine binding and reducing excessive action; when there is too little dopamine, it binds the receptor and exerts a dopamine-like effect.

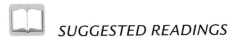

SUGGESTED READINGS

Van Os J, Marcelis M. The ecogenetics of schizophrenia: a review. *Schizophr Bull.* 1998;32 (20):127–135.

Krabbendam L, van Os J. Schizophrenia and urbanicity: a major environmental influence–conditional on genetic risk. *Schizophr Bull.* 2005;31(4):795–799.

Lichtenstein P, Björk C, Hultman CM, et al. Recurrence risks for schizophrenia in a Swedish National Cohort. *Psychological Med.* 2006;36(10):1417–1425.

Sullivan PF, Owen MJ, O'Donovan MC, et al. Genetics. In: Lieberman J, Stroup T, Perkins D, eds. *Textbook of Schizophrenia*. Washington, DC: American Psychiatric Publishing, Inc.; 2006:39–53.

"Mute and Immobile"

CC/ID: Mr. B. is a 17-year-old young man who is brought to the emergency room by ambulance. He is lying on a gurney, mute and immobile.

HPI: He is identified by his driver's license. He remains **absolutely still, with his eyes open,** refusing to say anything. While trying to take his blood pressure, the nurse comments that his arm feels unusual, and remains outstretched in a bizarre manner. He refuses to withdraw the arm, and is **resistant to passive motion.**

VS: Afebrile, BP 170/110, HR 65, RR 12

MSE: Unkempt; clothing is unclean and disheveled. He makes no eye contact and is unresponsive to all questioning. Waxy flexibility and negativism. Exam limited by mutism and lack of cooperation.

THOUGHT QUESTIONS

- What diagnosis are you considering?
- What tests would you like to have performed and why?

DISCUSSION

The differential diagnosis for mute and immobile patients must include both medical and psychiatric causes. Mutism may result from a variety of peripheral muscle and central nervous system lesions. Selective mutism may be seen in adjustment disorders and some personality disorders. **Catatonia is characterized by mutism, stupor, and motor symptoms.** This man exhibits the symptoms of catatonia.

Affective disorders: Catatonic states may occur in mania, a major depressive episode, and mixed episodes of bipolar disorder. It may respond to treatment of the underlying disorder. Contrary to popular belief, catatonia is more commonly found in affective disorders than in schizophrenia.

Schizophrenia: Catatonia can be seen in both acute and chronic cases of schizophrenia. Although Mr. B. may be responding to internal stimuli, we need further information to make this diagnosis.

Catatonia due to a general medical condition: The presence of catatonic signs and an etiologically related medical disorder may diagnose this condition.

Neuroleptic malignant syndrome (NMS): Research has recently shown that catatonia and NMS may be related. Both conditions tend to occur in those with psychiatric histories. Catatonia may be a risk factor for the development of NMS, and both may be related to deficits in dopamine.

Labs and investigations to consider should include the following:
1. CBC: Leukocytosis may indicate NMS or catatonia.
2. SMA 20: Abnormalities of electrolytes, creatine phosphokinase (CPK) in the tens of thousands, elevated LFTs, may indicate NMS or catatonia.
3. Urine and serum toxicology: A screen can rule out illicit substances.
4. CT scan of head: to rule out lesion.
5. Lumbar puncture: Fluid can be tested if a cerebral infection is suspected.

CASE CONTINUED

Mr. B.'s labs and head CT are negative. As organic causes have been ruled out, **he is given intramuscular lorazepam,** and he begins to slowly improve. He reluctantly gives permission to contact his family, who confirm that he left home a week ago after behaving in a bizarre manner for several weeks beforehand. He had become more withdrawn and was refusing to attend high school. He told his parents that the equipment in the radio station was emitting special rays which were affecting his brain. He has no significant medical history or allergies. Apparently, he has not experienced any recent significant stressors.

This patient probably has catatonia due to schizophreniform disorder. The history from his family suggests that he was becoming more withdrawn and paranoid for a few weeks prior to this evaluation. He has not had symptoms for longer than 6 months (which would suggest a diagnosis of schizophrenia), and apparently has had no symptoms of severe major depression or mania. In his continued evaluation, it would be important to assess for mood symptoms. He is hospitalized and treated with a neuroleptic, to which he responds well; he is then discharged home to his family and psychiatric followup.

 QUESTIONS

34-1. Which of the following is correct concerning the treatment of catatonia?
   A. It does not usually include a workup for possible organic causes.
   B. Catatonia rarely responds to ECT.
   C. Agents such as zolpidem and bromocriptine may be useful.
   D. The underlying psychiatric disorder does not influence treatment choice.
   E. Usually responds rapidly to treatment.

34-2. Which of the following is true of catatonia?
   A. Medical causes are usually found easily.
   B. Medical causes are very rarely found.
   C. Neurologic conditions are among the most rarely reported medical causes.
   D. It is not caused by metabolic conditions.
   E. Catatonic excitement is increasingly common.

34-3. Abnormal behaviors seen in catatonia do not include which of the following?
   A. Echolalia
   B. Waxy flexibility
   C. Negativism
   D. Excessive conversation
   E. Agitated excitement

34-4. Which of the following neurotransmitter systems are implicated in the pathophysiology of catatonia?
   A. Dopaminergic
   B. Noradrenergic
   C. Cholinergic
   D. Opioidergic
   E. Vasopressin

ANSWERS

34-1. C. Catatonia related to chronic psychiatric illness may not respond to high-dose benzodiazepines (the usual first line of treatment), and agents such as zolpidem (a GABA agonist) and bromocriptine (antiparkinsonian drug with NMDA antagonist and dopaminergic agonist properties) have been used with documented success in some cases. Treatment of the catatonic patient must include a workup for possible organic causes. Excited catatonia may require tranquilization and close monitoring. Catatonia may respond to ECT, particularly if it is associated with a mood disorder. Underlying psychiatric conditions should also be treated with appropriate medications.

34-2. D. In catatonic excitement, the patient may be extremely restless, agitated, disorganized, and hyperactive. This excess activity is not influenced by external stimuli and is apparently purposeless. This condition is seen less often since the development of antipsychotic medications. Waxy flexibility and bizarre behaviors (mannerisms) are also reported less often than in the past. The most common cause of catatonia is affective disorders with schizophrenia a close second, but it can occur in some medical illnesses. It can be extremely difficult to differentiate between medical and psychiatric causes based solely on symptoms. Catatonia from a medical etiology often occurs in those with psychiatric and medical risk factors: metabolic/toxic or drug-induced conditions (PCP, ketamine, etc.) are common causes, but neurological conditions are the most commonly reported medical cause and include degenerative, cerebrovascular, post-traumatic, and neoplastic lesions, seizure disorders, encephalitis, typhoid delirium, neurosyphilis, CNS infections, Wernicke's encephalopathy, multiple sclerosis, and SLE.

34-3. D. Catatonia covers a broad group of movement disorders usually seen in both psychotic conditions, and affective disorders. Motor abnormalities may include catalepsy (an immobile position constantly held), akinesia, stupor, rigidity, negativism (motiveless resistance to any instruction or attempt to move), posturing (voluntarily maintaining an unusual or bizarre position for extended periods of time), and waxy flexibility (partial passive resistance to movement, which may give way in a wax-like fashion, in combination with an ability to maintain the limb extended or in an unusual posture). Stereotypic movements may also occur; these are repetitive patterns of speech or behavior. Echolalia (repeating words or phrases) or echopraxia (copying movements of others) may also occur. In catatonic stupor, the patient is motionless and mute. There may be intermittent impulsive acts.

34-4. A. The dopaminergic system may be implicated. The treatment of choice is usually high dose benzodiazepines, implicating an abnormality of the GABAergic system, particularly the GABA$_A$ receptors. However, a few patients manifest paradoxical agitated reactions to lorazepam. Glutamate is implicated by the response of some patients to amantadine, an NMDA antagonist; however, amantadine is also a dopaminergic agonist, as is bromocriptine. There is no evidence that the cholinergic, opioidergic, or vasopressin systems play a role in the development of catatonia. The role of serotonin still needs clarification, but it may be associated via disequilibria of its receptor systems.

SUGGESTED READINGS

Carroll BT, Kennedy JC, Goforth HW. Catatonic signs in medical and psychiatric catatonias. *CNS Spectrums.* 2000;5(7):58–65.
Ungvari GS, Kau LS, Wai-Kwong T, et al. The pharmacological treatment of catatonia: an overview. *Eur Arch Psychiatry Clin Neurosci.* 2001;252(Suppl 1):31–34.

"Who Am I?"

CC/ID: 56-year-old man who comes into the ER after cutting his hand on some glass. Psychiatry is called after the triage nurse tries to take his demographic information, and he says, "I honestly don't know" to most questions.

HPI: D. D. states that about 3 months ago he **found himself in this town and couldn't remember his name.** When he passed a garage, he realized he knew how to fix cars, and began to work there in exchange for a room above the shop. He has been calling himself David Drier because on the floor of the shop there was an ad for Dave's Laundromat. He says that he has no memory of his name, his occupation, his marital status, or other details. He does have a clear memory of the 3 months since he started working at the garage. He reports that his **mood, sleep, energy, appetite, and concentration are all good.** He **denies any auditory or visual hallucinations,** or any paranoid ideations or delusions. He cannot explain why he hasn't sought help for his memory loss.

PMHx: Unknown

PPHx: Unknown

SHx/FHx: Unknown

THOUGHT QUESTIONS

- What is the differential diagnosis?
- What would be important in the workup?

DISCUSSION

He has complete **amnesia for personal details** starting 3 months ago. His **procedural memory is intact—he knows how to read, write, and fix cars.** Amnesia may be due to many "organic" causes, such as head trauma, other neurologic insults, complex partial seizures, dementia, substance-induced blackouts, uremia, benzodiazepines, or hallucinogens. "Organic" amnesia usually encompasses more than just personal history; it usually involves both memory and new learning. Malingering, dissociative amnesia, dissociative fugue, and dissociative identity disorder are in the psychiatric differential diagnosis.

 CASE CONTINUED

VS: BP 130/75, HR 60

PE: Exam unremarkable. *Gen:* no stigmata of chronic alcohol or other substance use. *Neuro:* nonfocal.

Mental status: *General:* well-related, appropriately dressed and groomed, bandage on left hand. Calm and cooperative demeanor. *Speech:* normal rate and tone. *Affect:* reactive, full range, neutral and with enigmatic appearance when questioned about personal information. *Thought process:* goal-directed, logical. *Thought content:* no suicidal or homicidal ideation, no psychotic symptoms.

D.D. was admitted to the hospital for a complete workup, and he gave the police permission to circulate his photograph. The workup, including EEG, neuroimaging, electrolytes, renal and hepatic functions, CBC, and urine toxicology, was unremarkable. Within a few days, the police from a town in a neighboring state responded that he resembled a businessman who had been missing for over 3 months. His wife was contacted, and she explained that they were in the process of a divorce, that he had recently been "downsized," and that he had lost a great deal of money in a risky business venture. One day he was supposed to appear at the lawyers' office, but he did not show up. His car was found at a train station. He had no significant past medical or psychiatric history. Upon seeing his wife, his memory of the past returned, and he could no longer remember the past 3 months. He said that when he was in college he may have "lost a weekend" after a stressful breakup with a girlfriend, but he did not have multiple periods of time that couldn't be accounted for. He denied symptoms of depersonalization (an altered experience of the self where one may feel unreal or detached from one's body), derealization (in which the external world seems different, unreal, distant, or disconnected), identity disturbance (e.g., having an inconsistent sense of self), substance use, or symptoms of another axis I or II disorder. He had worked in a garage in high school, fixing antique cars (Table 35-1).

TABLE 35-1   Table Reviewing Dissociative Disorders

Dissociative symptoms are manifest by a disruption in the usually integrated functions of

◼ Consciousness
◼ Memory
◼ Identity
◼ Perception of the environment

All the disorders below meet these criteria. **There is no evidence of a physical disorder or substance abuse that could explain the symptoms of any of these disorders. They are not better explained by another axis I disorder.** There is evidence of a temporal relation between **stressors/life events and the onset** of symptoms of these disorders. The symptoms cause significant impairment in functioning.

Dissociative amnesia	Amnesia (partial or complete) for recent traumatic or stressful events. Not explained by normal forgetting and may vary in detail at different examinations. Not due to PTSD, fugue, stress, somatization disorder, substances, or a medical condition. It is the most common dissociative disorder. Females > males and younger > older.
Dissociative fugue	An individual makes a sudden and unexpected move or trip away from his or her usual home or place of work. During this time, he or she maintains adequate self-care. Personal identity as well as the travel itself may be forgotten, and a new identity may be established. Prevalence of 0.2% in the general population. Persons with schizoid, borderline, and histrionic PDs may be at increased risk of developing the disorder.
Dissociative identity disorder	At least two or more distinct personalities that take over an individual's behavior in a recurring pattern. Difficulty remembering personal information is not due to forgetfulness. Chronic condition, usually with a history of trauma (often physical or sexual abuse in childhood). Studies report prevalence of up to 3% in psychiatric admissions. Females > males. Onset late adolescence or young adult. Can be difficult to differentiate from borderline PD; high rate of comorbid psychiatric disorders and suicide attempts.
Depersonalization disorder	Continuing or recurrent feelings of being detached from one's body; reality testing, however, remains intact. The person just feels disconnected as if he or she is walking/talking/functioning as an automaton. Does not happen during another axis I disorder (e.g.. panic disorder), nor is it caused by an underlying medical condition (e.g., epilepsy). As an isolated symptom (i.e., not recurrent or continuing), depersonalization may occur in normal individuals, especially under stress, and is commonly found in anxiety disorders and depression.

(Continued)

TABLE 35-1   Table Reviewing Dissociative Disorders (*continued*)

Dissociative disorder not otherwise specified (NOS)	Includes dissociative states that do not meet the criteria outlined above.
	Specifically, states in which the predominant feature is a dissociative symptom (i.e., a disruption in the usually integrated functions of consciousness, memory, identity, or perception of the environment) that does not meet the criteria for any specific dissociative disorder.
	■ Dissociative experiences not fulfilling criteria for an independent disorder are commonly experienced by psychiatric patients.
	■ Derealization without depersonalization.
	■ Dissociative trance disorder: An individual in a trance state is in an altered state of consciousness with diminished responses to environmental stimuli. There may be uncontrollable stereotyped behaviors. Alternatively a possession trance may occur where an individual's normal identity is temporarily replaced by a new identity. It must not fit the pattern of a usual cultural or religious practice.

Adapted from American Psychiatric Association. *Task Force on DSM-IV. Diagnostic and statistical manual of mental disorders: DSM-IV.* 4th ed. Washington, DC: American Psychiatric Association, 1994.

QUESTIONS

35-1. What is the most likely diagnosis for this patient?
A. Dissociative amnesia
B. Dissociative fugue
C. Dissociative identity disorder
D. Displaced identity disorder
E. Amnestic fugue

35-2. What techniques are *not* used in the treatment of this disorder?
A. Hypnosis
B. Sodium amobarbital interview
C. Systematic desensitization
D. Psychodynamic psychotherapy
E. Supportive psychotherapy

35-3. The epidemiology and course of this disorder includes which of the following:
A. People do not have recurrent episodes.
B. The prevalence is 10%.

   C. Spontaneous recovery is rare.
   D. It is not associated with childhood abuse or neglect.
   E. It usually happens in adulthood.

35-4. Which of the following is true about dissociative disorders?
   A. People with dissociative fugue always remember the time of their fugue when they return to their "normal" lives.
   B. Fugues typically last months.
   C. During a fugue a person will appear "weird" on casual inspection.
   D. Dissociative identity disorder probably accounts for most fugue states.
   E. Dissociative identity disorder is associated with a minimum of five "alternate" personalities.

ANSWERS

35-1. B. Dissociative fugue is the most likely diagnosis. Dissociative fugue involves one or more episodes of sudden, unexpected, purposeful travel away from home, coupled with an inability to recall portions or all of one's past and a loss of identity or the assumption of a new identity. The onset is usually sudden, and it frequently occurs after a severe stressor. Dissociative amnesia is defined as an inability to remember important personal information, usually of a traumatic nature, that is too extensive to be explained by forgetfulness and is not caused by a medical condition or substance use. An example would be forgetting the period of time surrounding a rape or a car accident. Dissociative identity disorder used to be called multiple personality disorder and is defined by the presence of distinct enduring personality states that control the person's behavior; in this illness each independent state of consciousness may manifest a different resting heart rate, a different blood pressure, and other idiosyncratic physiological parameters. Of note, this disorder may be associated with multiple fugues, as identities are usually not aware of the actions of other identities. Displaced identity disorder does not exist.

35-2. C. Systematic desensitization is usually used in the treatment of phobias, and consists of a progressive exposure to increasingly anxiety-provoking stimuli with the goal of erasing the phobic response (extinction, habituation). Hypnosis and the sodium amobarbital interview have been used in the evaluation of these patients and can help clarify the differential diagnosis. Essentially, hypnosis is a dissociated state marked by a narrowing of the field of consciousness. A possible mechanism by which the amobarbital interview is thought to function is by reducing levels of anxiety which are thought to produce the dissociated state in the first place; with the accompanying reduction in stress, the abnormal dissociative symptoms may briefly wane. The treatment of choice is usually psychodynamic psychotherapy or supportive psychotherapy, with an eye to the fact that there may have been a significant trauma that precipitated the fugue, which should be handled carefully.

35-3. E. Spontaneous remission of symptoms often occurs without treatment, and may last from a few hours to months. People may have recurrent fugues; one study suggests that 65% of people with fugues had experienced another. The prevalence is <0.3%. It may be associated with childhood abuse or neglect, and is usually first reported in adulthood.

35-4. D. Typically dissociative fugues last from a few days to a few weeks. During a fugue, a person usually does not appear confused or bizarre. People with dissociative fugue often have amnesia for the fugue state. Dissociative identity disorder does appear to be more prevalent than previously thought, and (as described in the answer to question 62) probably accounts for most fugue states. Interestingly, patients with dissociative identity disorder commonly may present with symptoms akin to the first rank symptoms of schizophrenia.

SUGGESTED READINGS

Simeon D, Guralnik O, Hazlett EA, et al. Feeling unreal: a PET study of depersonalization disorder. *Am J Psychiatry*. 2000;157(11): 1782–1788.

Simeon D, Guralnik O, Knutelska M, et al. Personality factors associated with dissociation: temperament, defenses, and cognitive schemata. *Am J Psychiatry*. 2002;159(3):489–491.

Simeon D, Guralnik O, Schmeidler J, et al. The role of childhood interpersonal trauma in depersonalization disorder. *Am J Psychiatry*. 2001;158(7):1027–1033.

CASE **36**

"Go Away! . . . Come Back!"

 CC/ID: 24-year-old single woman in the ER who has overdosed on "sleeping pills."

HPI: A.A. had been at a bar with her boyfriend. After she consumed about three bottles of beer, they had a fight, and she stormed out. She describes experiencing the **abrupt onset of "depression" while walking home, which led her to buy a bottle of sleeping pills and take a handful.** She then went to his house and waited for him to come home before telling him what she had done. He called EMS. Currently, she denies depressed mood or neurovegetative changes. She then says, **"I'm sick of talking to interns, I'll only talk to a real doctor,"** and she refuses to continue the interview.

PMHx: None

Meds: unknown, 1/2 bottle of diphenhydramine in bag.

VS: WNL

PE: *Gen:* WDWN, sedated. WNL except *Ext:* multiple superficial healed lacerations on left arm and both thighs.

MSE: *General:* eye contact fair, alcohol on breath, two visible tattoos on arm. Intermittently cooperative with interview. *Speech:* slurred. *Mood:* "crap." *Affect:* reactive, angry at times. *Thought process:* goal-directed. *Thought content:* no delusions, no hallucinations. "I don't think I want to die."

THOUGHT QUESTIONS

- What labs would you ensure she had?
- Would you hospitalize her?

DISCUSSION

Though she stated she had taken only sleeping pills, it is important to check urine and serum toxicology to look for other substances. She is intoxicated and won't disclose her alcohol history, so her vital signs should be closely monitored for alcohol withdrawal. She has just tried to kill herself, will not engage in a discussion, and thus requires admission.

CASE CONTINUED

Labs: WNL; serum, Utox negative; blood ethanol 250

You secure an inpatient psychiatric bed for her once she is medically cleared. In the morning, you complete her history. She has had no signs of withdrawal.

Meds: Outpatient: venlafaxine, clonazepam, valproate

PPHx: Describes **feeling depressed and empty her whole life**; never really feeling like herself. Two suicide attempts since college—one after a fight with a lover, one during a therapist's vacation. She **changes therapists frequently.** Her medication trials have included lorazepam, gabapentin, valproic acid, fluoxetine, and risperidone. She has binge alcohol use since age 14. She has "broken a few things" while drinking, including a car, which she smashed into a tree. Currently "gets wasted" about 3 times a month. She does not drink daily. **She went through "a bulimic phase"** and had group therapy with someone who cut herself instead of binging. She found if she felt empty, she could cut her arms or thighs, and feel better. No history of mania.

SHx: **Father was an alcoholic and left when she was 2 years old. Mother was hospitalized when the patient was 4 for a suicide attempt, and had many live-in boyfriends, two of whom sexually abused the patient at ages 6 and 11.** The patient finished college 2 years ago, and has had multiple jobs as a political canvasser, research assistant, advertising intern, sales clerk, and bartender. They "haven't worked out" because she found it hard to get along with her colleagues. At the end of the interview, she says, **"You're the best doctor; much better than Dr. [outpatient]. Can I come see you instead?"**

THOUGHT QUESTIONS

- What is in the differential diagnosis?
- What is the most likely diagnosis?
- How do you understand her reactions to you?

DISCUSSION

The differential includes major depressive disorder (MDD), dysthymia, bipolar disorder, cyclothymia, substance-use disorder, and substance-induced mood disorder. **All share symptoms with borderline personality disorder (BPD) (e.g., impulsivity in mania and suicidality in MDD).** Other personality disorders also have symptoms that overlap, though she does not meet criteria for any of these. **Unstable relationships, frantic attempts to avoid abandonment, identity disturbances, and alternation between idealization and devaluation** help make the diagnosis. (See Table 36-1 below for diagnostic criteria). Borderline patients are at risk for MDD, substance use, eating disorders, and PTSD. She previously had bulimia, and now has alcohol abuse.

Various theories regarding the pathogenesis of personality disorders can be found. Psychoanalytic theories describe a borderline personality as characterized by ego weakness (lack of impulse control, anxiety intolerance, blurred boundaries for self or others, occasionally distorted reality testing), **problematic object relations (seeing**

TABLE **36-1**   Criteria for BPD

Frantic efforts to avoid abandonment
A pattern of unstable and intense interpersonal relationships (idealization, devaluation)
Unstable self-image or sense of self
Marked impulsivity, which is potentially self-damaging (e.g., sex, spending, substance abuse, binge eating, etc.)
Recurrent suicidal or parasuicidal behavior (e.g., self-mutilating behaviors)
Affective instability, intense mood shifts (e.g., dysphoria, anxiety, irritability)
Chronic feelings of emptiness
Inappropriate, intense anger
Transient stress-related paranoia or severe dissociative symptoms

people as all good or all bad), a fragmented self-concept, and **immature defenses (e.g., splitting)**. Each of these is seen in normal development, but in PDs they persist into adulthood; essentially, the patient has not successfully completed various developmental stages or emotional milestones. Psychobiological theories present personality as an interaction of temperament (with a strong genetic component) with character (formed by family and environment). Thus, a person who is impulsive and novelty-seeking could be goalless, undisciplined, uncooperative, and have a PD, or be self-directed and cooperative, and become an entrepreneur. Maturation increases self-directedness and cooperation, leading to a decline in impulsivity and acting out with age; borderline patients tend to "burn out."

Her reaction to you is an example of classic behavior in BPD: she first sees you as all bad (devaluation) and then as all good (idealization). **Patients with BPD have difficulty maintaining a steady internal image of people in their environments.** Combined with impulsivity, this feature makes for their profound disruptive behavior on psychiatric units.

 QUESTIONS

36-1. Which is a diagnostic symptom of BPD?
   A. Auditory hallucinations
   B. Anhedonia
   C. Recurrent self-mutilatory behavior
   D. Pressured speech
   E. Inappropriately sexually seductive or provocative behavior

36-2. Which of the following is true about this illness?
   A. BPD is seen in 10% to 12% of the population.
   B. First-degree relatives have no increased risk of BPD.
   C. The mortality rate is >25%.
   D. The M/F ratio is 1:1.
   E. The greatest instability and impulsivity is in early adulthood.

36-3. Which is true concerning the psychobiology of BPD?
   A. Medications are not appropriate for treating the symptoms of BPD.
   B. Impulsive aggression is linked to serotonin.
   C. Antipsychotics are not used for the transient psychotic symptoms.

    D. Acetylcholine mediates cognitive distortions in BPD.

    E. Comorbid axis I disorders should be treated only with psychotherapy as this is a personality disorder.

36-4. Which is *not* recommended in the psychological treatment of BPD?

    A. Dynamic psychotherapy

    B. Behavior therapy

    C. Dialectical behavioral therapy

    D. Classic psychoanalysis

    E. Cognitive behavioral therapy

ANSWERS

36-1. C. BPD is a pervasive pattern from early adulthood of unstable relationships, self-image, and affect, with marked impulsivity. There must be ≥5 of the following: (i) frantic efforts to avoid abandonment, (ii) relationships that swing from idealizing to devaluing, (iii) unstable self-image, (iv) possibly dangerous impulsivity (e.g., sex, substance abuse, bingeing), (v) recurrent suicidal or self-mutilatory behavior, (vi) marked affective instability, (vii) chronic feelings of emptiness, (viii) inappropriate intense anger, and (ix) stress-related paranoia or dissociative symptoms. While inappropriately seductive or provocative behavior may be manifest in a patient with BPD, it is not a core feature of the disorder. These patients may manifest auditory hallucinations (in so-called "micropsychotic episodes"), but their presence tends to be more transient and stress related than it is in psychotic disorders.

36-2. E. The greatest instability and impulsivity in BPD is seen in early adulthood, often improving in the 30s and 40s. The mortality is closer to 10%. From 2% to 3% of the population has BPD. The M/F ratio is 1:3. It is five times more common in first-degree relatives than in the general population.

36-3. B. Acetylcholine is a neurotransmitter that is affected in Alzheimer's disease and is involved in memory. It is not implicated in cognitive distortions in BPD. Comorbid axis I disorders are common and should be treated, and medications are an appropriate part of that treatment. Medications may also address aggression/impulsivity, affective symptoms/mood dysregulation, anxiety, and cognitive/perceptual disturbances; for example, impulsive aggression is associated with low CSF 5-hydroxyindole acetic acid (5-HIAA, a serotonin metabolite). With medications and psychotherapy, the cycle of maladaptive behaviors may be broken. For example, patients with BPD may have transient psychotic symptoms in response to a stressor, fostering avoidance. By using an antipsychotic, the patient may be able to confront and integrate the stressor, breaking a maladaptive pattern.

36-4. D. Dynamic psychotherapy sees symptoms as external manifestations of internal conflicts. Behavior therapy finds ways to control symptom manifestations. Cognitive therapy addresses distorted cognitions, and helps reframe and understand cues (environment, thoughts, and emotions). Dialectical behavioral therapy is based on helping patients control emotional dysregulation—finding ways to self-soothe, instead of self-mutilate. These may be used together to mature and develop a patient's character by helping him or her to change responses to and understanding of internal and external cues. Classic psychoanalysis requires better ego function and boundaries (what is internal and felt or thought vs. what is external and perceived) than are seen in BPD.

SUGGESTED READINGS

Rinne T, van den Brink W, Wouters L, et al. SSRI treatment of borderline personality disorder: a randomized, placebo-controlled clinical trial for female patients with borderline personality disorder. *Am J Psychiatry*. 2002;159(12):2048–2054.

Golier JA, Yehuda R, Bierer LM, et al. The relationship of borderline personality disorder to posttraumatic stress disorder and traumatic events. *Am J Psychiatry*. 2003;160(11):2018–2024.

Lieb K, Zanarini MC, Schmahl C, et al. Borderline personality disorder. *Lancet*. 2004;364(9432):453–461.

Verheul R, Van Den Bosch LM, Koeter MW, et al. Dialectical behaviour therapy for women with borderline personality disorder: 12-month, randomised clinical trial in The Netherlands. *Br J Psychiatry*. 2003;182:135–140.

"Something's Wrong with My Baby"

CC/ID: 30-year-old married mother of two whom you have been asked to see by a colleague in the pediatrics ER.

HPI: Mrs. B. came to the ER claiming there was "something really wrong" with her baby. She had delivered a healthy full-term daughter 2 weeks ago. In the immediate postpartum period, there were no problems of note, and she and her baby had been discharged home. She had chosen not to breast-feed. Her husband reported that she had begun to act peculiarly a few days ago, telling him that she was **unsure if this was in fact their baby.** Her behavior became more **bizarre,** and her husband found Mrs. B. **trying to "exorcise" the infant** that evening, leading him to bring them to the ER. **She had not been sleeping properly** for the preceding week, and her **appetite had been poor.** Her husband described her to be "a little spacey" at times, and Mrs. B. herself admits to feeling at times as if she is "not really there." Upon direct questioning, she describes a general concern for the family's well-being. **She denies symptoms of depressed mood.** She has not had similar symptoms in the past.

PMHx/PSHx: None

Meds: None

PPHx: Mrs. B. was **diagnosed as bipolar at the age of 20.** In the past, she had an episode of major depression and two episodes of mania, both of which responded to treatment. She has received prophylactic lithium therapy in the past, and this was restarted recently. During her pregnancies, she had been maintained on antipsychotics alone. She has no history of suicidal or homicidal behaviors or of substance abuse.

FHx: Sickle cell anemia in a cousin. Major depression in a maternal aunt.

SHx: Mrs. B. and her husband live in their own apartment. Until the recent delivery she had worked part-time as an office manager in an accounting firm. She has a degree in business administration.

VS: WNL

PE: *Gen:* appears her stated age, medium build, and good hygiene.

Labs: CBC, SMA 20, UA and Utox all WNL. Li 0.2 μmol/liter, TSH 1.3 (0.5–5.0).

MSE: *General:* eye contact is limited, and she appears to be irritable and suspicious at times during the interview. *Affect:* labile and fearful. *Mood:* "Fine . . . there's nothing wrong with me. The problem is in my baby." *Thought process:* flight of ideas. *Thought content:* illogical, delusional, and paranoid. She believes that this is not her baby and that "someone" has switched her real baby at the hospital. She admits to hearing voices telling her the same and that the child is "evil." She denies other perceptual abnormalities. She denies suicidal or homicidal ideations. *Insight:* little insight into her current symptoms and becomes hostile on further questioning. *Judgment:* poor. *Cognitive:* alert and oriented.

THOUGHT QUESTIONS

- What do you think is happening to Mrs. B.?
- What is your differential diagnosis?
- What are your treatment recommendations?

DISCUSSION

Mrs. B. is suffering from a **postpartum psychosis.** The incidence is about 1.5 per 1000 childbirths (0.15%). Up to **60% of episodes occur in primiparous women.** It is associated with perinatal complications or a family history of affective disorders. Psychosis is defined as grossly impaired reality testing, evidenced by delusions or hallucinations, and a lack of insight into their pathological nature. (Neurosis refers to a chronic nonpsychotic disorder, characterized mainly by anxiety.) The presentation of postpartum psychosis is usually that of a manic or depressive episode with psychotic features. Mrs. B has been experiencing insomnia, poor appetite, and episodes of both confusion and depersonalization. Patients may also be restless, agitated, or emotionally labile. These early symptoms can rapidly change to a floridly psychotic state with prominent hallucinations (25%), suspiciousness, and delusions (50%). Mothers may worry obsessively about their babies. A manic presentation can shift rapidly to depression within a couple of days. Symptoms often begin within days of the delivery but can start up to 8 weeks postpartum.

Differential diagnoses of her condition can also include the following: Acute manic or depressive episodes are possible in this patient with a history of bipolar disorder, despite the fact that she has been maintained on medications. However, the present lack of mood symptoms makes this much less likely a cause of her current distress. **Organic causes of a postpartum delirium** need to be ruled out and include latent infection, hemorrhage, toxemia, neoplasms, Sheehan syndrome (postpartum infarction of the pituitary), thyrotoxicosis, hypothyroidism, Cushing syndrome, or medication effects (meperidine, pentazocine, or scopolamine). Her labs and vital signs are normal, and she is not experiencing any unusual physical symptoms, but these should continue to be monitored. **Substance-induced mood disorder** was ruled out with a careful history and the serum toxicology screen. Inquiry should always be made about the use of over-the-counter and herbal preparations.

CASE CONTINUED

Mrs. B.'s lithium level is low and needs to be carefully titrated up to a therapeutic level of at least 0.5 μmol/L. She is admitted and is also treated with antipsychotics, supportive psychotherapy, and psychoeducation (also provided to her husband). She responds quickly to these treatments. She is discharged home a week later to the care of her family with close followup.

QUESTIONS

37-1. Which of the following is correct about the postpartum period?
  A. Lithium is not contraindicated in breast-feeding.
  B. Studies have shown different incidence rates of psychopathology among those who breast-feed and those who do not.

   C. There is no increased risk of developing lithium-induced hypothyroidism.

   D. Rapid cycling is very rarely induced by hypothyroidism.

   E. All psychopharmacological agents should be avoided if breast-feeding.

37-2. Which of the following is true of postpartum psychosis?

   A. Early treatment can decrease episode length, and it may last less than a week.

   B. In general, those who have this disorder have a poor prognosis.

   C. Women with this illness are at no increased risk of later psychiatric admission.

   D. Antipsychotics are contraindicated.

   E. It does not occur in men.

37-3. Which of the following is accurate concerning the use of psychiatric medications during pregnancy and the postpartum period?

   A. Women should be treated with usual doses of lithium during pregnancy.

   B. Higher doses may be needed postdelivery.

   C. Lithium should never be used in pregnancy.

   D. If lithium is used, the fetus should have a special ultra-sound exam before delivery.

   E. Treatment of postpartum psychosis may require a combination of a mood stabilizer, an antipsychotic, and an antidepressant.

37-4. Which of the following is correct concerning postpartum psychosis?

   A. The risk is about 1 in 500.

   B. If there was a previous episode, the risk increases to approximately 1 in 2 for subsequent pregnancies.

   C. Approximately 30% of these episodes are due to mood disorders.

   D. Approximately 10% of those with this disorder commit infanticide.

   E. Diagnostic criteria are well defined in the DSM-IV-TR.

ANSWERS

37-1. E. All psychopharmacological medications should be avoided if breast-feeding. If the medications are vital, breast-feeding should be avoided. Breast-feeding has not been shown to confer any difference in risk of psychopathology for the mother or infant, but the infant does glean beneficial immunologic and attachment/ bonding effects. Lithium can cause hypothyroidism and goiter development in the neonate, and thus should be avoided when breast-feeding. Neonatal hypothyroidism may cause mental retardation but is preventable if detected at birth. The rate of lithium-induced hypothyroidism is approximately 3% per year in those taking lithium. Women themselves seem to be extra sensitive to developing hypothyroidism from lithium in the postpartum period and need careful monitoring. Patients with rapid cycling may have increased rates of hypothyroidism.

37-2. **A.** If early intervention is instituted, symptoms may resolve fairly rapidly, and these women usually have a good prognosis. Evidence from large epidemiological studies suggest that these women are at increased risk for psychiatric admission for the next 2 years. Women with histories of postpartum depression or recurrent major depressive disorder are at high risk for postpartum episodes, and prophylaxis should be considered. Those with histories of depression during pregnancy, bipolar I or II disorder, or puerperal psychosis are at the highest risk and specific prophylaxis should be given. Although care is needed with antipsychotics in breast-feeding women, small doses may be used and the neonate should be monitored for any adverse effects. Although extremely rare, postpartum psychosis has been reported to occur in men. These men probably already have a psychiatric disorder, which may be exacerbated by the stress of becoming a father.

37-3. **E.** The treatment of postpartum psychosis may require a combination of a mood stabilizer (usually lithium), an antipsychotic, an antidepressant (if significantly depressed), and psychosocial interventions. During pregnancy, women may need higher doses of lithium to achieve the desired therapeutic level due to their altered physiology with increased glomerular filtration rates and plasma volume. Care must be taken at delivery, as there is a rapid loss of fluids that may affect the serum level, causing toxicity; the lithium dosage should be halved approximately 1 week prior to delivery. If possible, lithium should be avoided in pregnancy, due to the possible teratogenic effects, particularly Ebstein anomaly. However, lithium may be used during the last trimester. Lithium freely crosses the placenta and may cause goiter and hypothyroidism in the fetus, which should be evaluated with ultrasound

37-4. **B.** As mentioned in the text, the incidence of postpartum psychosis is about 1.5 per 1000 childbirths. The risk of having another episode in subsequent pregnancies may run as high as 50%. Approximately 4% of women with postpartum psychosis may commit infanticide; the risk of suicide is also elevated. Command hallucinations may tell the mother to kill the baby. Care must be taken to spot symptoms early and instigate treatment as soon as possible. If the woman needs to be hospitalized, supervised access to care for her baby should be allowed to facilitate the vital bonding between mother and child. Approximately 90% of these episodes are mood disorders, and 40% are manic in presentation. The short-term treatment includes antipsychotic medications and a mood stabilizer as appropriate; ECT may be needed. Some authors recommend stopping antipsychotic medications when psychotic symptoms clear, whereas others suggest continuing, as these women are at increased risk for up to a year. Mood stabilizers should be continued beyond the resolution of active symptoms to prevent relapse. These disorders usually have a good prognosis, clearing within a few weeks to months, but some patients may continue to experience occasional psychotic symptoms.

SUGGESTED READINGS

Harlow BL, Vitonis AF, Sparen P, et al. Incidence of hospitalization for postpartum psychotic and bipolar episodes with and without prior prepregnancy or prenatal psychiatric hospitalizations. *Arch Gen Psychiatry*. 2007;64(1):42–48.

Sit D, Rothchild AJ, Wisner KL. A review of postpartum psychosis. *J Womens Health*. 2006;15(4):352–368.

"Mute with a Fever"

CC/ID: 28-year-old single white man suffering from paranoid schizophrenia who has been brought to the ER from a sheltered housing program because "he isn't right."

HPI: Mr. T. is **mute and appears very stiff, lying on a gurney**. He is **not responsive** to questioning. Information from the facility confirms that Mr. T. had been diagnosed as **schizophrenic** at the age of 19 and is currently maintained on haloperidol decanoate injections every 4 weeks with benztropine (Cogentin). This afternoon he returned early from his part-time job as a messenger complaining of **feeling feverish** and stiff. When staff went to check on him a short time later, they found him mute, rigid, and with a fever of 40°C. He has no other recent symptoms or complaints.

PMHx: None

Meds: Haldol decanoate, 150 mg IM monthly; benztropine, 1 mg PO BID.

PPHx: First psychiatric contact occurred at age 19 when he required hospitalization for 6 months. Since then he has been hospitalized twice, once for 4 months (age 22), and most recently for 1 year (age 27) at a state facility. He went through a rehabilitation program, and has been managing to function relatively independently in this sheltered housing program over the past year. He has been compliant with medications. His symptom history consists of chronic low-level auditory hallucinations, social isolation, and a moderate amount of paranoia that minimally impacts his job as a messenger. However, during acute episodes he has become grossly paranoid and has refused food and water. No history of suicide attempts. No history of substance abuse.

SHx: Youngest of six children, graduated high school and had begun to attend a local junior college when he had his first episode of illness. He did not return to college, but has held several part-time jobs between episodes. Parents and siblings are alive and well.

FHx: One cousin has schizophrenia. One sister has a seizure disorder.

VS: **Temp 40° C**, BP 130/90, **HR 120**, RR 16

PE: *Gen:* no evidence of trauma. *HEENT:* PERRLA, mucous membranes dry. Diaphoretic. *Lungs:* fields clear to auscultation and percussion, but with tachypnea. *CV:* tachycardia with a rate of 120, regular rhythm, no murmurs. *Abdomen:* soft, nontender, normal bowel sounds. *Neuro:* generalized **muscle rigidity throughout body**. Fluctuating level of consciousness. Intermittently responding to painful stimuli. No focal signs. Babinski reflexes normal.

MSE *General:* Lying in hospital pajamas, appears stated age, hygiene good. *Behavior:* mute, unresponsive to questioning; eyes are closed and he is drooling; no negativism or purposeless movements.

THOUGHT QUESTIONS

- What is your differential diagnosis?
- How should his symptoms be managed?
- What are your recommendations for labs and his psychiatric condition at this time?

DISCUSSION

The differential diagnosis includes the following.

Lethal catatonia: Rapid onset of a hyperactive manic delirium, rigidity, elevated temperature, and a catatonic stupor. It has a mortality rate of over 50%. There may be a considerable overlap between this condition and NMS. Many patients experience a behavioral prodrome as well as hyperthermia in the prestuporous phase (unlike in NMS where this is seen in the stuporous phase).

Neuroleptic malignant syndrome (NMS): This patient is likely suffering from NMS, a life-threatening complication of antipsychotic treatment with a reported **mortality of up to 20%**. The characteristic features include autonomic instability (hyperthermia), altered consciousness, and muscle rigidity. However, there have been cases reported without muscle rigidity or hyperthermia. It has been reported with both typical and atypical antipsychotics.

Signs and symptoms: Severe muscle rigidity, hyperthermia, alternating levels of consciousness (agitated confusion to mutism and coma), and autonomic instability (diaphoresis, tachypnea, tachycardia, and elevated or labile blood pressure). May also include dysphagia, tremor, and incontinence. Laboratory findings may include leucocytosis (up to 40,000 cells/mm³ +/− a left shift, elevated CPK (up to 60,000 IU/L), LFTs, myoglobin, and myoglobinuria.

Epidemiology: It most commonly occurs within the first 10 days of starting or changing antipsychotic treatment but it can occur at any time. It occurs in approximately 1% of those taking these medications. NMS might also occur in patients with Parkinson disease who have their levodopa dose decreased or withdrawn quickly, but it is not thought to be dose related.

Risk factors: Although it is believed to be mainly a medication effect, certain individuals may be at increased risk. Risk factors include dehydration, hot weather, cognitive impairment, and brain damage.

Etiology: NMS is thought to be caused by an acute hypodopaminergic crisis, particularly in the hypothalamus and the basal ganglia (Fig. 38-1). Glutamate, acetylcholine, norepinephrine, and serotonin may also be involved.

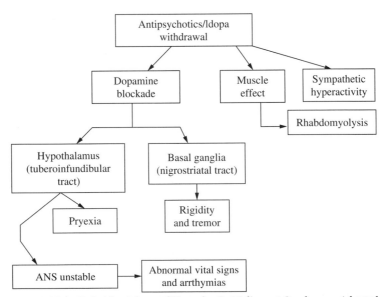

FIGURE 38-1. Pathophysiology of Neuroleptic Malignant Syndrome. *Adapted from Bhanushali and Tuite, 2004.*

TABLE 38-1 Medication Changes Implicated in NMS

Taking	Antipsychotics, antinausea medications that are also dopamine antagonists (e.g., metoclopramide and prochlorperazine), amphetamines, cocaine, and lithium
Removing	L-Dopa, dopamine agonists (e.g., amantadine, pramipexole), and catechol-o-methyltransferase (COMT) inhibitors (e.g., entacapone, tolcapone)

Workup: In addition to CBC (looking for leukocytosis), serum chemistry (looking for increases in BUN and creatinine signaling worsening renal function), CPK, LFTs, and myoglobin, workup should also include TFTs, blood cultures, UA, ECG, lumbar puncture, and CXR. CT scan for underlying brain pathology.

Morbidity/Mortality: Rhabdomyolysis can lead to acute renal failure which is the most common cause of mortality. Other causes of death include cardiac arrthymias/failure, DVTs with pulmonary embolism, or DIC. Other complications include aspiration, infection, and respiratory failure. Electrolyte abnormalities should be monitored closely.

Further differential diagnoses include any CNS infection/vasculitis, malignant hyperthermia (if recently had anesthetic), heat stroke, dystonic reactions, and serotonin syndrome (see Tables 38-1 and 38-2 for details).

TABLE 38-2 Serotonin Syndrome

Features	Toxic effect of combining serotonin-modulating antidepressants (e.g., SSRIs, MAOIs, TCAs); MAOIs inhibit the breakdown of serotonin and TCAs inhibit serotonin reuptake. Thought to be caused by over-activity of 5-HT-1a receptor. Altered mental status (40%, may appear agitated/manic), autonomic instability, hyperreflexia, neuromuscular effects (primarily myoclonus, but also tremor and rigidity), GI upset (nausea and vomiting), pyrexia, and sweating. Rare complications reported include rhabdomyolysis, renal failure, DIC, and seizures.
Treatment	Usually resolves with removal of offending agent. Supportive measures are similar to those for NMS and require plenty of IV fluids. Benzodiazepines are useful for helping muscle rigidity and even myoclonus. Other possible treatments include serotonin antagonists (e.g., cyproheptadine), diphenhydramine, and chlorpromazine (unlike NMS).

Adapted from Bhanushali MJ, Tuite PJ. The evaluation and management of patients with neuroleptic malignant syndrome. *Neurol Clin.* 2004;22(2):389–411.

CASE CONTINUED

Mr. T's lab results reveal leucocytosis, elevated BUN, CPK, and myoglobin. The LFTs are WNL, serum toxicology is negative, and hemoglobin and platelets are WNL. He is admitted to intensive care with a diagnosis of NMS, where he is monitored carefully. His baseline medications are stopped, and he is treated with IV fluids, cooling blankets, dantrolene, and benzodiazepines. After 8 days, his lab results return to normal values, and there are no neurologic sequelae. He is started on a low dose of an atypical antipsychotic and discharged to the care of the staff at the program; psychiatry followup is arranged.

QUESTIONS

38-1. Which of the following conditions that cause hyperthermia is correctly matched with a medication or substance-inducing cause?

    A. Malignant hyperthermia .... Lidocaine
    B. Malignant hyperthermia .... Tricyclic antidepressants
    C. Autonomic hyperreflexia .... Lead poisoning
    D. Autonomic hyperreflexia .... Amphetamines
    E. Lethal catatonia .... Antipsychotics

38-2. Those at increased risk of NMS include which of the following?

    A. Individuals treated with metronidazole
    B. Individuals with a history of schizophrenia or mood disorders
    C. Children
    D. Individuals with cataplexy
    E. Individuals with psychogenic polydipsia

38-3. Which of the following is correct concerning the management of NMS?

    A. ECT is contraindicated.
    B. Treatment usually continues for up to 10 days.
    C. Agitation may be treated with haloperidol.
    D. Intravenous bromocriptine is the treatment of choice.
    E. Anticholinergic agents should be stopped immediately.

38-4. Which of the following helps to differentiate serotonin syndrome from NMS?

A. Serotonin syndrome is more likely to present with EPS.
B. NMS is more likely to present with ataxia, hyperreflexia, and myoclonus.
C. NMS is more likely to present with EPS.
D. Serotonin syndrome is more likely to present with very high fevers.
E. Serotonin syndrome is more likely to present with dysphagia and incontinence.

ANSWERS

38-1. D. There are several other causes of hyperthermia other than neuroleptic malignant syndrome: lethal catatonia, which can be caused by lead poisoning and may be fatal if not treated (supportive care, benzodiazepines, and avoid antipsychotics). Autonomic hyperreflexia can be caused by CNS stimulants (e.g., amphetamine) and is reversible with IV trimethaphan. Cocaine and tricyclic antidepressants can cause a hyperthermia due to increased heat production. This is treated with physostigmine and sodium bicarbonate (if needed for arrhythmias, under careful cardiac monitoring). Malignant hyperthermia may be caused by the anesthetic halothane or neuromuscular blockers like succinylcholine, and may be fatal if untreated (with dantrolene and supportive care).

38-2. B. NMS appears to be rare in children. The cause of this disorder is unknown, but it is more common in men than in women, in younger patients, and in those with mental retardation, a history of schizophrenia, mood disorders, or catatonia. Many consider it a severe form of neuroleptic-induced catatonia. The 1-year prevalence is reported to be between 0.02% and 2.4% among those exposed to antipsychotics. It is more often seen with high potency antipsychotics and when the dosages have been rapidly increased, but it can occur at any time while on neuroleptic treatment. NMS has rarely been reported with the use of atypical antipsychotics such as clozapine, risperidone, olanzapine, and quetiapine. It may also occur while using other dopaminergic antagonists, such as metoclopramide (Reglan) or prochlorperazine (Compazine), but not the antibiotic metronidazole (Flagyl). Cataplexy is a sudden loss of muscle tone that occurs in narcolepsy. Psychogenic polydipsia is found in some patients with schizophrenia and is an excessive consumption of water which can lead to water intoxication and clinical hyponatremia. It is the reverse of dehydration which is a risk factor for NMS.

38-3. B. Treatment for NMS usually continues for up to 10 days, but may need to be longer if long-acting depot preparations of antipsychotic medications have been used. If there has been no response after a few days, ECT may be considered, but succinylcholine should be avoided in those with rhabdomyolysis. Care must be taken with the reintroduction of antipsychotic medications; low potency or atypical agents may be preferable. Anticholinergic agents should be tapered slowly, as they may interfere with thermoregulation. Management includes supportive treatment in an intensive care unit with careful monitoring of vital signs and renal function. Treatment is symptomatic. Antipsychotic medication must be stopped; agitation may be treated with benzodiazepines, which may be an effective treatment in and of itself. Treatment includes dantrolene, a direct-acting muscle relaxant that blocks calcium release from the sarcoplasmic reticulum. It is initially given intravenously and then orally when the patient can swallow. It should not be used in conjunction with calcium channel blockers. Side effects include impaired respiratory or hepatic function, and LFTs should be monitored. Bromocriptine or amantadine (an NMDA receptor antagonist and dopamine agonist) may also be used orally. Other possible treatments remain controversial.

38-4. C. NMS is more likely to present with extrapyramidal features, high fevers, incontinence, difficulty swallowing, and drooling. Patients with serotonin syndrome are more likely to present with ataxia, nausea, vomiting, diarrhea, hyperreflexia, myoclonus, and diaphoresis. However, if symptoms are mild, it can be difficult to differentiate between the two, and a careful history is vital.

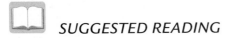 *SUGGESTED READING*

Carbone JR. The neuroleptic malignant and serotonin syndromes. *Emergency Med Clin N Am.* 2000;18(2):317–325.

Bhanushali MJ, Tuite PJ. The evaluation and management of patients with neuroleptic malignant syndrome. *Neurol Clin.* 2004;22(2):389–411.

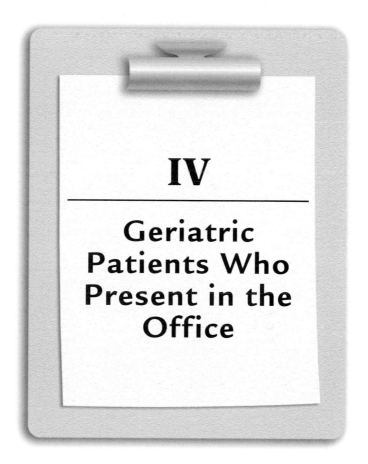

IV

Geriatric Patients Who Present in the Office

"I Can't Sleep"

CC/ID: 70-year-old married man comes in for evaluation of insomnia.

HPI: CS was in his usual state of health until 6 months ago when he sold his business and retired. He was initially happy and hopeful, but now he states that his sleep has been worsening: "now I'm a wreck." He has no difficulty falling asleep but has **multiple awakenings throughout** the night and needs to read for 30 minutes before he can return to sleep. **Though he has never slept that well, this is clearly a change from his baseline and is accompanied by** "horrible nightmares." He will not describe the dreams but says they are incredibly vivid.

THOUGHT QUESTION

- Why might someone have a sleep disturbance?

DISCUSSION

The differential of a sleep disturbance is long. Sleep hygiene (e.g., taking long naps close to bedtime) or medications (e.g., caffeinated beverages or diuretics at night) may interfere with sleep. Sleep apnea causes multiple awakenings and interferes with daytime functioning. Certain medications are associated with vivid dreams (e.g., antimalarials). Psychiatric syndromes like mania, depression, generalized anxiety disorder, and PTSD often interfere with sleep.

CASE CONTINUED

The patient sold his business because his factory was on a valuable piece of land, and a developer offered him "more than I could turn down." **Prior to retirement, he was a "workaholic"** and a "bear with a temper." He was known for saying, "I came to this country with nothing. Of course I work, I had a family to support!" **He was reluctant to discuss his history.** Eventually, he explained that he came to the United States in 1945. He was born in Austria, and **at age 10 he watched helplessly from a neighbor's window while his mother and sister were taken away by the Nazis.** A man tried to help them but was shot. He and his brother were hidden by the neighbor for 6 months in the storeroom of a shoe store. He states that he can remember nothing about his time in the store, only that they were smuggled to England. No one else in his family survived. He refuses to watch anything about WWII, and will not enter a shoe store or wear leather shoes as the smell reminds him of the storeroom. He does not know his family's fate: "I cannot bear to think of what happened to them. Every war movie or memorial just cements what I know must have happened. I cannot and will not think of my mother or sisters in the hands of a Mengele."

PMHx: Hypertension, no prostatic disease or snoring.

Meds: Lisinopril

PPHx: None

SHx: As above, two sons.

VS: BP 130/80

PE: *Gen:* thin WM in NAD. Noncontributory.

Labs: Noncontributory.

MSE: *General:* elderly man, direct eye contact and intense expression, though looks fatigued. Cooperative with interview. *Affect:* constricted and angry. *Mood:* "exhausted and fed up." *Speech:* pained and slow, but deliberate. *Thought process:* linear and goal-directed. *Thought content:* preoccupied with insomnia. No delusions or hallucinations. No suicidal or homicidal ideations. *Cognition:* intact

 ## *THOUGHT QUESTION*

- What is your working diagnosis?

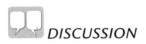 ## *DISCUSSION*

PTSD is a pathological response that occurs in approximately 20% of people exposed to severe trauma. The nature, severity, and duration of the trauma affect the incidence of PTSD. **Individual**

characteristics that increase risk include an early history of
trauma or pre-existing anxiety or depression, or substance
abuse. Four factors are needed for a diagnosis of PTSD:

1. trauma
2. re-experiencing phenomena
3. avoidance
4. hyperarousal

These symptoms must last at least 1 month and cause significant distress or functional impairment. PTSD that first occurs 6 months after
the trauma is termed "delayed-onset." A trauma is "experiencing or
witnessing an event that involved actual or threatened death or serious injury to self or others," and feeling fear, helplessness, or horror.
Re-experiencing refers to intrusive recollections, nightmares, or feeling
as if the traumatic event were reoccurring. Avoidance includes avoiding things associated with the trauma, inability to recall important
aspects of the event, feelings of detachment, a restricted range of
affect, or a sense of a foreshortened future. Hyperarousal includes difficulty falling or staying asleep, irritability or anger outbursts, exaggerated startle, poor concentration, or hypervigilance. This man meets
these criteria. His symptoms have increased since retiring; it is not
uncommon that with aging—retirement, loss of purpose or structure,
death of friends, or illness— a reawakening of symptoms may occur.

CASE CONTINUED

He denies prominent symptoms of depression or mania. He does
not awaken to urinate, nor does he nap during the day. His wife
confirms that he does not have apneic episodes during sleep. He
asks, "Can't you give me something for these damn nightmares?"
You review medications used for sleep (Table 39-1) and start pra-
zosin 2 mgs QHS. This alpha-1-antagonist has shown some effect
against nightmares in PTSD. You refer him to a PTSD psychotherapy program.

QUESTIONS

39-1. Which of the following medications is considered a first
line treatment for PTSD?
  A. Imipramine
  B. Haloperidol

TABLE 39-1   Agents used for Insomnia

Benzodiazepines	Lorazepam (0.5–2 mg) Temazepam (7.5–15 mg) Diazepam (5–10 mg) Flurazepam (15–30 mg) Clonazepam (0.5–1 mg) Written in order of increasing half-life. May cause ataxia, sedation, headache, leg pain (in elderly), and amnesia if taken in large doses. Note that diazepam may have the longest functional half-life, as active metabolites can build up in elderly individuals.
Antidepressants	Trazadone (25–400 mg): May cause sedation, nightmares, hypotension or priapism. Mirtazapine (7.5–15 mg): Sedation, nightmares and weight gain. Higher doses than 15–30 mg may be activating and interfere with sleep. Tricyclics (e.g., amitriptyline 10–50 mg): Anticholinergic side effects, arrthymias and postural hypotension. Avoid in cardiac patients.
Anticholinergic agents	Diphenhydramine (25–100 mg): Sedation, anticholinergic side effects, and may cause paradoxical excitement in some.
Antipsychotics	Quetiapine (25–50 mg): May cause sedation, orthostatic hypotension, or weight gain.
Miscellaneous	Zolpidem (5–10 mg): May cause ataxia, dizziness or hangover effects. Chloral hydrate (500 mg): May cause rashes and decreased effect with chronic use.

    C. Sertraline
    D. Chlordiazepoxide
    E. Clonidine

39-2. Which of the following techniques is recommended in the treatment of PTSD?
    A. Implosion therapy
    B. Group therapy
    C. Light boxes
    D. Regression therapy
    E. Aversion therapy

39-3. Which trauma is most likely to result in PTSD?
    A. Rape
    B. Being shot or stabbed
    C. Severe physical assault
    D. Serious car accident
    E. Death of a close friend

39-4. Which of the following statements is accurate concerning the psychobiology of PTSD?
  A. There are decreased circulating catecholamines.
  B. Amygdalar size is negatively correlated with symptom severity.
  C. Hippocampal size is positively correlated with symptom severity.
  D. The opioid system may be overactive
  E. The corpus callosum is hypertrophied.

ANSWERS

39-1. C. Antidepressants attenuate some of the core symptoms of PTSD. Most of the research has been done with tricyclics and SSRIs, and SSRIs are considered first line agents in this disorder. Clonidine may address hyperarousal symptoms, and clonazepam anxiety symptoms. There may be a limited role for antipsychotics, especially if there is severe agitation or psychotic features. Chlordiazepoxide (Librium) is a benzodiazepine, which is used primarily in alcohol detoxification protocols.

39-2. B. As a trauma undermines one's sense of safety and reconfigures one's outlook on the world, the best treatment may be to intervene immediately after the trauma and help the person integrate and accept what has happened. Debriefing techniques may not be helpful for civilian victims. Relaxation training can reduce physiological arousal. Group therapy provides mutual support, addresses avoidance, and allows for processing of intense affects that are brought up. Graded exposure can address avoidance and has been successfully studied in rape victims. Implosion therapy may be suitable for some phobic disorders but not for PTSD. Light boxes are used to treat seasonal affective disorder. In regression therapy, the patient is encouraged to regress to earlier developmental stages; it is not used in psychiatric practice, and is not a validated therapy. Aversion therapy has been used to treat pedophiles; an aversive stimuli is applied (e.g., apomorphine to induce vomiting or electric currents) when undesired thoughts or fantasies are imagined. This too has fallen out of favor in psychiatry.

39-3. A. Studies have examined the likelihood that various traumas will cause PTSD. In descending order: physical torture (>75% will develop PTSD), rape, severe physical assault, other sexual assault, shootings or stabbings, sudden unexpected death of a close friend or relative, being threatened with a weapon, flood, fire, or other natural disaster, and serious motor vehicle accident (approximately 3%). Although there are no specific reported "risk factors," certain individuals may be at increased risk of developing PTSD: those with histories of childhood traumas, poor support systems, female gender, recent alcohol abuse, and those who subscribe to an external locus of control (meaning that they perceive experiences that occur to be beyond their power [e.g., force of deity, or the like]) as opposed to an internal locus of control (in which they can script their destinies and experiences).

39-4. D. The corpus callosum is not affected. Patients have increased levels of circulating catecholamines (dopamine, norepinephrine), which are associated with a hyperactive sympathetic nervous system (involved in the fight or flight response to a stressor). Cortisol secretion, while initially helping to activate the stress response, eventually serves to feed back and shut off the sympathetic system. Studies of cortisol levels in the acute aftermath of trauma suggest that people with lower levels may go on to develop PTSD. Essentially the stress response system is activated and cannot be terminated, leading to inappropriate levels of fear, as the person continues to experience a trauma long after it has passed. The opioid system may also be overactive, and studies have shown that PTSD symptoms may be helped by opioid receptor antagonists. Hippocampal volume is negatively correlated with symptom severity, and the shrinkage may be due to elevated glucocorticoids and glutamate excitotoxicity. As the neuroanatomical site of fear memories and charged with initiating the stress response, the amygdala is hypertrophic in PTSD.

SUGGESTED READINGS

Yehuda R. Post-traumatic stress disorder. *N Engl J Med.* 2002; 346(2):108–114.

Golier JA, Harvey PD, Legge L, et al. Memory performance in older trauma survivors: implications for the longitudinal course of PTSD. *Ann N Y Acad Sci.* 2006;1071:54–66.

Davidson JR, Stein DJ, Shalev AY, et al. Posttraumatic stress disorder: acquisition, recognition, course, and treatment. *J Neuropsychiatry Clin Neurosci.* 2004;16(2):135–147.

"Why Is My Husband Fighting with Me?"

 CC/ID: 72-year-old married white man who is brought in by his wife because "he's been so angry."

HPI: The wife reports the patient was a healthy, partially retired businessman until 1 year ago, when he fell and had weakness on his left side. Since then, he "has not been right," is somewhat **forgetful, repeats stories,** and is **no longer able to participate meaningfully** in the business (though he does still enjoy talking about business with his daughter). She thinks he may have had a stroke. He was initially cooperative with care, but after another "bad spell" 6 months ago, he has been **volatile, irritable,** and **combative** at times, especially around bathing. She is worried that when they try to help him bathe he will strike her or one of the recently hired aides. She notes that he is often confused and disoriented. **The patient says, "Why am I here? I'm fine."**

THOUGHT QUESTIONS

- At this point what is the differential diagnosis?
- What would be important to look for on his physical examination?
- What would be important to look for on his mental status examination?

DISCUSSION

By this history it is clear that this patient meets the **criteria for dementia.** He is forgetful, repetitive, and has difficulties with executive functioning. Given the progression of his illness, and the history of what sounds like possible cerebrovascular accidents (CVAs), it is probable that there is a vascular cause of his dementia. **He needs a careful neurologic exam.** In addition he has a **worsening behavioral disturbance,** and it is important to **look for signs of acute medical illness, delirium, depression, anxiety, or psychosis,** all of which could fuel his agitation. It is crucial that a mental status exam include a test of memory and cognition.

PMHx: Hypertension, prior coronary angioplasty, hypercholesterolemia.

Meds: Lisinopril; lovastatin; aspirin, 81 mg QD

PPHx: None

FHx: Mother died age 62 of a CVA; father died age 77 of MI.

SHx: Owned a successful manufacturing company, married, two children. No ETOH or other substance use.

VS: BP 150/85, HR 70, and RR 12

PE: *HEENT, Lungs, and Abdomen:* all unremarkable. *CV:* regular, no murmurs. *Neuro:* mild left facial droop. *Ext:* strength 4/5 left upper extremity, 5/5 right; 4/5 left lower extremity, 5/5 right.

MSE: *General:* appears older than his stated age, in a wheelchair, appropriately dressed. *Behavior:* irritable, impatient, and somewhat confused. *Speech:* normal rate and tone. *Mood:* "I'm fine," and denies depression or anxiety when specifically questioned. *Affect:* reactive, somewhat labile. *Thought process:* perseverative, repetitive, with decreased rate of thinking. *Thought content/perceptions:* no suicidal or homicidal ideation, no abnormal perceptions. *Insight:* poor. *MMSE:* 16/30 (−4 time, −2 place, −2 delayed recall, −4 world, −1 repeating, −1 pentagons). Difficulty following directions.

THOUGHT QUESTIONS

- How did his history, physical examination, and mental status examination affect your thinking?
- What laboratory tests should be ordered and why?

DISCUSSION

He has **focal neurologic signs,** and a clear temporal relationship between his probable strokes and his dementia symptoms, and thus

TABLE 40-1   Differentiating Delirium from Dementia

Parameter	Dementia	Delirium
Level of consciousness	Normal	Impaired, waxing and waning
Rate of onset	Usually insidious (except in vascular dementia)	Acute or subacute
Stability of symptoms	Generally stable	Marked fluctuation
Reversibility	Rarely reversible	Most often reversible
Autonomic function	Intact	May have autonomic dysfunction (e.g., in alcohol withdrawal delirium)

meets the criteria for vascular dementia. His MMSE reveals difficulties in multiple areas. He **should have neuroimaging** (MRI) to evaluate the extent of the cerebral damage. Patients with dementia may become agitated for many reasons. He could have an **infection** (e.g., a UTI); an exacerbation of an underlying medical condition; a pain syndrome which he is not able to describe; a **depression secondary to a stroke** causing irritability; psychotic symptoms due to the dementia which are making him agitated; frustration due to his inability to complete tasks; or nonspecific agitation due to his dementia. His physical examination does not suggest an acute medical illness, although lab testing, including UA, should be done to rule out possible causes such as electrolyte abnormalities and infection (Table 40-1). In addition, reversible causes of dementia that might be complicating his condition should be ruled out.

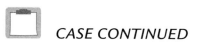

CASE CONTINUED

Serum chemistries, CBC, B_{12}, folate, RPR, and TSH WNL. His MRI revealed an old right hemisphere stroke and some lacunar infarcts in the thalami bilaterally. His wife asks, "What can we do?"

QUESTIONS

40-1. All of the following are useful nonpharmacologic interventions *except*:
  A. Activity planning
  B. Providing familiar objects
  C. Restraining the patient in bed

   D. Family education, support groups
   E. Reminiscence therapies

40-2. Which of these medications are used to treat agitation in dementia?
   A. Haloperidol
   B. Diphenhydramine
   C. Diazepam
   D. Chlorpromazine
   E. Amitriptyline

40-3. Which of the following is true about agitation in dementia?
   A. Agitation is narrowly defined as behaviors that are physically or verbally threatening.
   B. Sleep disturbance is uncommon.
   C. Psychotic symptoms are uncommon.
   D. The most common delusions are erotic.
   E. It occurs in >50% of community dwelling patients with dementia.

40-4. What is correct concerning the evaluation of behavioral disturbance?
   A. Infections may rarely cause behavioral disturbance.
   B. Psychiatric drugs have few drug–drug interactions.
   C. Lighting and isolation are not important.
   D. Anxiety may present as hypersomnia.
   E. Anticholinergic drugs may increase confusion and agitation.

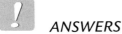

ANSWERS

40-1. C. Restraints may increase agitation and confusion. Supervision is recommended rather than restraints. Activity planning can provide daytime activities, exercise, socialization, and routines. As patients may become agitated because of frustration or inability to complete tasks (e.g., brushing teeth), one remedy is to break the task into smaller units (e.g., take toothbrush, wet it, squeeze toothpaste, etc.). It is always crucial to ensure safety (e.g., hand-held showers, bath seats), and safety may decrease conflict in the bathroom. Adequate illumination, restoration of vision and hearing aids, reorientation, and providing familiar objects may help. Unfamiliar or unstructured environments can increase confusion. Family education, support groups, and reassurance can also help decrease conflict. Reminiscence therapy allows patients to be reminded about events in their pasts by using old photos or relevant literature.

40-2. A. All of the other listed medications may cause sedation, anticholinergic effects, confusion, or orthostasis and are not recommended. Some considerations: (a) If the symptoms are not causing distress or problems functioning, there is no need to treat. (b) Remember cost. Most people on Medicare do not have prescription coverage, so always ask. (c) Any med used may cause worsening symptoms or cognition. (d) There are many classes of medications used for agitation. The only ones with randomized clinical trials are risperidone and haloperidol. Other medications that have been studied are trazodone, carbamazepine, valproic acid, and gabapentin. In uncontrolled studies and case reports, these all have benefit. Remember the rule of "start low, go slow" when treating geriatric patients. Along these lines, it is advisable to use medications with short half-lives as the elderly have reduced renal clearance and hepatic metabolism. They are also sensitive to the sedating effects of medications, and ataxia and falls are common.

40-3. E. Agitation is seen in >50% of community dwelling patients with dementia. Agitation encompasses a multitude of symptoms, such as wandering, pacing, purposeless behaviors (e.g., packing, hoarding), irritability, hitting, yelling, threatening, sleep-wake disturbance, "sundowning," sexually inappropriate behavior, self-injurious behaviors (e.g., head banging), paranoia, visual or auditory hallucinations, and resisting care. Sleep difficulty is common (approximately 50%). Psychotic symptoms usually occur in moderate dementia. Depending on the sample, prevalence has been estimated at over 50%. The most common delusions are paranoid (approximately 40%), such as suspicion about caregivers or others stealing or hiding things.

40-4. E. Psychiatric drugs may cause many drug–drug interactions (e.g., SSRIs may inhibit the p450 enzymes and increase certain drug levels). Anticholinergic agents may cause confusion or delirium. In general, it is crucial to look for medical causes of behavioral disturbance, such as delirium, pain or other distress from a medical condition, side effects of medications, substance use or withdrawal, or even a UTI or constipation. Look for new medications, interactions, or changes in excretion or metabolism. Evaluate for psychiatric syndromes such as depression, anxiety, or psychosis. Evaluate the environment—changes in routine, temperature, lighting, noise, over- or understimulation—and look at time course. Psychological factors include inability to channel energy, anger or fear about the disease, frustration at not being able to complete tasks, anxiety about being bathed or toileted, or response to the anger or frustration of the spouse. Psychiatric syndromes—for example, anxiety and psychosis—may complicate the course of dementia and lead to behavioral disturbances.

 SUGGESTED READINGS

Alexopoulos GS, Jeste DV, Chung H, et al. The expert consensus guideline series. Treatment of dementia and its behavioral disturbances. Introduction: methods, commentary, and summary. *Postgrad Med.* 2005;Spec No: 6–22.

Grossman H, Bergmann C, Parker S, et al. Dementia: a brief review. *Mt Sinai J Med.* 2006;73(7):985–992.

Guermazi A, Miaux Y, Rovira-Canellas A, et al. Neuroradiological findings in vascular dementia. *Neuroradiology.* 2007;49(1): 1–22.

"Is My Husband Depressed?"

 CC/ID: 72-year-old retired physician, is brought in by his wife for evaluation of possible depression.

HPI: G.P.'s wife says **he stays home "doing nothing,"** and she worries that he is depressed. This has been going on for "months." He says he is "Okay . . . I like staying home. I'm catching up on reading." She agrees that his **sleep and appetite are fine,** and he has **no complaints of sadness.** He is not doing bills or chores, and she says he hasn't read a book in months. They deny recent stressors. She admits that for about a year he has been **forgetting conversations,** which she attributes to his poor hearing. She admits that this may be getting worse. Also, at a party 6 months ago, he was repeating stories, which she attributed to "his second glass of wine." He gave up his position as secretary of the local club last year because the minutes were "too much."

THOUGHT QUESTION

- At this point what is the differential diagnosis?
- What would be important to look for on his physical examination?
- What would be important to look for on his mental status examination?

PMHx: Hypertension, high cholesterol, chronic atrial fibrillation.

Meds: Lisinopril, lovastatin, diphenhydramine PRN for insomnia.

PPHx: None.

SHx: Internist, worked until 2 years ago when HMO bought his practice. No transfusions, use of ETOH, tobacco, drugs, or unsafe sexual practices.

VS: BP 150/85, HR 72, RR 12

PE: Unremarkable. *CV:* irregularly irregular. *Neuro:* nonfocal, no cogwheel rigidity, tremor, or bradykinesia.

MSE: *General:* well groomed. *Behavior:* cooperative but impatient. *Speech:* WNL. *Mood:* "fine," and denies dysphoria when specifically questioned. *Affect:* blunted and neutral. *Thought process:* somewhat repetitive. *Thought content:* no suicidality, no abnormal perceptions. MMSE: 25/30 (−2 time, −3 delayed recall).

THOUGHT QUESTIONS

- How did his history, physical examination, and mental status examination affect your thinking?
- What laboratory tests should be ordered and why?

DISCUSSION

Though this patient presents with amotivation, and his wife is concerned about depression, neither endorses depressive symptoms. He has a **decline in functioning,** is not participating in activities or in the financial management of the home, and is forgetful. **He meets the criteria for dementia as manifest by a problem with memory and executive function** (the bills, the minutes). These cognitive deficits are stable and persistent, unlike those seen in patients with delirium. Areas of cognitive functioning that may be affected in dementia include attention and concentration, language, problem solving, executive functioning, learning, memory, language, IQ, and orientation. **Personality may also be affected and is commonly an early sign.** It is crucial that a test of cognition (e.g., Folstein's mini-mental) be done. On examination, it is important to look for significant medical illness (e.g., hypothyroidism), focal neurologic abnormalities, and so on. The cause of dementia can usually be identified (Table 41-1). About **5% to 15% of patients with dementia may have an underlying reversible cause,** which must be identified and rectified as soon as possible (e.g., B_{12} deficiency).

TABLE 41-1   Causes of Dementia and some Features

Alzheimer disease	Exact etiology remains unknown. Abnormal processing of the amyloid precursor protein. Cerebral atrophy is seen, particularly in temporal and parietal regions. Senile amyloid plaques, neurofibrillary tangles (hyperphosphorylated tau). Neuronal and synaptic loss (greatest in hippocampus and temporal lobes). Loss of cholinergic (nucleus basalis of Meynert) and noradrenergic (locus ceruleus) neurons. Corticotrophin and somatostatin may also be depleted. Course is manifest by a slow progressive decline.
Vascular dementia	Multi-infarct type (more common in men, affects small and medium sized vessels) or Binswanger disease (subcortical atherosclerotic encephalopathy with subcortical white matter lesions). Course is manifest by a stepwise progressive decline coinciding with clinical infarcts. Focal neurological deficits are also present.
Lowy body	Characterized by extreme sensitivity to antipsychotics, hallucinations (n.b visual), history of falls, extrapyramidal symptoms and parkinsonian features.
Drugs/toxins	Alcohol and illicit substances
Trauma	Head injuries or repetitive injuries such as dementia pugilistica (seen in boxers)
Infection	AIDS (direct effects of virus on brain and secondary to various infections/lesions), encephalitis, meningitis, Creutzfeldt-Jakob, and syphilis
Inflammation	Systemic lupus erythmatosus and multiple sclerosis
Neurological	Huntington disease (subcortical type with less language but more motor abnormalities and high rates of depression and psychosis), Parkinson disease (40% develop dementia and 50% become depressed), Pick disease (Pick bodies in frontotemporal areas, men > women, onset 4th decade), Wilson disease
Nutritional	B$_{12}$, folate, and thiamine (Korsakoff syndrome) deficiencies, pellagra
Metabolic	Thyroid and parathyroid disorders, Cushing syndrome, hepatic and renal failure (and dialysis).

There are several diagnoses to consider in this patient.

Major depression disorder (MDD) with secondary cognitive decline: Though MDD may cause a reversible cognitive decline (termed pseudodementia), he does not meet criteria for MDD. Pseudodementia can be differentiated from dementia by the presence of significant depressive symptoms. Additionally, demented patients may give approximate or grossly wrong answers to factual questions while depressed patients with pseudodementia put forth little effort and are content to say, "I don't know."

Dementia due to a medical condition or medications: Medications that may affect cognition (e.g., diphenhydramine) should be stopped. One must also rule out metabolic, nutritional, or infectious causes or chronic illnesses like severe anemia. His physical did not suggest an acute process, nor Parkinson disease. He has no HIV risk factors.

Vascular dementia: His risk factors include hypertension, atrial fibrillation, and high cholesterol. His neurologic exam is nonfocal, and he has no history of a CVA or TIA.

Alzheimer disease (AD): A gradual onset of dementia that progresses over time. Other possible causes should be ruled out. Clinical diagnosis may be made using consensus criteria but can only be confirmed at postmortem. His cardiologist started him on Warfarin.

CASE CONTINUED

His diphenhydramine was stopped with no change. CBC, TSH, RPR, chemistries, B_{12}, and folate were WNL. MRI showed scattered white matter hyperintensities.His cardiologist started him on warfarin.

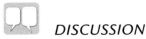

THOUGHT QUESTIONS

- What is the most likely cause of his dementia?
- What is the relevance of his white matter disease in diagnosing dementia?
- What nonmedical advice would you give regarding management of dementia?

DISCUSSION

Scattered white matter changes are common with aging, are associated with hypertension, and are not diagnostic of vascular dementia. 5% of patients over age 65 and ~20% over age 85 have a dementia; 60% of these are caused by AD, 15% by vascular dementia, 15% mixed AD and vascular dementia, and 10% "other." **Dr. P. has a gradually progressive course with no other**

cause for his symptoms, and thus probably has early AD. The patient and family should be counseled about assigning a health-care proxy, advanced directives, and possible consultation with an elder care attorney for financial planning. Another concern for the future is caregiver stress. The Alzheimer's Association is a good resource for workshops, education, and support groups.

QUESTIONS

41-1. Which is true about the genetics of AD?
- A. Most cases of AD are associated with a known mutation.
- B. The Apo E4 allele is associated with an increased risk of AD.
- C. The mutation associated with late onset AD has autosomal recessive inheritance.
- D. Genetic testing is necessary for making an accurate diagnosis.
- E. 10% of patients have a family history.

41-2. Which is diagnostic of vascular dementia?
- A. Scattered areas of decreased attenuation in the subcortical white matter on CT
- B. A well-defined CVA followed by cognitive decline
- C. A gradually progressive dementia with a new CVA with left-sided weakness and no worsening of cognition
- D. A sudden onset of right-sided weakness without decline in memory
- E. Slow gradual decline in functioning

41-3. Which of the following is accurate concerning AD?
- A. The average duration of illness is 2 to 3 years.
- B. It is the fourth leading cause of death in the United States
- C. AD occurs in 10% of people over 65.
- D. Early signs include disorientation and getting lost.
- E. Patients should not be told their diagnosis.

41-4. Which has been significantly studied in the treatment of Alzheimer disease?
- A. Acetylcholinesterase inhibitors
- B. Vitamin D
- C. Alkylating agents
- D. Testosterone
- E. Kava kava

ANSWERS

41-1. B. Most AD is sporadic. There are three known types of mutations in familial AD, which often presents with onset before age 60. Mutations in the presenillins on chromosome 1 and 14 and the APP gene on chromosome 21 are associated with autosomal dominant, variable penetrance inheritance. The Apo E gene is on chromosome 19, and exists in three isoforms (E2, E3, E4); E4 confers risk and E2 is protective. Apo E testing is not used clinically because the absence of E4 does not preclude AD, and as its presence does not inevitably lead to AD, thus it is not predictive. There is no reliably sensitive and specific genetic test for AD. However, it has been reported that up to 40% of patients have a family history of Alzheimer disease. Rarely transmission may occur in an autosomal dominant pattern. Definitive diagnosis can be made only on autopsy. In centers that specialize in memory disorders, the autopsy-confirmed accuracy in diagnosis is approximately 90% to 95%.

41-2. B. Vascular dementia often progresses in a stepwise manner, as opposed to a slow gradual decline as in AD, and presents with focal neurological signs. It is seen in patients with CVAs and a temporally associated cognitive decline. Patients may have CVAs that affect other areas but have no cognitive sequelae; this is not dementia. Binswanger disease is another type of vascular dementia that is caused by severe confluent microinfarctions of white matter with sparing of the cortex.

41-3. B. AD occurs in approximately 4% of people over 65. Its course begins with losing things, repetitiveness, forgetting conversations, and progresses to disorientation, first to time then place, getting lost in unfamiliar and then familiar places, and later needing assistance with dressing, bathing, then feeding and toileting. In the final stages, patients are unable to sit up and are nonverbal. It is the fourth leading cause of death in the United States, and about half die of pneumonia, often from aspiration. The duration of illness depends on how early the diagnosis is made, but is estimated at about 8 to 10 years. Research has shown that patients respond fairly well to learning their diagnosis. This allows the patient to be involved in the planning of his or her care, legal matters, and future wishes.

41-4. A. Alkylating agents are used in antineoplastic therapy. FDA-approved treatments for AD are cholinesterase inhibitors such as donepezil (Aricept), galanthamine (Reminyl), tacrine (Cognex), and rivastigmine (Exelon). Common side effects are GI upset and diarrhea from pro-cholinergic effects. They afford a 6-month improvement in functioning, but do not prevent progression. Antioxidants may slow progression, and given its benign side effect profile, vitamin E is often added to the medication regimen. This patient was on *warfarin,* and as vitamin E can cause platelet dysfunction, it probably would not be used. Other potentially neuroprotective agents that have been studied include estrogen (in women) and anti-inflammatory agents, but the literature does not yet support their use. Memantine (Namenda) is a glutamate antagonist that may be neuroprotective and is used in moderate to severe AD, unlike the cholinesterase inhibitors which are used in mild to moderate disease. Other agents under investigation include serotoninergic agents, calcium channel antagonists, MAO-B inhibitors (selegiline), and NSAIDs. COX-2 inhibitors have been studied for their potential neuroprotective effects but have recently caused serious concern as results have shown an increased incidence of CVAs. Herbal preparations of ginkgo biloba have been studied in AD with controversial findings. Kava kava (another herb) may help anxiety symptoms, but it has not been studied for the treatment of AD.

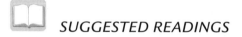 *SUGGESTED READINGS*

Marksteiner J. Schmidt R. Treatment strategies in Alzheimer's disease with a focus on early pharmacological interventions. *Drugs Aging.* 2004;21(7):415–426.

Caselli RJ, Beach TG, Yaari R, et al. Alzheimer's disease a century later. *J Clin Psychiatry.* 2006;67 (11):1784–1800.

Goedert M. Spillantini MG. A century of Alzheimer's disease. *Science.* 2006;314(5800):777–781.

"He Won't Leave the Neighbors Alone"

CC/ID: 70-year-old divorced man who is accompanied by his daughter to your clinic for assessment.

HPI: The daughter reveals that Mr. D. is increasingly **difficult to manage.** He telephones her several times a day and at night to complain about his neighbors in the downstairs apartment. He believes that they have a special "noise machine," which he can hear. He thinks that these neighbors are working "for the government" and are **trying to spy on him.** He has been complaining to the building superintendent, and his daughter is concerned that he will be evicted. This behavior began about 2 months ago and is getting worse. He is **easily agitated** and shouts loudly at the neighbors and his daughter. There are no symptoms of depressed mood, neurovegetative symptoms, or physical complaints.

PMHx: Hard of hearing, COPD, hypertension.

Meds: Diuretic, potassium, inhaler PRN

PPHx: None

FHx: His mother died from Alzheimer disease and his father from a stroke.

SHx: Mr. D. is divorced and lives alone in a rent-controlled apartment. He retired 5 years ago. He has one daughter who lives nearby. He used to smoke one pack per day for 25 years but gave up about 25 years ago. He denies alcohol or illicit substance abuse.

VS: Afebrile, BP 130/90, HR 72, RR 14

PE: *Gen:* hard of hearing. *Lungs:* B/L wheezes on auscultation. Otherwise exam normal.

MSE: *General:* appears his stated age; clothing unkempt with food stains. He is quite hard of hearing, and questions have to be repeated several times during the interview, though he is cooperative with the exam. *Speech:* loud at times, but normal rate and rhythm. *Affect:* labile and angry at times. *Mood:* "fine," though upon further elaboration states that he feels angry. *Thought process:* linear. *Thought content:* delusional, paranoid. Auditory hallucinations, but no visual or somatic hallucinations. No suicidal or homicidal ideation. *Cognitive function:* intact, MMSE 30/30. *Insight:* very limited.

THOUGHT QUESTIONS

- What is your differential diagnosis?
- What investigations would you like to order, if any?
- What is your plan for management?

DISCUSSION

The differential diagnosis for this patient may include the following:

Delusional disorder: Delusions tend to be nonbizarre and last at least 1 month and are not caused by another axis I disorder. This is a relatively stable diagnosis with few patients receiving a later change in diagnosis (e.g., to one of schizophrenia). The delusions can be persecutory, somatic, erotomanic, or grandiose in nature. Delusional disorder is rare, with a prevalence of 0.03%, usually presents in the fourth and fifth decades, and is slightly more common in women. It can be **differentiated from schizophrenia by the absence of prominent hallucinations and a lack of functional deterioration** (not related to delusional thinking). Patients with this disorder can be very difficult to manage. Males tend to develop paranoid delusions, while females tend to develop erotomanic delusions. There are increased rates of delusional disorder in the families of these patients.

Psychosis due to a general medical condition: The appearance of new onset psychotic symptoms in an older person warrants careful consideration of medical conditions such as neoplasms, metabolic or endocrine disorders, infections (including syphilis, HIV), medications, toxic agents, and seizure disorders or other neurologic disorders. If IQ has been affected by the underlying condition, more simple delusions may be evident. See below for a list of delusional subtypes and their associated conditions and causes.

TABLE 42-1   Medical Conditions Associated with Delusions

Types of Delusion	Associated Medical Condition
First rank symptoms (delusions of control, etc.)	Hypothyroidism, hepatic encephalopathy, cerebrovascular disease, temporal lobe epilepsy (TLE), and neoplasms
Misidentification syndromes	Capgras syndrome (belief that a familiar person has been replaced by an impostor): hypothyroidism, hepatic encephalopathy, and B_{12} deficiency Doppelganger syndrome (belief that another person has been transformed into oneself): migraine Fregoli syndrome (opposite of Capgras; belief that a stranger is actually a familiar person): TLE Intermetamorphosis syndrome: (person A becomes B, and B becomes C, etc): cerebral palsy
Jealousy (Othello syndrome)	Alcohol, Alzheimer disease, Huntington disease, MS, seizure disorder, and tumors
Erotomania (de Clerambault syndrome)	Seizure disorder, toxic psychoses, or tumors (e.g., meningiomas)
Infestation	Anemia (B_{12} deficiency, iron deficiency) or toxic psychoses
Persecution	Anticholinergic agents, heavy metal toxicity (e.g., manganese, thallium, and mercury), medications (tuberculosis agents, cortisone, cimetidine, levodopa, and tricyclic antidepressants), and Parkinson disease.

Dementia: Mr. D.'s mother had Alzheimer disease, and first-degree relatives are at greater risk. During their illness, approximately **one-third of patients with Alzheimer disease develop psychotic symptoms** such as delusions and hallucinations. Other causes of dementia include vascular lesions or alcohol. Mr. D. does not have evidence of cognitive impairment on exam and does not meet criteria for this disorder.

Late-onset schizophrenia: The "late onset" term may be used to describe the type of schizophrenia that appears after the age of 45. The lifetime risk of schizophrenia is equal in both genders but the peaks of age of onset differ between the sexes, with women having a second peak at age 62 years. Studies have shown that approximately **15% of schizophrenic patients may present over 45 years of age,** with approximately 12% presenting over 65 years. Risk factors for late schizophrenia include psychosocial factors such as bereavement, death of peers, retirement, financial stressors, and physical illness. Patients with late onset schizophrenia meet DSM-IV-TR criteria for schizophrenia with at least 6 months duration of symptoms and the onset of symptoms (including prodromal symptoms) at or after age 45 years. It usually has a chronic course, and patients are more likely to manifest delusions of persecution and auditory hallucinations (made worse by trouble hearing) and less likely to have affective flattening or thought disorder.

Evaluation: Laboratory tests to consider include ECG, CBC, SMA 20, UA, B$_{12}$, folate, TFTs, RPR, and Utox. A CT scan or MRI may be considered to out rule any vascular or neoplastic lesions. Any further investigations may be prompted by physical complaints such as a cough in a smoker.

CASE CONTINUED

Mr. D.'s labs and investigations are normal. **A diagnosis of late onset schizophrenia is made.** His management consists of a combination of neuroleptic agents and psychosocial interventions. Mr. D. is started on risperidone, and his symptoms decrease; he is monitored for extrapyramidal symptoms and tardive dyskinesia, as older persons are at increased risk. He is referred for audiometric assessment and is **fitted with a hearing aid.** He attends a local senior citizen's program, and his daughter attends a caregiver group.

QUESTIONS

42-1. Which of the following are the defense mechanisms used in delusional disorder?
   A. Reaction formation, sublimation, and repression
   B. Reaction formation, sublimation, and denial
   C. Reaction formation, projection, and denial
   D. Magical undoing, ambivalence, and isolation
   E. Repression, reaction formation, and displacement

42-2. Which of these is true of patients with late-onset schizophrenia?
   A. Premorbid personality traits may include dependent and histrionic types.
   B. Specific abnormalities are found on brain imaging.
   C. Those with sensory deficits are at increased risk.
   D. There is a greater prevalence of this disorder in their first-degree relatives.
   E. There are increased rates of delusional disorders in their relatives.

42-3. Which of the following is correct concerning the symptoms of late-onset schizophrenia?
   A. Auditory hallucinations are usually in the first person.
   B. Auditory hallucinations may be in the form of a running commentary.
   C. The delusions are mostly nonbizarre in nature.
   D. Mild depressive symptoms are rarely present.
   E. Generally, insight is not impaired.

42-4. Which of the following is accurate about late-onset schizophrenia?
   A. It occurs most frequently in older men.
   B. The rate of negative symptoms is the same as in early onset forms of the disorder.
   C. Neuropsychological testing may reveal deficits.
   D. It does not respond to the usual treatments.
   E. Noncompliance is the general rule.

 ANSWERS

42-1. C. The defense mechanisms displayed in delusional disorder include denial, reaction formation, and projection. Denial is the conscious refusal to acknowledge reality, reaction formation is feeling or behaving in a manner that is opposite to the underlying innate urges, and projection involves the assignment of unacceptable thoughts or emotions to others. The defense mechanisms associated with paranoia include projection and splitting. Repression, isolation, magical undoing, reaction formation, ambivalence, and displacement are all involved in OCD.

42-2. D. First-degree relatives of those with late-onset schizophrenia have a greater risk of developing this disorder than does the general population. Premorbid personality traits may include schizoid or paranoid types (cluster A). Nonspecific findings such as increased white matter abnormalities or slightly enlarged ventricles may be found on imaging. Although sensory deficits such as visual or auditory impairments have been found to be associated with this disorder, they have not been found to be specific risk factors. There is no increased rate of delusional disorder in relatives of probands with late-onset schizophrenia.

42-3. B. Although patients may present without auditory hallucinations, they tend to be derogatory in nature or in the form of a running commentary. The delusions are mostly bizarre in nature and are often persecutory in content. There is no difference between the earlier and later onset types regarding the lack of insight; that is, it is variable but frequently extremely limited. Though patients may also have some depressive symptoms and may be demoralized, depression is minor compared with the primary psychotic symptoms.

42-4. C. Late-onset schizophrenia usually responds to antipsychotics, psychosocial interventions, and behavioral treatments with the same frequency as early onset forms of the disorder. It may also require long-term, low-dose maintenance therapy, as many patients relapse when medications are stopped. It is reported to occur more frequently in older women than men. Symptoms commonly consist of organized and systematized persecutory delusions and auditory hallucinations. In comparison with those with earlier onset, these patients tend to have fewer negative symptoms, loosening of associations, or inappropriate affect. Neuropsychological testing may reveal deficits in those with late onset schizophrenia including impaired executive functioning, verbal ability, and complex perceptual, motor, abstraction, attention, sensory, and motor skills; however, memory is not usually impaired. Overall cognitive skills are similar to those found in earlier onset schizophrenia. In fact noncompliance is not the general rule, unlike in delusional disorder where depot medications may be necessary.

SUGGESTED READINGS

Riecher-Rossler A, Rossler W, Forstl H, et al. Late-onset schizophrenia and late paraphrenia. *Schizophr Bull.* 1995; 21(3): 345–354.

Howard R, Rabins PV, Seeman MV, et al. Late-onset schizophrenia and very-late-onset schizophrenia-like psychosis: an international consensus. The International Late-Onset Schizophrenia Group. *Am J Psychiatry.* 2000;157(2):172–178.

"Should Mom Be in a Home?"

CC/ID: An 82-year-old married female is brought in by her family to be evaluated for possible placement in a nursing home.

HPI: The family note that the patient was at her usual state ("an unhappy person" but functioning well) until approximately 2 years ago, when she sustained a compression fracture to her spine and was in **significant pain.** Her internist prescribed Fioricet (acetaminophen and **butalbital**) which allowed a fair amount of relief. Around the same time, she also complained of **depressed mood,** not enjoying anything, **poor sleep,** and **decreased energy** and concentration. She went to see a psychiatrist who prescribed **nefazodone,** but felt no significant relief despite doses of 750 mg per day (usual adult range 400 to 600 mg). Her family states that she is still depressed, with **anhedonia,** and poor energy, sleep, appetite, and concentration. They do not describe her as sedated, rather as amotivational, spending long periods of time on the couch. She has **difficulty with memory,** forgets conversations, repeats herself, and has lost interest in her activities of daily living (ADLs, e.g., toileting, feeding herself, hygiene) and instrumental activities of daily living (IADLs, e.g., shopping, managing finances). She is **not suicidal** and has no psychotic symptoms.

THOUGHT QUESTIONS

- At this point what is the differential diagnosis?
- What would be important to look for on physical examination?
- What would be important to look for on mental status examination?
- What laboratory tests should be ordered and why?

DISCUSSION

This patient has poor energy, appetite, and concentration, depressed mood, anhedonia, forgetfulness, and problems with ADLs and IADLs. This suggests a large range of differential diagnoses.

Major depression with secondary cognitive decline (so-called pseudodementia): She meets criteria for major depression. She may be a nonresponder to nefazodone and might require augmentation or a medication change.

Could there be another cause for her symptoms?

Dementia: She is forgetful, repetitive, and unable to manage ADLs and IADLs. This is a decline from her previous functioning. Is this dementia with depression? See Table 43-1 below to contrast features of dementia and pseudodementia.

Dementia or depression due to a general medical condition or medication: She is on a **high dose of nefazodone and an unknown amount of Fioricet**. Could either of these be a cause of her symptoms? Both are **sedating**, and the latter is specifically **cognitively dulling** (barbiturate). Could she have an **electrolyte imbalance** from a diuretic? Could she have **anemia** from a chronic illness? It is important to check labs, thyroid function, and vitamin levels. On physical examination you should look for illnesses such as thyroid disease, a CVA, severe CHF, severe anemia, hepatic or renal failure, or delirium (e.g., shifting levels of attention), any of which could explain some symptoms.

CASE CONTINUED

PMHx: Hypertension

Meds: "Water pill," nefazodone 250 TID, Fioricet PRN (unclear how many)

PPHx: None

SHx/FHx: Daughter treated for depression.

VS: BP 150/80, HR 72, and RR 12

PE: *HEENT:* WNL. *Lungs:* clear. *CV:* regular, no murmurs. *Abdomen:* soft, nontender, and no masses. *Neuro:* nonfocal.

TABLE 43-1   Depression vs. Pseudodementia

Parameters	Dementia	"Pseudodementia" due to depression
Awareness of onset	Family vaguely aware of onset, patient usually not aware or minimizes	Family usually aware of onset of symptoms; patient vaguely aware
Progression of symptoms	Slow	Slow
Specific complaints	Usually no complaints or vague	Tend to complain in detail of deficits and symptoms
Types of memory affected	Memory deficits usually affect short-term memory and learning of new material	Memory deficits appear to affect both short term and long term memory
Insight	Minimize their failures	Highlight failures, emphasize difficulties, and communicate distress
Behavior at psychological testing	Dismissed as unimportant; may confabulate	May manifest little effort to perform on testing, often answering "I don't know"
Results of psychological testing	Show consistent trouble on similar tasks	Marked variability in performance of similarly difficult tasks
Nocturnal excaerbation	Confusion may occur	Uncommon
Neuroimaging and neurophysiology	May have areas of cortical atrophy; EEG may show increased slow waves	No cortical atrophy or EEG changes consistent with dementia
Physical exam	May have focal findings, particularly in vascular dementias	Generally do not have focal findings

MSE: *General:* cooperative, pleasant, and approachable. *Speech:* spontaneous, with normal rate and tone. *Mood:* "I don't know." *Affect:* constricted, neutral. *Thought process:* somewhat repetitive. *Thought content/perceptions:* no suicidal ideation, no abnormal perceptions. *MMSE:* 21/30 (-3 time, -2 delayed recall, -3 world, -1 three-step command).

THOUGHT QUESTIONS

- How did her history, physical, and mental status examination affect your thinking?
- What would you do now?
- What level of care does she need?

 DISCUSSION

Laboratory tests are ordered. Because the antidepressant is an unusually high dose, especially for her age, the patient is instructed to taper it over 2 weeks. She has been taking Fioricet for $1^1/_2$ years, possibly multiple times per day, and the indication is no longer clear. It should be tapered off, and will require the help of her husband. She does not require hospital-level care because she is not suicidal or homicidal and has a supportive family to help with her medications, ADLs, and IADLs. You check her labs that afternoon, and they are unremarkable.

When she returns 2 weeks later she is brighter, still complains of decreased energy and motivation, but eats and sleeps better. Her concentration is fair and she is mildly repetitive. Her repeat MMSE is 27/30 (–1 time, –2 world). As she is brighter and her cognition has improved, you elect to have her return in 3 more weeks, and keep her off medications. When she returns, she looks even better. She is gardening, attending the senior center, going to lunch and lectures, and socializing. Her MMSE is now 30/30.

 QUESTIONS

43-1. In this case, which of the following is the most probable diagnosis?
   A. Major depressive disorder
   B. Dysthymia
   C. Alzheimer disease
   D. Substance-induced cognitive disorder
   E. Vascular dementia

43-2. What is an "adequate trial" of an antidepressant in the elderly?
   A. 1 week
   B. 2 weeks
   C. 4 weeks
   D. 12 weeks
   E. 24 weeks

43-3. Which of the following does not have potential cognitive or psychiatric side effects?
   A. Propranolol
   B. Prochlorperazine
   C. Nadolol
   D. Diphenhydramine
   E. Levofloxacin

43-4. Which of the following symptoms can be caused by medications?
   A. Depressed mood
   B. Anxiety
   C. Mania
   D. Paranoia
   E. Hallucinations
   F. Confusion
   G. All of the above

ANSWERS

43-1. D. At the time of presentation, this woman's symptomatology was due to side effects of medications. While elderly patients are more susceptible to the cognitive effects of medications, barbiturates can have profound effects on cognition even in young patients; they can affect attention, memory, and concentration. Further, as an addictive substance, chronic use of a barbiturate can result in anhedonia, apathy, amotivation, and depressed mood. Substance-induced cognitive disorders may take weeks to months to completely clear, especially in elderly patients with more fragile underlying cognitive states.

43-2. D. In the elderly, an adequate medication trial may be up to 12 weeks. This patient originally had a major depression, which likely resulted from the stress of fracturing her vertebrae and the associated pain. Although antidepressant and analgesic medications may have been indicated at the time, they should not have been continued and increased over such an extended period. It is often difficult to decide if an antidepressant has not worked because of an inadequate dose, or because the depression is not responsive to that medication. Once a person has had an adequate dose (e.g., sertraline up to 100–150 mg) for an adequate time, it is prudent to try another medication. The patient should show at least some minor response in the first few weeks. In a younger patient with a partial response after 4 weeks at a higher dose, it may be warranted to try an augmentation strategy. These decisions should be made in conjunction with the literature and with experience. As a rule, monotherapy is preferable in the elderly.

43-3. C, 43-4. G. Many medications have potential psychiatric side effects. Every year *The Medical Letter* publishes a list of these medications which fills four pages in a tiny font. It is important to recognize that medications commonly have psychiatric side effects, and to be aware of available resources to consult should one of your patients present with a new psychiatric complaint. Case reports, the *Physician's Desk Reference*, *The Medical Letter*, and the drug companies are all possible resources. Nadolol is potentially without psychiatric effects because it does not cross the blood brain barrier.

SUGGESTED READINGS

Drugs that may cause cognitive disorders in the elderly. *Med Lett.* (1093) Nov 27, 2000.

Drugs that may cause psychiatric symptoms. *Med Lett* (1134) July 8, 2002.

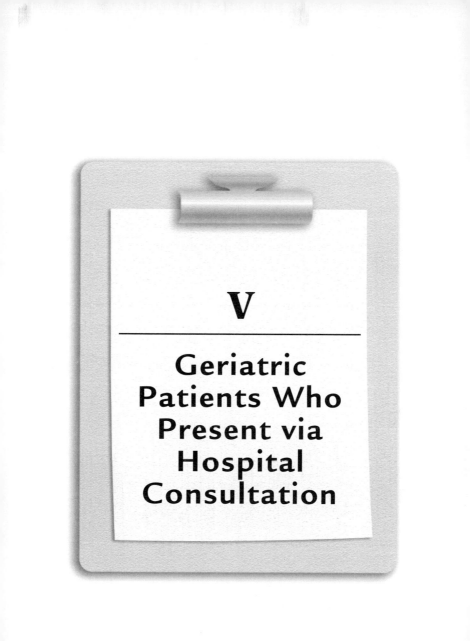

V

Geriatric Patients Who Present via Hospital Consultation

CASE 44

"We Can't Find Anything Wrong"

CC/ID: You are called to see a 75-year-old single man who is hospitalized on the medicine service. He has been complaining of abdominal pain, but the workup is negative. He is willing to have the consultation, but denies any concerns.

HPI: He was "fine" until 6 months ago when he was admitted for CHF, and then 3 months ago, for gastritis. Since then he hasn't felt "right"—he is **weak, sleepless, and uninterested in everything. His appetite is fair, but he has lost 10 lb.** He has **diffuse abdominal pain** that "comes and goes" but is "always there." Nothing makes it better or worse. He worries about constipation, and moves his bowels daily. He has had an endoscopy, an abdominal CT, a colonoscopy, and angiography, all of which were WNL.

THOUGHT QUESTIONS

- What is in your differential diagnosis at this point?

The differential diagnosis includes medical etiologies despite the negative workup, depression, somatization disorder, and substance-induced mood disorder.

CASE CONTINUED

PMHx: CHF, gastritis, hypertension, mild COPD

Meds: Propranolol, furosemide, digoxin, ranitidine

SHx/FHx: Lives alone, retired dockworker. Never married, one sister, no contact. Tobacco: 80 pack years, quit 6 months ago. EtOH: "a few beers," until 3 months ago.

PPHx: None

VS: Afebrile, BP 145/80, HR 72

PE: *CV, Lungs, and Neuro:* noncontributory. *Abdomen:* soft, mild diffuse tenderness

MSE: *General:* cooperative, frequently pointing to and holding his belly. *Speech:* normal rate and tone. *Mood:* "If it weren't for my stomach. . . ." *Affect:* reactive, pained. *Thought process:* logical and linear. *Thought content:* occasional suicidal ideation ("I won't lie to you doc, the way I feel, sometimes I wish I wouldn't wake up," "Sometimes I think of my service revolver . . . no, things aren't that bad"). No homicidal ideation, no auditory or visual hallucinations. *Insight:* fair. *MMSE:* 28/30 (transposed 2 letters on world).

THOUGHT QUESTIONS

- What did you learn from the history and physical examination?
- What laboratory tests would you order?

DISCUSSION

Depression may present with somatic symptoms, particularly in the elderly. This may be a cohort effect. **Medical illnesses can cause or exacerbate depression.** CHF can present as poor exercise tolerance, which may mimic poor motivation and energy. COPD may exacerbate or mimic anxiety. From the physical examination, it is clear that this patient is not acutely ill. His concentration is decreased on MMSE. His medications raise questions; for example, propranolol may cause depressive symptoms. He lives alone, has few social supports, and a possible history of EtOH abuse. His diet may be inadequate. Thus, check thyroid, B_{12}, folate, CBC, liver function, and chemistries. Other conditions should be considered as well.

Substance-induced mood disorder: This patient "stopped" his EtOH use after the gastritis. Was or is his substance use worse than described? How long has he been taking his current medications?

Nutritional disturbances can also lead to depressive symptoms: 3% to 18% of the elderly have low B_{12} levels. If the B_{12} level is less than 350 ng/L in a geriatric patient, check methylmalonic acid

(MMA) and homocysteine (Hc). MMA is elevated because B_{12} is a cofactor in its transformation to succinic acid. Hc is elevated because B_{12} is a cofactor in transforming Hc to methionine while turning methyltetrahydrofolate (mTHF) to THF. In folate deficiency, Hc is elevated.

Somatization disorder: This diagnosis requires a history of complaints in multiple organ symptoms since before the age of 30. There is no evidence to support this diagnosis in this patient. Major depression can also present as somatic complaints.

CASE CONTINUED

Labs: TSH WNL, CBC, SMA 7, LFTs WNL, B_{12} 395, folate 675.

You obtain further information from the patient and, with his consent, from his landlady who "keeps an eye on him." He was a heavy drinker but has been sober for 6 months. He was on propranolol for 10 years. It was supposed to have been stopped because of a reactive component to his COPD.

THOUGHT QUESTIONS

- What is your diagnosis?
- Would you start an antidepressant? When?
- What are your concerns about discharge?

DISCUSSION

With the further history and lab results, his **most likely diagnosis is major depression.** An antidepressant should be started now. He must be counseled that it may take up to 12 weeks to have a full effect. Medications are safe, tolerated, and efficacious in the elderly, as is psychotherapy. **The elderly are prone to side effects, but can tolerate medications if you "start low and go slow (Table 44-1)."** Given his cardiac concerns, a medication that does not affect cardiac conduction (e.g., an SSRI) should be chosen. He will need to be followed to evaluate the efficacy of and titrate the medication as needed. He also may benefit from psychotherapy. The most important thing in considering his discharge planning is his suicide risk.

TABLE **44-1**   Review of Antidepresants in the Elderly

Agent	Starting dose	Usual max dose	Supplied	Precautions/ Comments
SSRIs				
Citalopram (Celexa)	10 mg	20–40 mg	20, 40 mg tabs	Half life ~36h
Escitalopram (Lexapro)	5 mg	20–30 mg	5, 10, 20 mg tabs	Smaller dosing range –10 mg may well be effective dose
Sertraline (Zoloft)	25 mg	50–150 mg	25, 50, 100mg	Half-life in elderly ~34 h; sig. decreased clearance with liver dysfunction.
Fluoxetine (Prozac)	10 mg	20–40 mg	10, 20 mg capsules; 20 mg/ 5mL liquid	Very long half-life (1–4 days) with active metabolite (half life 7–15 days); sig. decreased clearance with liver dysfunction
Paroxetine (Paxil)	5 mg	20–30 mg	10, 20, 30 mg tabs	Half-life is prolonged in the elderly ranging from 36 to 90 h; decreased clearance with liver dysfunction More sedating/ anticholinergic effects than other SSRIs
SNRIs				
Venlafaxine (Effexor)	12.5 to 37.5XR	150 mg	25, 37.5, 50, 75, 100 mg tabs XR: 37.5, 75 or 150 mg	May be associated with hypertension. May need to go up to 225 mg. Acts like an SSRI until doses over ~200 mg. Short half-life for drug and active metabolite. Decreased dosage with hepatic or renal impairment. Not highly protein bound.
Duloxetine (Cymbalta)	20 mg	60 mg	20, 30, 60 mg caps	Elimination half-life ~17 h, metabolized by CYP 2D6 and 1A2.

(Continued)

TABLE **44-1**   Review of Antidepresants in the Elderly (*continued*)

Agent	Starting dose	Usual max dose	Supplied	Precautions/ Comments
Duloxetine (Cymbalta) (*Cont.*)				Not recommended in ESRD or hepatic insufficiency. Cimetidine and quinolones may increase levels (they inhibit 1A2). Highly protein bound.
SNRIs				
Bupropion (Wellbutrin)	37.5– 75 mg	200–300 mg	75, 100 mg tabs SR: 100, 150, 200 mg tabs XL: 150, 300 mg tabs	Half-life of parent ~20 h, but multiple active metabolites. Hepatically metabolized and excreted by the kidney so use with caution in hepatic or renal dysfunction. Extra caution in those on L-DOPA.
Mirtazapine (Remeron)	7.5 mg	15–45 mg	15, 30, 45 mg tabs	Half-life ~40 h, clearance decreased in elderly, particularly men. Metabolism and clearance decreased with hepatic and renal insufficiency so lower doses recommended.

QUESTIONS

44-1. What is the prevalence of major depression in the elderly?
- A. 1%
- B. 25%
- C. 50%
- D. 75%
- E. 90%

44-2. Which is associated with increased risk of suicide in the elderly?

    A. Good social supports
    B. African American
    C. Married
    D. Low level of education
    E. Male

44-3. After stopping alcohol, how long does it take to be sure that a depression isn't secondary to the alcohol?

    A. 2 days
    B. 1 week
    C. 4 weeks
    D. 6 months
    E. 1 year

44-4. Which of the following is not likely to directly cause or mimic depression?

    A. Iron deficiency anemia
    B. Pancreatic cancer
    C. Multiple sclerosis
    D. CVA
    E. Poliomyelitis

ANSWERS

44-1. A. The prevalence of major depression in the elderly is 1% (less than in adults), but 15% of elderly people have depressive symptoms. In nursing home residents and hospitalized elderly, this increases to approximately 40%. Elderly depression is more often chronic and recurrent, but it is treatable in 70% to 80% of cases. Mental health services are underused, especially among people over 65, and suicide rates in the elderly are higher than in other adults.

44-2. E. In the overall population, the rates of suicide are about 12 in 100,000; in the elderly they are about 20 in 100,000; in elderly men they are 41 in 100,000. Very frequently, elderly people who commit suicide are not receiving psychiatric care, but have communicated their distress to someone, frequently an internist. Being white, male, single, and having medical problems, few social supports, and access to a weapon are all risk factors.

44-3. C. It takes at least 1 month free of alcohol to reverse all potential mood symptoms. Depression diagnosed within 4 weeks of significant alcohol abuse may be diagnosed as substance induced. After 4 weeks, other etiologies must be sought.

44-4. E. Depression can be caused or mimicked by many medical illnesses. Strokes (especially left hemisphere near frontal pole), Parkinson disease (50%), and dementing illnesses are common causes. Dementia may mimic depression; for example, in Alzheimer disease, patients complain of decreased interests, apathy, poor concentration, and decreased energy. Hypothyroidism and certain cancers (e.g., pancreatic) can also present as depression. Anemia or CHF can mimic depression because of overlapping symptoms of weakness, fatigue, and anxiety. Although patients with poliomyelitis may become depressed, it does not directly cause or mimic depression.

SUGGESTED READINGS

Roose SP, Sackeim HA, et al. Antidepressant pharmacotherapy in the treatment of depression in the very old: a randomized, placebo-controlled trial. *Am J Psychiatry*. 2004;161(11): 2050–2059.

Alexopoulos GS, Jeste DV, et al. The expert consensus guideline series. Treatment of dementia and its behavioral disturbances. Introduction: methods, commentary, and summary. *Postgrad Med*. 2005;Spec No: 6–22.

Sirey JA, Bruce ML, et al. The Treatment Initiation Program: an intervention to improve depression outcomes in older adults. *Am J Psychiatry*. 2005;162(1):18418–6.

"He Refuses to Eat"

CC/ID: 57-year-old married man who you are asked to see by the inpatient medical team because he is refusing to eat and has lost over 20 lb.

HPI: When questioned Mr. A. reveals that **he has stopped eating because he believes that his bowels have ceased to function and are rotting.** According to his wife, these symptoms started insidiously about 5 weeks ago and have become progressively worse. Until recently he was taking liquid preparations of food, but now he believes his urinary system is also rotting. His wife has been crushing his medications into these liquids, which he has been refusing for the past 2 days. His wife also confirmed that he has become increasingly **withdrawn** over the past month, with **low energy, decreased libido, poor sleep with early morning awakening,** and decreased interest and pleasure in his usual activities.

PMHx: Hypertension controlled on medications.

Meds: ACE inhibitor

PPHx: One episode of major depression in his late 20s that responded to tricyclics. No history of suicidal or homicidal behaviors.

FHx: Significant for hypertension and CVD. Parents died from MIs.

SHx: Was in the military for 3 years, no combat. Worked as a mechanic, retired earlier this year. Two daughters live nearby. Married for 35 years. No EtOH or illicit substance use.

VS: Afebrile, BP 130/92, HR 90, RR 14

PE: *Gen:* thin, paucity of subcutaneous fat, on IV fluids. *HEENT:* tongue coated, PERRLA. *CV:* no murmurs. *Lungs:* clear to auscultation and percussion. *Abdomen:* scaphoid, soft, nontender, and no masses, positive for bowel sounds. *Neuro:* nonfocal.

Labs: Elevated BUN and creatinine, low albumin. CBC, UA, TFTs, B_{12}, folate, VDRL, ECG, all WNL. CT scan and GI workup negative.

MSE: *General:* appears older than stated age, poor eye contact, withdrawn, *Speech:* low volume and tonality. Intermittent deep sighing. *Affect:* blunted, dysphoric, suspicious. *Mood:* "Bad." PMR+. *Thought process:* linear. *Thought content:* somatic delusions, guilty, hopeless, and pessimistic. Perceptual disturbances: Olfactory and somatic hallucinations, says he can feel and smell his bowels disintegrating. Denies active suicidal ideations, but admits to passive ideations. *Cognitive function:* attention and concentration are impaired, but fully oriented. *Insight:* very limited, refusing to consider that there could be any psychiatric problem or treatments.

THOUGHT QUESTIONS

- What is your differential diagnosis at this point?
- What investigations would you like to have seen performed?
- How would you treat this man?

DISCUSSION

Several differential diagnoses should be considered.

Mood disorder due to a general medical condition: Although weight loss and anorexia are important features of major depression, these symptoms could be caused by a medical condition such as an occult cancer. There are many conditions and medications that are associated with the development of depression. To make this diagnosis, there must be evidence from the history, physical examination, or labs that the mood disorder is caused directly by the physiological consequences of a medical condition.

Major depressive disorder (MDD), recurrent: Mr. A. meets the criteria for this disorder; **he has melancholic features typified by loss of pleasure in almost all activities, lack of reactivity to usually pleasurable events, diurnal mood variation (mood worse in the morning), early morning wakening, psychomotor retardation, anorexia, weight loss, and inappropriate guilt.** Prodromal periods may last weeks to months. Mr. A. has experienced these symptoms for over 2 weeks. About **15% of patients with melancholic depression develop psychotic features.** Mood disorders may be specified by severity, presence of psychotic features, remission status, and with or without full recovery between episodes. Additional specifiers include descriptors such as melancholia, atypical features, catatonia, seasonal onset pattern, rapid cycling, or with postpartum onset. Atypical features include increased appetite, weight gain, hypersomnia, hypersensitivity to rejection, and low energy, but with mood reactivity.

CASE CONTINUED

His condition is cause for serious concern. Given his physical and laboratory findings, you are convinced that this is a recurrence of his mood disorder. The treatment options are medications

TABLE 45-1   Electroconvulsive Therapy (ECT)

Indications	Treatment-resistant major depression, or major depression in a patient who cannot tolerate medications
	Major depression with severe suicidal ideation, agitation, psychosis, or serious medical compromise
	Bipolar disorder: mania, mixed episodes, or depressed
	Schizophrenia: treatment resistant or catatonic subtype
	Schizoaffective disorder
	Schizophreniform disorders
	Psychosis NOS with similar symptoms to above disorders
	Depression in Parkinson disease ($+/-$ psychosis)
	Neuroleptic malignant syndrome
	Intractable seizures
Predictors of response	**Lower response**
	Medication resistant depression
	Major depression with personality disorders
	Better response
	Elderly with psychotic depression
	Catatonic symptoms
	Shorter illness and less medication nonresponse
Side effects	Mortality rate of general anesthesia is 0.002%. Transient autonomic disturbances (BP, pulse) or arrhythmias. Rare reports of MI, tardive seizures/status. Common nonserious side effects include headaches, muscle aches, and nausea. Cognitive impairment includes acute confusion at time of treatment and both anterograde and retrograde amnesia (most serious)
Contraindications	Acute MI, significant arrhythmias, severe CHF, and raised intracranial pressure (especially if intracranial mass)

TABLE 45-2   Treatment Strategies for Resistant Depression

Ensure compliance with medications
Adequate therapeutic doses for at least 6–8 weeks
Consider change of class of medication (e.g., from SSRI to a SNRI)
Reconsider diagnosis
Add additional antidepressant agent (e.g., bupropion to an SSRI, a TCA to an SSRI)
Add augmenting agent such as antipsychotic, lithium or other mood stabilizer, methylphenidate (Ritalin), or thyroid supplement T3 (25–50 μg per day)

(an antidepressant in combination with an antipsychotic) or ECT. After talking to his wife, he agrees to transfer to the psychiatric unit for a course of ECT. Pre-ECT workup includes routine labs and an ECG. After three treatments and low-dose antipsychotics, he begins to improve. Psychotherapy is begun, and he completes his course of ECT with good effect. See Table 45-1 for review of ECT and Table 45-2 for treatments for resistant depression.

 QUESTIONS

45-1. Which of the following is correct about MDD?
A. About 25% develop psychotic symptoms.
B. Suicide risk should be monitored throughout treatment.
C. Suicide rates may reach 50%.
D. About 5% of patients seen in primary care clinics have MDD.
E. Prophylaxis may be considered if there has been one episode in the past 5 years.

45-2. Which of the following may have depression as a presenting symptom?
A. Laryngeal carcinoma
B. Cellulitis
C. Osteoporosis
D. Guillain-Barré syndrome
E. Addison disease

45-3. Which of the following statements is correct concerning ECT?
A. It has no effects on motor symptoms in Parkinson disease.
B. Initial response rates for depression are usually 50%.
C. Reported results in cerebrovascular disease are mixed.

    D. Relapse of depression after ECT is less than 25%.
    E. Psychoactive medications need to be stopped during a course of ECT.

45-4. How does the seizure relate to the efficacy of ECT?
    A. Response is directly related to the length of the seizure.
    B. The supra threshold stimulus may be most important in unilateral ECT
    C. Seizures with a higher amplitude spike and wave activity have worse outcomes.
    D. Retrograde amnesia is less significant with bilateral compared with unilateral electrode placement.
    E. The seizure threshold may increase by as much as 200% over the course of an ECT treatment.

ANSWERS

45-1. B. Major depression has a lifetime prevalence of about 15%, but this may reach 25% in women. Suicide is always a concern at every stage of the depressive illness, particularly as medication begins to take effect and the patient is more energized prior to becoming euthymic. Rates of suicide in major depression are approximately 15%. Up to 10% of primary care patients may have MDD, and this increases to about 15% of hospital inpatients (nonpsychiatric). About 15% of patients with depression may develop psychotic features (hallucinations or delusions). Medications may take 2 to 4 weeks to show an effect and up to 12 weeks for a maximum effect. ECT is often successful in patients with delusional depression and has a more rapid onset of action than medications. Prophylaxis should be considered if there have been two or more episodes in the preceding 5 years, particularly in a patient with a family history.

45-2. E. Addison's disease the list of pharmacologic agents and diseases associated with depressive symptoms is long, but important causes may include medications (steroids, reserpine, thiazides, cimetidine, indomethacin), some chemotherapeutic agents, endocrine disorders (diabetes mellitus, Cushing disease, Addison disease, hypo/hyperthyroid, hyperparathyroid, hypopituitarism), infections (syphilis, HIV/AIDS, mononucleosis, viral hepatitis, toxoplasmosis, influenza), collagen disorders (SLE, rheumatoid arthritis), cancers (abdominal or metastatic), nutritional causes (pellagra, pernicious anemia), and many neurological conditions (multiple sclerosis, Parkinson disease, head injury, seizures, cerebrovascular disease).

45-3. C. Reported results in cerebrovascular disease are mixed and may reflect issues of study design. Overall, those with significant confluent white matter lesions on MRI or several lesions in the basal ganglia/reticular formation or the frontal cortex affecting functioning are usually associated with poor medication outcome, but ECT studies are unclear. Poststroke depression is common with reported rates of up to 23% depending on the location of the lesion. There are case reports of ECT being helpful in these cases. ECT may not only treat the significant depression reported in Parkinson disease (rates reported up to 50%), but it has been reported to improve motor function independently of its effects on mood or psychosis; these effects may last weeks to months. Response rates of up to 80% to 90% have been reported but this falls to 50% to 60% in those who have failed an adequate trial of medications. Relapse rates after ECT may reach over 50% in the year following treatment; this is particularly evident in those who have failed a trial of TCAs before ECT. Others at a higher risk of relapse include older patients with psychotic depression. Previously it was believed that most if not all psychoactive medications should be stopped during ECT. Now, most medications may be given except those that significantly alter the seizure threshold such as benzodiazepines, barbiturates, or anticonvulsants. Lithium should be stopped or given in very low doses to avoid increased the risk of confusion or increased seizures. Antipsychotics are now thought be safe and may be beneficial in some cases, as may be most antidepressants. These agents may help prevent relapse after ECT.

45-4. B. Stimulus dosing relative to seizure threshold can affect recovery in both unilateral and bilateral ECT. It is the intensity of supra threshold stimulus, not the actual stimulus dose, that appears to affect the outcome with unilateral ECT and also cognitive side effects in both types of ECT. It has been reported that there is a strong dose-response relationship for unilateral ECT. In fact, if unilateral ECT is given at markedly supra threshold levels it can be as efficacious as bilateral ECT, but the risk of cognitive deficits also increases. The length of seizure is monitored during treatment and seizures that last less than 15 seconds are less likely to be therapeutic. Extended seizures may also be harmful and those >3 minutes should be terminated using IV medications such as lorazepam. It has also been reported that seizures with higher amplitude spike and wave activity are associated with better clinical outcomes. Relapse rates may reach 50% up to 1 year after ECT. Maintenance ECT may be used to prevent relapse or to maintain euthymia. Tapering of treatments may also help prevent relapse. There are several types of amnesia described as being associated with ECT: (i) Confusion around the actual treatment itself; (ii) anterograde amnesia (impaired formation of new memories after the treatment); and (iii) retrograde amnesia (impaired memory for material before the treatment). This latter type of amnesia can be the most impairing of the three. However, severe depression or psychosis prior to ECT treatment may also affect an individual's cognitive function. Patients with delirium or dementia are at increased risk of developing acute confusion. There is a higher rate of relapse in those who had had two or more episodes of depression, with rates of up to 85% at 3 years reported from placebo studies. Patients can continue with maintenance ECT on an outpatient basis, or antidepressants could be started during or after a course of ECT. Maintenance ECT is usually reserved for those who have failed trials with or are too sensitive to medications. There is evidence that this type of depression responds better to tricyclics or combinations of tricyclics and antipsychotics, which appear to be successful in both younger and older patients. Medication should be continued for 6 to 9 months to avoid relapse. Continued symptoms would warrant ongoing and more aggressive treatment. Medications should be tapered slowly to avoid unpleasant withdrawal phenomena.

SUGGESTED READINGS

Alexopolous GS , Katz IR, Reynolds CF III, et al. The expert consensus guideline series. Pharmacotherapy of depressive disorders in older patients. *Postgrad Med.* 2001 Oct:1–86.

Alexopolous GS, Streim J, Carpenter D, et al. Using antipsychotic agents in older patients. *J Clin Psychiatry.* 2004;65(Suppl 2): 5–99.

Ganguli, M. For debate: the evidence for electroconvulsive therapy (ect) in the treatment of severe late-life depression. *Int Psychogeriatric.* 2007;19(1):9–10.

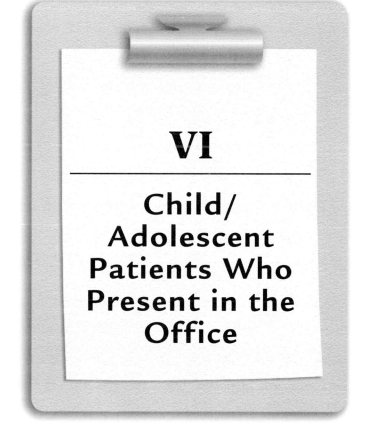

VI

Child/ Adolescent Patients Who Present in the Office

"My Son Isn't Doing Well in School"

 CC/ID: 7-year-old boy brought in by his mother at the school's recommendation.

HPI: Mrs. R. describes T.R. as exuberant and "always running." He did well at a preschool where "free play was encouraged." Since he started 1st grade, he has had difficulty sitting still, and he gets up multiple times during class. There have been some complaints from the teachers, and his mother is concerned that the school is too strict or isn't the right environment for him.

THOUGHT QUESTION

- What other information do you need to complete your evaluation?

DISCUSSION

You obtain written permission to speak to the teacher, who describes T.R. as "on the go." He always **fidgets** and frequently leaves his seat. On a class trip he had a great deal of difficulty staying with the group and was frequently running around the exhibit hall. She says that he is a nice child who at times has difficulty with peers because he is **unable to wait** his turn and blurts out answers. He has had a couple of playground **accidents** because of inattention to what he is doing.

CASE CONTINUED

PMHx: None

Meds: None

FHx: Father had a "hard time in school," stopped after 11th grade, and owns a house painting business. Grandfather used EtOH.

DevHx: Unremarkable pregnancy, delivery, milestones, toilet training.

VS: WNL

PE: Unremarkable

Labs: Unremarkable

MSE: *General:* Appears his age; shirt half tucked in, shoes untied; well-related. *Behavior:* **Restless,** trying to climb on file cabinets and **easily distracted** by noises outside. *Speech and language:* unremarkable. *Mood:* no depressed mood or anxiety, no elatedness. His favorite thing about school is recess. No signs consistent with delusions or hallucinations.

 THOUGHT QUESTIONS

■ What is the differential diagnosis for this constellation of symptoms?

■ What risk factors are important in this case?

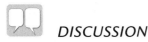 *DISCUSSION*

To make a diagnosis of ADHD, there must be at least 6 months of either six inattentive or six hyperactive/impulsive symptoms (Table 46-1). The symptoms must be maladaptive, inconsistent with the child's developmental level, and must cause functional impairment. ADHD is not usually diagnosed until the child enters school; this is probably because of more stringent behavioral expectations than are present at home. **It is important to differentiate the normal, age-appropriate exuberance and attention span of a toddler/preschooler from a developmentally inappropriate problem.** It is crucial to get corroborative information from the school or other programs which the child attends.

TABLE **46-1**   Criteria for ADHD

Inattention	Hyperactivity
Fails to give close attention to details or makes careless errors in schoolwork, etc.	Fidgets or squirms Talks excessively
Has difficulty sustaining attention in tasks or play	Has difficulty playing quietly
Does not seem to listen when spoken to directly	Is "on the go," as if "driven by a motor"
Does not follow through on instructions and fails to finish chores or work (not because of opposition or not understanding)	Runs or climbs excessively in inappropriate situations (adolescents may be subjectively restless)
Avoids or dislikes tasks that require sustained mental effort	Leaves seat in class or when sitting still is expected
Has difficulty organizing tasks and activities	Is impulsive
Loses necessary things (toys, books, etc.)	Blurts out answers
Is easily distracted by extraneous stimuli	Has difficulty awaiting turn
Is forgetful in daily activities	Interrupts or intrudes on others

Adapted from American Psychiatric Association. *Task Force on DSM-IV. Diagnostic and statistical manual of mental disorders: DSM-IV.* 4th ed. Washington, DC: American Psychiatric Association, 1994.

In this case, the **family history is suggestive of possible ADHD** in the father; this would be important to assess, as a family history is a risk factor. It is also important to assess the child's hearing and vision, and whether he has a nutritional deficiency, thyroid abnormality, or substance-induced problem. For instance, he might be on a medication that makes him akathetic (e.g., antihistamines), or he might be drinking large amounts of caffeinated soda. The differential diagnosis also includes oppositional defiant disorder (a pattern of defiant behavior associated with arguing with adults, blaming others, and spitefulness) or conduct disorder (persistent pattern of behavior in which the basic rights of others or age appropriate norms are violated; e.g., physical cruelty, torturing animals, destroying property). The symptoms of ADHD have considerable overlap with other disorders. Therefore, it is crucial to see the symptoms in the context of the child's developmental stage, and to look for other possible causes. This child meets criteria for ADHD, hyperactive impulsive subtype.

CASE CONTINUED

After careful discussion with his parents and teachers, you recommend a trial of medication in combination with individual and family therapy sessions. Other treatment interventions include psychoeducation and general support. Three months later his parents and teachers report a significant improvement in his behavior and schoolwork.

QUESTIONS

46-1. Which of the following is a risk factor for ADHD?
A. Family history of schizophrenia
B. Family history of OCD
C. Family history of alcohol abuse
D. High socioeconomic status
E. Female gender

46-2. Which of the following is a correct statement about ADHD?
A. Twin studies show 15% concordance across studies.
B. Major depression is seen less often in ADHD than in the general population.
C. Heritability is not supported by adoption studies.
D. Genetic studies show a two- to eightfold increased risk for ADHD in families with the disorder.
E. Schizotypal personality disorder is seen more often in families with ADHD than in the general population.

46-3. Which of the following has been evaluated as a genetic mechanism of ADHD?
A. Dopamine transporter and receptor genes
B. Nondisjunction of chromosome 21
C. 45X0
D. Trinucleotide repeat on the short arm of chromosome 4
E. A point mutation on chromosome 11

46-4. Which of the following is correct about ADHD?
A. The prevalence of ADHD is 15% in the United States.
B. The sex ratio is 2:1 female to male.
C. Comorbid psychiatric illnesses are rare.
D. The incidence of Tourette syndrome is elevated.
E. Children with ADHD are no more likely to have a serious accident than the general population.

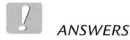

ANSWERS

46-1. C. Family history of ADHD, family history of alcohol abuse, family discord, low socioeconomic status, and male gender are risk factors for ADHD. Family history of OCD has not been associated with ADHD.

46-2. D. Genetic studies show a two- to eightfold increased risk for ADHD within families, and twin studies show a 60% to 80% concordance rate. Heritability is supported by adoption studies, with the most probable model being polygenic. Disorders seen comorbid with ADHD include bipolar disorder, conduct disorder, learning disabilities, and major depression. Schizotypal personality disorder is more frequent in family members of patients with schizophrenia, not ADHD.

46-3. A. Many biological studies of ADHD have examined catecholamines, and the dopamine transporter gene has been most implicated. Hyperdopaminergic animal knockout models produce hyperlocomotion. Other studies have found a mutation in the dopamine receptor D_4 gene (associated with novelty seeking and impulsivity). The molecular genetics of ADHD are not consistently replicated, and most models account for a minority of cases. It is interesting that mutations in the thyroid receptor–b gene cause resistance to thyroid hormone and hyperactivity. Nondisjunction of chromosome 21 is a cause of Down syndrome, and trinucleotide repeats on chromosome 4 are found in Huntington disease. 45X0 is the genotype of Turner syndrome (ovarian dysgenesis, short stature, webbed neck, and cardiac abnormalities).

46-4. D. Tourette syndrome is seen in about 2% of children with ADHD, which is much higher than the general population; reciprocally 50% of people with Tourette syndrome have ADHD. The prevalence of ADHD is 3% to 5% in the United States. It is lower in the United Kingdom because of narrower criteria. The sex ratio is at least 2:1 male to female. Comorbid psychiatric illnesses are very common and include oppositional defiant disorder (a pattern of defiant behavior associated with arguing with adults, blaming others, and spitefulness, without meeting criteria for conduct disorder), conduct disorder (persistent pattern of behavior in which the basic rights of others or age-appropriate norms are violated; e.g., physical cruelty, torturing animals, and destroying property), anxiety disorders, mood disorders, and learning disorders. ADHD is associated with increased accidents. Excessive activity, impulsivity, and inattention make children accident prone and increase their risk of car accidents in adolescence.

SUGGESTED READING

Daly BP, Creed T, Xanthopoulos M, et al. Psychosocial treatments for children with attention deficit/hyperactivity disorder. *Neuropsychol Rev*. 2007;17(1)73–89.

CASE 47

"My Daughter Isn't Doing Well in School"

CC/ID: 8-year-old girl brought in by her mother at the school's recommendation.

HPI: Mrs. E. describes her daughter as "spacey." She says that she **doesn't seem to listen** and won't follow through on chores or tasks. She frequently can't find her homework, bus pass, and knapsack when preparing for school. She has **difficulty with organization,** and since the time homework was first assigned in 2nd grade, the evenings have been tense. She is often distracted. For example, she goes for a glass of water and doesn't return, having found some crayons or a comic book on the table. You obtain permission to call the school and speak to the teacher, who describes D.E. as "off in her own world." She **frequently makes careless errors** in her work, and has **difficulty completing projects,** often starting one thing and ending up in another group doing something else. She has a hard time staying in her seat; she fidgets and may blurt out answers. Recently she has had more difficulty, because the projects require more focused attention.

PMHx: None

PSHx: None

Meds: None

FHx: Younger brother, 4 years old, is "a bit wild."

DevHx: Unremarkable pregnancy and delivery, slightly delayed gross motor skills, "a little clumsy."

VS: WNL

PE: Unremarkable

Labs: Unremarkable

MSE: *General:* Appears stated age, glasses awry, shoelaces untied, pleasant, well-related. *Behavior:* Restless in chair, going from one game to another in the office. *Speech and language:* WNL. *Mood:* denies depressed mood or anxiety, no elation is evident. Her least favorite thing about school is reading time. No psychotic symptoms and not internally preoccupied.

THOUGHT QUESTIONS

- What is your differential diagnosis?
- What might you want to clarify?

DISCUSSION

Girls with ADHD are more often diagnosed with the inattentive than hyperactive subtype. This may reflect variability in magnitude of symptoms in boys and girls. D.E. has more than six inattentive symptoms, as well as impulsive and hyperactive symptoms (see previous case for symptoms).

The teacher describes her as "being in her own world." This may be seen in a number of disorders, including absence seizures, which can interfere with attention, concentration, and school performance. Absence seizures are characterized by sudden unresponsiveness that may be accompanied by automatisms. They rarely last more than 10 seconds, and are not associated with an aura or postictal confusion. They may be mistaken for daydreaming or inattention. Another possibility is Asperger syndrome, which is characterized by poor interpersonal interactions and emotional reciprocity, and repetitive stereotyped interests or activities. Autistic disorder shares these characteristics, but is also associated with severe language impairment and impaired intellectual functioning. In autistic disorder, the abnormalities are usually noted in infancy, whereas in Asperger syndrome they may be picked up later, may not need as extensive interventions, and usually have a better outcome. Severe depression or psychotic disorders may also make a child look withdrawn.

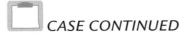

CASE CONTINUED

Although D.E. sometimes has had difficulty with peers because of impulsive behavior, she was well-related and formed normal attachments with family. She did not have episodes of staring into space or those resembling absence seizures. She had no evidence of psychotic symptoms and her mood has been euthymic, especially during the school holidays. Her teacher provided further clarification, saying that D.E. was easily distracted, often looking out the window, getting up for a drink of water, or doodling in class. She received a full educational assessment and was found to be quite bright, but with a degree of dyslexia.

THOUGHT QUESTION

- How would you treat this child?

DISCUSSION

D.E. was treated with methylphenidate (Ritalin), a stimulant. Approximately 75% of children manifest improved attention with stimulant medications (e.g., methylphenidate or dextroamphetamine). Side effects are usually very mild. See Table 47-1 for medication options for ADHD. D.E.'s parents attended training sessions to learn to use behavior modification techniques and reward good behavior, and to make clear and consistent rules. Her teachers, as part of a larger state funded project, were given behavioral training as well. She was also tutored individually for dyslexia. She did well, and was able to interact better with her peers.

TABLE 47-1   Medication Options for ADHD

Medication	Brands	Mechanism of Action	Side Effects
Methylphenidate	Ritalin, Concerta	Releases dopamine (DA) and norepinephrine (NE)	Decreased appetite, headache, weight loss, irritability, decreased growth rate, mild increase in BP and pulse, exacerbation of tics or psychosis

(Continued)

TABLE 47-1 Medication Options for ADHD (*continued*)

Medication	Brands	Mechanism of Action	Side Effects
Dextroamphetamine	Dexedrine, Adderall	Blocks DA and NE reuptake from the synapse, inhibits monoamine oxidase, and facilitates release of catecholamines	Same as above
Atomoxetine	Strattera	Inhibits NE reuptake	Decreased appetite, nausea, vomiting, fatigue, slowed rate of growth, mild increase in BP and pulse; rare hepatic injury
Buproprion	Wellbutrin	Unclear, but probably inhibits dopamine reuptake and seems to enhance NE functional activity	Weight loss, insomnia, anxiety, and seizure; not approved by FDA for children

 QUESTIONS

47-1. Which of the following is used as first line pharmacotherapy for ADHD?
  A. Imipramine
  B. Diazepam
  C. Haloperidol
  D. Bupropion
  E. Dextroamphetamine

47-2. Which of the following is an example of a nonpharmacological treatment used in ADHD?
  A. Contingent reinforcement
  B. Psychoanalytic psychotherapy
  C. Commercial video games
  D. Agreement to not have school report to parents
  E. Studying with TV on

47-3. Which of the following best describes the course of ADHD?
- A. Hyperactive symptoms increase with age.
- B. Inattentive symptoms are correlated with depression in adulthood.
- C. Problems with executive function do not persist into adulthood.
- D. Changing jobs multiple times could represent impulsivity in adulthood.
- E. Inattentive symptoms are correlated with substance abuse in adulthood.

47-4. Which of the following is correct about comorbid disorders in ADHD?
- A. 1 out of 20 has a learning disorders.
- B. 1 out of 5 has psychotic symptoms.
- C. 1 out of 3 suffers from depression.
- D. 1 out of 25 has an anxiety disorder.
- E. 1 out of 2 has a personality disorder.

ANSWERS

47-1. **E.** Stimulants are the most effective and extensively studied treatment for ADHD. They are safe in children, generally not addictive in patients with ADHD, and effective in up to 90% of cases. They increase performance, vigilance, attention, social appropriateness, and organization. Other drugs that affect catecholamines (e.g., tricyclic antidepressants, bupropion, α_2 agonists) have also been used. Benzodiazepines are not used in this disorder. Possible adverse effects of stimulants include initial insomnia, poor appetite, headaches, irritability, and dysphoria. In people with comorbid tic disorders, stimulants may increase tics. Stimulants have been shown to decrease the incidence of substance use disorders, frequently comorbid in ADHD.

47-2. **A.** Contingent reinforcement implies that the desired response or behavior (e.g., finish homework) is related in time or frequency pattern to the reinforcement (e.g., reward). Many helpful treatments are taken from behavior theory. Parents are taught principles of behavior management and social learning, such as using time outs, rewards, consequences, and home-to-school communication and reporting. Teachers are also taught to use behavioral strategies. Psychoanalytic psychotherapy is not used in this disorder.

Counseling can address the child's difficulties in peer relations, expecting to fail, and poor self-esteem. Educational remediation targets learning disabilities and underachievement.

47-3. D. Impulsivity in adults with ADHD may take characteristic forms, such as changing jobs frequently or problems driving. The symptoms that most frequently persist into adulthood include problems with attention and executive function. Inattentive symptoms are not correlated with depression in adulthood. Hyperactive symptoms decline with age, although restlessness may persist.

47-4. C. About one-fourth of patients with ADHD have anxiety disorders and one-third suffer from depression, which may be induced by clumsiness and poor interpersonal skills, which may lead to teasing, not being picked for sport teams, and low self-esteem. These patients do not have an increased risk of psychosis. 20% to 25% of children with ADHD have comorbid learning disorders.

SUGGESTED READINGS

Biederman, J. Impact of comorbidity in adults with attention-deficit/ hyperactivity disorder. *J Clin Psychiatry*. 2004;65(Suppl 3):3–7.
Bobb AJ, Castellanos FX, et al. Molecular genetic studies of ADHD: 1991 to 2004. *Am J Med Genet B Neuropsychiatr Genet*. 2005; 132(1):109–125.

CASE **48**

"I'm Having Trouble in School"

CC/ID: 18-year-old male college freshman comes in complaining, "I can't get my work done."

THOUGHT QUESTION

- Before knowing anything else, what differential diagnosis are you considering?

DISCUSSION

There are many reasons why someone complains of not being able to get work done. It could be as simple as a time management problem or preoccupation with life events. Psychiatric disorders like ADHD, major depression, or anxiety disorders can affect concentration. In schizophrenia, hallucinations can impede concentration; or a thought disorder may cause disorganized thinking or impair executive function. OCD may interfere with task completion. Primary obsessional slowness is an uncommon subtype of OCD, in which a person spends many hours doing tasks of daily living. Additionally, the first time away from home in the context of greater independence may trigger the manifestation of personality traits which, in a self-defeating way, lead to work problems, failure, and ultimately result in returning home with concomitant greater dependence and attachment.

CASE CONTINUED

HPI: With the increased reading in college, J.B. is having **difficulty finishing** his work. He denies depressed mood, or any change

327

in energy, appetite, or sleep. He denies other difficulties, although admits that he and his roommate have been arguing about the bathroom: "He complains that I take too long in the shower, so I shower when he's out." On examination of his study habits, he admits to reading each sentence exactly three times, underlining the nouns and circling the verbs. He started doing this in 5th grade when they learned about parts of speech; now he cannot read without doing it. He has tried "to skim"; it makes him nervous, so he goes back to his usual way. "I know this sounds nuts, but I have this feeling that if I don't do it, **something bad will happen** to my mom." He is concerned about **cleanliness,** and showers for 33 minutes twice a day. In addition, he washes his hands for 6 minutes after he uses the bathroom and 3 minutes if he touches a doorknob. He also **checks** that his computer is off and the door is locked 12 times before leaving his room. He has recently had **intrusive worries** about lead poisoning after he found peeled paint around his radiator.

PMHx: None

Meds: None

SHx: No tobacco, illicit substances, or EtOH use

**VS/PE/
Labs:**   WNL

MSE: *General:* Well-related, pleasant, neatly dressed. *Speech:* slightly rapid. *Mood:* "Fine," but upon greater clarification is relayed as "concerned." *Affect:* reactive and slightly anxious. *Thought process:* logical, goal-directed. *Thought content:* no delusions, no hallucinations, no suicidal ideation. No gross cognitive impairments.

THOUGHT QUESTIONS

- What exactly defines an obsession and a compulsion?
- What is the differential diagnosis of obsessions and compulsions?

DISCUSSION

Obsessions are recurrent persistent thoughts, impulses, or images experienced as intrusive and causing distress. They are not experienced as thought insertion. They are **not excessive worries about real problems.** Usually the person attempts to neutralize them (by compulsions). These thoughts are often associated with anxiety, guilt, or shame. As a response to the feelings generated by the thoughts, the person may perform compulsions, which temporarily decrease the negative affect. **Compulsions are repetitive behaviors or mental acts** that the person feels driven to perform in response to an obsession or according to rigid rules. The acts are **aimed at reducing anxiety** or preventing a dreaded event, and may include repetitive checking, washing, cleaning, or rearranging, or mental rituals like repeating phrases or counting. The obsessions and compulsions may consume hours each day. A patient does not have to have both obsessions and compulsions to have OCD. See Table 48-1 below. Obsessive-compulsive symptoms may also be seen in anorexia nervosa, generalized anxiety, depression, and early stages of dementia.

This patient has no depressive or psychotic symptoms. He meets criteria for OCD.

In further sessions, it would be important to explore his obsessions more fully. People are often reluctant to talk about their obsessions or compulsions, and using a structured instrument and being nonjudgmental are helpful. In fact, people usually suffer with their symptoms for more than 7 years prior to seeking help. Questions that help define symptom severity include determining the amount of time spent in each ritual, the amount of distress experienced, the amount of difficulty in not performing the ritual, and the extent to which the compulsions limit social and occupational functioning (Table 48-1).

TABLE **48-1**   Common Types of Obsessions and Compulsions

Obsessions	**A**ggressive (impulses toward others)
	Sexual
	Symmetry (need for)
	Orderliness
	Religion
	Dirt/**D**isease (fears of contamination)
	Infection
	Doubt
Compulsions	Checking, cleaning, counting, rearranging, repeating phrases, washing

CASE CONTINUED

On the following visit, you do a semistructured interview and discover that he is spending at least 4 hours a day **performing compulsive rituals.** He admits to some intrusive thoughts but doesn't want to talk about them, feeling embarassed. He says, "I never realized that other people do these things too," and asks what treatments are available. He elects to try behavioral therapy first to avoid medication side effects.

QUESTIONS

48-1. Which of the following is used in the first line treatment of OCD?

A. Avoidance of stressful stimuli
B. Neurosurgery
C. Exposure and response prevention
D. Lithium
E. Haloperidol

48-2. Which of the following best describes the course and prognosis of OCD?

A. The prevalence is approximately 13% of the population.
B. OCD is not a disabling illness.
C. Onset is usually in middle adulthood.
D. OCD symptoms may occur after a brain injury.
E. Approximately 75% of cases are severe.

48-3. Which of the following can cause similar symptoms to OCD?

A. Schizophrenia
B. Major depression
C. OC personality disorder
D. Simple phobias
E. All of the above

48-4. Which of the following is a common theme of obsessions?

A. Thoughts of causing harm to others
B. Being controlled
C. Alien threats
D. Rotting inside
E. Worthlessness

ANSWERS

48-1. C. Exposure and response prevention (e.g., shaking the patient's hand and not letting him wash for 5 minutes) is a type pf behavioral therapy and is used as a first line treatment. As it takes quite a commitment on the part of the patient, about 25% of patients refuse this form of treatment; however, those who proceed to successful completion experience a 75% symptom reduction. Medications are also effective for OCD: clomipramine (a tricyclic antidepressant that primarily affects serotonin reuptake) and SSRIs reduce symptoms by 30% to 40%; the norm is that residual symptoms remain even with effective medication treatment, and discontinuation is associated with high relapse rates. Neurosurgery, often involving the anterior cingulated (cingulotomy), has been used in patients with very severe treatment refractory disease, and has shown good success.

48-2. D. OCD may be seen in association with brain injury or after encephalitis, although these are rare causes. OCD is often a very disabling disorder. The prevalence is 2% to 3% of the adult population, and approximately 0.6% of the general population has severe OCD. The onset is often in adolescence or young adulthood, and the course is often chronic, with residual symptoms remaining even with effective treatment. In patients with OCD, the lifetime prevalence of major depression approaches 60%.

48-3. E. Isolated obsessive and compulsive symptoms are not unique to OCD and are seen in all of the psychiatric disorders included in this question. In major depression, there may be ruminations about real life events, perceived failures, and so on, which generally take on a negative or self denigrating quality. These ruminations must be differentiated from obsessive compulsive *disorder*, and may be present in an isolated major depressive episode. People with OC personality disorders require enormous order and control and pay great obsessive attention to minutiae, generally impairing their ability to complete certain tasks. They are often rigid and perfectionistic, but they do not have compulsions and obsessions and are usually able to function without severe impairments. In schizophrenia, delusional systems may seem similar to severe obsessions, and rituals may be driven by psychotic beliefs. Phobias are irrational fears of a specific thing (e.g., blood, snakes, heights) and do not have associated compulsions. In OCD there may be phobic avoidance associated with an obsession (e.g., avoiding subway travel because of fear of contamination), but not avoidance because of the thing itself as in a phobia.

48-4. A. Common themes of obsessions include contamination, order and symmetry, thoughts of causing harm to others, and harm that may befall others. Thoughts of being controlled are usually associated with psychotic disorders. For example, a kind and gentle patient may experience a sudden impulse to stab an old lady with his pen; this impulse may be associated with an unbidden but persistent vivid visual image in his mind's eye of his lodging the pen in the old woman's eye socket. Such experiences make the patient extremely anxious, and are not acted upon.

SUGGESTED READINGS

Ipser JC, Carey P, Dhansay Y, et al. Pharmacotherapy augmentation strategies in treatment-resistant anxiety disorders. *Cochrane Database Syst Rev*. 2006;(4):CD005473.

Mataix-Cols D, Rosario-Campos MC, Leckman JF. A multidimensional model of obsessive-compulsive disorder. *Am J Psychiatry*. 2005;162(2):228–238.

Oakley-Browne M, Hatcher S, Churchill R, et al. Cochrane Depression Anxiety & Neurosis Group. In: *The Cochrane Library*, Issue 4, 2001. Oxford: Update Software.

Pato MT, Pato CN, Pauls DL. Recent findings in the genetics of OCD. *J Clin Psychiatry*. 2002;63 (Suppl 6):30–33.

What's Wrong with My Son?

  CC/ID: Mr. and Mrs. Q. come to your clinic with their first-born son, Peter, who is 3 years 1 month old. They are concerned that he is not doing as well as other children his age.

HPI: Mrs. Q. had a normal pregnancy and delivery, and neonatal screening in the hospital revealed no abnormalities. Peter has always been at the 50th percentile for height, weight, and head circumference. However, his parents note that it is his **language skills** about which they are the most concerned. Other concerns include his very **flexible joints** and the lack of success with potty training.

PMHx: There is no significant past medical or surgical history. He received all his vaccinations to date.

Allergies: NKDA

FHx: There is a male cousin on the maternal side who has mental retardation.

SHx: Peter is the first-born. His father and mother both work in the family dry cleaning business.

Examination: He appears shy at first, but then babbles away non-sensically to himself. He appears to have a long, narrow face and large ears. Otherwise his physical exam is normal.

THOUGHT QUESTIONS

- What is the cause of his developmental delay?
- What tests may aid in the diagnosis of mental retardation, after usual neonatal screening?

DISCUSSION

Global developmental delay affects between 1% and 3% of children in the United States, and, by definition, includes delay in two or more of the following skill areas: **activities of daily living, cognitive functioning, language/speech, social skills, and motor skills (gross and fine).** Significant delay is defined as two or more standard deviations below that of peers on standardized testing. Not every child with developmental delay will manifest mental retardation when appropriate formal cognitive testing can be performed at about 5 years of age (for example, a child with a neuromuscular disorder may have a normal IQ on formal testing: **Weschler Preschool Primary Scale of Intelligence** or the **Stanford-Binet IQ scale**). However, developmental delay—and specifically language impairment—is a significant risk factor for later mental retardation.

It is important to attempt to identify any underlying cause(s) of impairment to plan for possible treatments (medical and psychiatric), as well as to be able to advise and support families regarding the risk of recurrence in subsequent children. Thus, it is vital to take a comprehensive **history from both parents** and to perform a thorough medical and neurological examination of the affected child. Remember that parents who work in chemically toxic environments (e.g., dry cleaning) may inadvertently expose their young children. Neonatal screening programs usually identify most children with metabolic and thyroid disorders; other features, such as physical abnormalities (e.g., hepatosplenomegaly) and other symptoms (e.g., failure to thrive) make it unlikely that these children remain undiagnosed. However, in those children where history, examination, and routine screenings have failed to identify a cause of the global developmental delay/mental retardation, newer molecular techniques such as fluorescence in situ hybridization (FISH) or microstellite markers may be used to identify subtelomeric chromosomal rearrangements. Imaging techniques, either CT or MRI scanning, are not used for general screening but may identify the cause of global developmental delay when physical findings such as microcephaly or focal motor problems have been found. MRI is reported to be more sensitive than CT in detecting abnormalities associated with global developmental delay.

Fragile X syndrome: This disorder is also known as Martin Bell syndrome and is caused by a mutation in the FMR1 gene on the long arm of the **X chromosome.** The function of the FMR1 gene is still unknown. It is the **second most common genetic cause of**

global developmental delay after Down syndrome. The fragile site was identified at Xq27.3 when cells were grown in a folate-deficient medium. This original site is referred to as FRAXA, and other more recently described sites are referred to as FRAXB through E. It is caused by a CGG **trinucleotide repeat** and the full mutation (200 or more CGG repeats) is associated with global developmental delay. The premutation or **carrier state** (between 55 and 200 CGG repeats) has been estimated to be 1 per 246 to 468 **females** in the general population. Overall, the incidence of the full fragile X syndrome is reported to be approximately **1 in 1000 males and 1 in 2000 females,** and it is reported across all ethnic and racial groups. About 80% of the males affected are mentally retarded, with IQs in the 35 to 45 range; up to 70% of affected females are mentally retarded but show milder levels of retardation. Features to look for when considering this diagnosis include

- Family history of mental retardation
- Long jaw
- High forehead, narrow face
- Large, long, protuberant ears
- Testicular enlargement (post-puberty)
- Hyperextendible joints
- Soft, velvety palmar skin

Children with fragile X syndrome may also be described as initially shy, with poor eye contact, but this presentation may be followed by friendliness and overtalking. Other features may include autistic behaviors, attention deficit–hyperactivity disorder, speech and language disorders, and rarely seizures (Tables 49-1 and 49-2).

TABLE **49-1**   Diagnostic Tests for Global Developmental Delay

Genetic studies	Cytogenetic studies, subtelomeric deletions (e.g., fragile X and Rett syndrome)
Neuroimaging	MRI/CT scans
Metabolic testing	Blood amino acid levels, lactate and ammonia levels, urinary organic acids
Thyroid screening	TSH and T$_4$
Serum lead levels	Above 10 μg/dL is toxic
EEG	For myoclonic epilepsy, Lennox-Gastaut syndrome, or Rett syndrome

TABLE 49-2 Causes of Global Developmental Delay/Mental Retardation

Chromosomal Abnormalities

Trisomies	Trisomy 13–15 (Patau syndrome)
	Trisomy 17–18 (Edwards syndrome)
	Trisomy 21(22) (Down syndrome)
Deletions	Short arm 5p (cri du chat)
	Short arm 4p (Wolf-Hirschhorn syndrome)
Sex chromosomes	XXX
	XXY (Klinefelter syndrome)
	XYY
	XO (Turner syndrome)
	Fragile site Q 27–28 (fragile X)

Other Genetic Abnormalities

Autosomal dominant	Neurofibromatosis
	Tuberous sclerosis
	Sturge-Weber
Autosomal recessive	Microcephaly
	Laurence-Moon-Biedl syndrome
X-linked	Lesch-Nyhan syndrome (inborn error of metabolism)
	Hunter syndrome (inborn error of metabolism)
	Rett syndrome
	Albright syndrome
Other genetic causes	Cornelia de Lange syndrome
	Prader-Willi
	Autism

Inborn Errors of Metabolism

	Phenylketonuria
	Homocystinurea
	Maple syrup disease
	Hartnup disease
	Galactosemia
	Tay-Sachs
	Niemann-Picks
	Gauchers
	Refsum disease
	Hurler syndrome
	Sanfilippo syndrome
	Hypothyroidism (cretinism)

CASE CONTINUED

You suspect with a high probability that Peter has fragile X syndrome and arrange for cytogenetic testing. The test comes back confirming your diagnosis. You explain the condition to his parents and arrange to see them again soon to help plan for his future care. You refer his parents to a geneticist to advise them about the risk in future pregnancies.

 QUESTIONS

49-1. The parents of a 2-year-old girl present to your clinic, concerned about their daughter. Her speech has deteriorated, and she has begun to show some unusual stereotypical hand-wringing movements as well as an unbalanced gait. What other features would aid you in making the diagnosis in this child?

    A. Macrocephaly
    B. Microcephaly
    C. A male sibling with similar features
    D. Short stature with webbed neck
    E. Shield-like chest

49-2. New parents who have just moved into a renovated home ask you if they should be concerned about lead poisoning in their child. Which of the following do you tell them?

    A. Lead is the least common environmental neurotoxin.
    B. Markedly elevated serum lead levels definitely cause mental retardation.
    C. Average blood lead levels have fallen dramatically since the 1970s in the United States.
    D. Each 1 μg/dL increase in blood lead levels may decrease a child's IQ by 1 to 3 points.
    E. Not to worry if their home was built before 1950.

49-3. Neonatal screening revealed an elevated phenylalanine level of 30 mg/dL. Which of the following do you tell the parents?

    A. If the condition remains untreated, mild mental retardation invariably follows.
    B. The condition is caused by the build up of phenylketones in the body.
    C. The phenylalanine-free diet is recommended for the first 12 years of life.
    D. Overtreatment can lead to serious consequences.
    E. The prevalence of this autosomal dominant disorder in the United States is 1 in 14,000 to 20,000 live births.

49-4. Which of the following metabolic disorders is correctly paired with its reported enzyme defect?
- A. Lesch-Nyhan syndrome — Cystathionine B synthase
- B. Galactosemia — Hypoxanthine phosphoribosyltransferase
- C. Homocystinuria — Galactose-1-P-uridyl transferase
- D. Lesch-Nyhan — Hypoxanthine phosphoribosyltransferase
- E. Fructosuria — Fructose 1-phosphate aldolase

ANSWERS

49-1. B. Microcephaly is caused by a deceleration in head growth in Rett syndrome. Importantly, affected girls manifest a deterioration and loss of previously gained developmental milestones. This disorder is one of the leading causes of global developmental delay/mental retardation in females, with prevalence in the general population estimated at between 1 and 3 per 10,000 live births. The prevalence of this disorder in males or milder forms in females is unclear at this time. Rett syndrome is caused by mutations in the X-linked gene that encodes for methyl-CpG-binding protein 2 (MECP2). However MECP2 mutations can occur without the clinical features of Rett syndrome. Other clinical features include: hand-wringing, autistic behaviors, ataxia, periods of hyperventilation, and seizures. Short stature, webbed neck, shield-like chest, low set ears, and sexual infantilism are associated with Turner syndrome, caused by the sex chromosome abnormality XO.

49-2. C. Although the average blood lead levels have fallen significantly since the 1970s, some children remain at higher risk of developing lead poisoning. This high-risk group includes those children living in communities where the average blood serum lead level is greater than 10 μg/dL or where the majority of housing was build before 1950, children who may have been exposed to folk medicines containing lead, immigrants from countries where lead poisoning is endemic, and children with socioeconomic disadvantages. Recently reports of lead paint used in the manufacture of childern toys have led to large recalls of the implicated models. Though low-level lead poisoning is associated with mild cognitive impairments, even markedly elevated serum lead levels have not been reported to definitely cause mental retardation. Lead is the most common environmental neurotoxin. Each 10 μg/dL increase in blood lead levels may decrease a child's IQ by 1 to 3 points.

49-3. D. Overtreatment of phenylketonuria (PKU) can cause phenylalanine deficiency, which can cause anemia, anorexia, diarrhea, failure to thrive, lethargy, and even death. Classic PKU is caused by a deficiency of p-hydroxyphenylalanine hydroxylase or its cofactor tetrahydrobiopterin, causing an accumulation of phenylalanine in body fluids and the CNS. The excess phenylalanine is metabolized to phenylketones, which can be detected in the urine. The presence of phenylalanine in the brain interferes with the transportation of other amino acids into the brain. The aim of treatment is to keep phenylalanine levels low in the body, and infants should be started on formulae that are low or free of this amino acid. A certain amount of this essential amino acid is very important. Stopping the diet in adulthood is associated with deterioration in cognitive function and IQ, and the diet is currently recommended for the life of the individual. Pregnant women with hyperphenylalaninemia who do not follow the diet have a very high risk of having infants with heart disease, microcephaly, and mental retardation. The prevalence of classic PKU and autosomal recessive condition in the United States is 1 in 14,000 to 20,000 live births. It is more common in Whites and Native Americans and less common in Blacks, Hispanics, and Asians. The gene for phenylalanine hydroxylase has been located on chromosome 12q22-q24.1 and over 400 mutations have been reported.

49-4 D. Lesch-Nyhan is an X-linked condition causing neurological impairment and self-mutilatory behaviors (e.g., chewing and biting off one's own lips and fingertips). It is caused by a defect in the enzyme hypoxanthine phosphoribosyltransferase. Galactosemia is an autosomal recessive condition caused by a defect in the galactose 1-P-uridyltransferase enzymes leading to mental retardation, cataracts, liver dysfunction, sepsis, and even death. Homocystinurea is caused by an autosomal recessive defect in the cystathionine B synthase enzyme causing mental retardation, Marfan features with lens dislocation, and arterial thrombosis. Fructosuria is a benign condition caused by an autosomal recessive defect in the enzyme fructokinase.

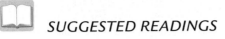 *SUGGESTED READINGS*

Volkmar F, Cook EH Jr, Pomeroy J, et al. Practice parameters for the assessment and treatment of children, adolescents, and adults with autism and other pervasive developmental disorders. *J Am Acad Child Adolesc Psychiatry*. 1999;38 (12 Suppl):32S–54S.

McDonald L, Rennie A, Tolmie J, et al. Investigation of global developmental delay. *Arch Dis Child*. 2006;91(8):701–705.

CASE **50**

"My Son Is Twitching"

CC/ID: 7-year-old boy who is brought to your clinic by his parents who are concerned that he is developing a "twitch."

HPI: About 2 weeks ago, G.S.'s parents noticed a relatively **sudden onset of a facial "twitch,"** described as intense **blinking of both eyes.** At first they thought it might be related to fatigue, as he has recently started an extended day program at school, and it was more pronounced late in the day. Additionally, this twitch seemed to get **worse when he was excited or anxious** and was not present at sleep. When asked by his parents, G.S. denied any specific worries or concerns. His parents reported that he was eating, drinking, sleeping, eliminating, and socializing as usual. They also report that they had called the school to check if there had been any recent events that may have upset him in any way, but none were discovered. There has been **no other change in his behavior,** including new onset ritualistic behaviors or routines. G.S. tells you that he is fine, and describes that he knows he is blinking a lot, but that it does not appear to be causing him any particular distress.

PMHx: G.S. was born by normal delivery at term and weighed 8 lb. He achieved all his milestones on time and was fully continent by age 3. He received the usual recommended vaccines. No surgical history.

FHx: His paternal uncle has OCD.

Allergies: NKDA

Meds: MVI daily

SHx: G.S. is the oldest of 3 boys (7, 4, 2 years). He currently attends first grade, where he is an average student with normal socialization. His father runs his own accounting firm, and his mother is a homemaker.

MSE: *General:* pale and **anxious appearing** young boy who clings to his mother's side. *Motor:* intermittent multiple intense blinking movements of both eyes simultaneously. No other abnormal movements are noted. *Speech:* normal rate, rhythm, and tone. No abnormal vocalizations. *Affect:* neutral, reactive, and full range. *Mood:* described as "okay," and appears euthymic. *Thought process:* logical and goal-directed. *Thought content:* no evidence of psychosis or thoughts of self-harm. *Cognitive:* intact and age appropriate.

THOUGHT QUESTIONS

- What is a tic?
- What do you think is this boy's differential diagnosis?
- What treatments are available for these disorders?

DISCUSSION

A tic is a sudden, rapid, quasiresistible, nonrhythmic stereotyped movement or verbalization. **Patients tend to describe their tics as akin to "itches," in which there is a strong desire to "scratch" or enact the movement, which initially they can resist.** However, their anxiety builds to such an extent that relief is only found in activating the movement (or scratching the itch). This neutralizes the anxiety, which then only returns in exaggerated intensity, thus perpetuating a vicious cycle. Tics may occur in any muscle group, but are most commonly found in facial muscles.

Differential diagnosis is as follows:

Dystonia: The abnormal movements may be repetitive or may reflect a sustained contracture of a single or multiple muscle groups. Primary types of dystonia are not associated with other neurological complaints or cognitive impairments (i.e., the pathology is limited to the motor system). If severe enough, they can cause significant discomfort and even muscle breakdown. Tremors may also coexist with this condition. Cerebral palsy is a common cause of secondary dystonia, in which cognitive impairments may be found as well. Some dystonic movements may be situation specific (e.g., when using the computer). Decreases in norepinephrine levels in the hypothalamus and red nucleus have been reported in those with certain types of dystonia. Dopa-responsive dystonia is a genetic cause of dystonia that responds to either dopamine agonists or anticholinergic medications. Other causes of dystonias in children include thyrotoxicosis, reflux, various metabolic disorders, and MS. Treatment of dystonias in children should include trials of L-dopa, anticholinergic agents, pimozide, or tetrabenzine. Botulism toxin may be used in more focal dystonias, and neurosurgery is reserved for those who have exhausted or failed to respond to conventional treatments.

Stereotypies: repetitive, purposeless movements such as chewing, sucking, touching, and rocking. They may occur in normal children or in those with autistic disorders or mental retardation. These movements may present in those less than 3 years of age, and they may be attenuated with cuing and exacerbated by anxiety, stress, or excitement. There may be a family history of stereotypies and comorbid ADHD or learning disorders.

Tourette syndrome (TS): should be differentiated from transient tics, the latter of which may occur in up to 25% of children. In TS, the tics generally occur throughout the day (though usually in bouts) nearly every day, or they may occur intermittently over a period of more than 1 year; during this period there is never a tic-free interval of more than 3 consecutive months. Tics seen in TS may be simple (e.g., blinking, grimacing, shrugging the shoulders, or jerking the head) or more complex (e.g., kicking, jumping, scratching, or bizarre gait), but the **tics in TS must include both motor and vocal versions.** Vocal tics may include echolalia (repeating a word of part of a sentence), palilalia (repeating the last syllable of a word with increasing speed), or coprolalia (obscene words; occurring in ~10% of patients with TS). Echopraxia (copying movements or gestures of another) and copropraxia (obscene gestures) may also occur. **In both TS and simple tic disorders, tics may wax and wane, are usually exacerbated by stress or anxiety,** and may occur during sleep. Patients with Tourette syndrome usually continue to be symptomatic into adulthood. Tics may initially be resisted at the expense of rising tension, which is relieved after the movement has been performed (somewhat like scratching an itch).

Transient tic disorder: includes single or multiple vocal or motor tics that occur many times per day, nearly every day for at least 4 weeks, but for no longer than 12 consecutive months. In contrast, **Chronic tic disorder** is defined by the presence of either vocal or motor tics (not both) present for longer than 1 year.

Genetic causes of tics: Tourette syndrome, Huntington's chorea, dystonia, and neuroacanthocytosis. Tics may also develop **secondary to other medical and neurological** disorders (Table 50-1). It has been reported that children and adults with Tourette syndrome have increased antistreptolysin O titers and antibodies to basal ganglia neurons.

TABLE 50-1   Secondary Causes of Tics

Developmental	Mental retardation and chromosomal abnormalities
Infection	Sydenham chorea (rheumatic fever), encephalitis, Creutzfeldt-Jakob disease
Medications	Carbamazepine, levodopa, phenytoin, phenobarbital, stimulants (methylphenidate and dextroamphetamine)
Toxins	Carbon monoxide
Miscellaneous	Head injury, schizophrenia, neuroacanthocytosis, stroke

Treatment of tics: Dopamine (D_2) antagonists such as fluphenazine, pimozide, and haloperidol. Pergolide is an agonist at D_1, D_2, and D_3 receptors and also may be useful in those with more severe tics; however, its use is limited by reports of increased cardiac valve disease in those taking the medication. Another dopamine agonist, ropinirole, may also prove to be helpful. Although SSRIs may help behavioral problems in those with tic disorders (e.g., obsessive-compulsive symptoms, impulse dyscontrol, rages), in a certain population they may actually exacerbate tics. Treatment of comorbid ADHD with stimulants may also exacerbate symptoms.

CASE CONTINUED

After a thorough evaluation, you diagnose G.S. with a transient tic disorder. You reassure his parents that this presentation may be normal in children but educate them to observe for any exacerbation or change in symptoms. Six months later, G.S. returns with his parents, and there is no evidence of a tic.

QUESTIONS

50-1. Which of the following movement disorders is correctly paired with its causal lesion?

A. Hemiballismus   ipsilateral subthalamic nuclei
B. Chorea   contralateral putamen
C. Hemidystonia   contralateral subthalamic nuclei
D. Sydenham chorea   basal ganglia and cerebellum
E. Wilson disease   Kaiser-Fleischer rings

50-2. Which of the following best describes TS?
  A. It is an autosomal dominant disorder.
  B. Imaging studies have revealed decreased right frontal white matter volumes compared to controls.
  C. Imaging studies have revealed decreased left frontal gray matter volumes compared to controls.
  D. The average age of onset of tics is 2 years.
  E. Vocal tics tend to present before motor ones.

50-3. Which of the following best describes the course and prognosis of TS?
  A. Self-injurious behavior is rare.
  B. Affective dyscontrol and anger are rare.
  C. There is an increased risk of depression in those with tics.
  D. Boys are more likely than girls to present with comorbid OCD.
  E. Girls are more likely than boys to first present with vocal or motor symptoms.

50-4. Which of the following is most commonly found in Wilson disease?
  A. Psychiatric complaints usually include anxiety and feelings of impending doom.
  B. Psychiatric complaints usually include psychotic features.
  C. Memory complaints are common.
  D. Decreased levels of copper are found in the urine.
  E. It is an autosomal dominant condition.

ANSWERS

50-1. D. Sydenham chorea is caused by rheumatic fever and is one of the most common causes of chorea in children. The choreiform movements including dance-like, rapid, jerky, nonstereo-typed, and involuntary movements, generally appearing after the associated arthritis and carditis. Emotional changes (e.g., lability) may also occur. Lesions have been reported in the basal ganglia, cerebellum, and the cortex. The chorea generally improves slowly and should be treated with penicillin. If the choreiform movements are causing distress, antipsychotics, benzodiazepines, carbamazepine, or valproic acid may be used for relief, but these medications do not affect the disease course. Conversely, corticosteroids may shorten the course of Sydenham chorea. Hemiballismus is a severe form of chorea caused by lesions in the contralateral subthalamic nuclei and adjacent areas. In cerebral palsy, the choreiform movements are caused by hypoxia in utero or at birth, with lesions generally occurring in the contralateral basal ganglia; the cortex may be involved which would usually lead to cognitive impairment. Hemidystonia occurs with vascular or traumatic lesions of the contralateral basal ganglia, mostly the putamen. Wilson's disease, though associated with Kaiser-Fleischer rings (copper deposits in the eye), is actually caused by decreased serum ceruloplasmin leading to copper deposits throughout the body and in the brain.

50-2. C. Imaging studies of TS have revealed decreased volumes of left frontal gray matter, which reflects a loss of the usual cortical asymmetry (left is usually larger than right). Though initially TS was thought to be transmitted via an autosomal dominant mechanism, now a more complex pattern of inheritance seems likely. The onset of TS is usually between 2 and 15 years of age, with the average age of onset at approximately 6 years, but cases of later onset have been described. Males are affected more than females. The character of a single individual's tics (e.g., location, number, frequency, complexity, and severity) usually changes over time. Simple and complex motor tics may affect any part of the body, with simple motor tics being rapid, meaningless contractions of one or a few muscles (e.g., eye blinking), and complex motor tics involving touching, squatting, deep knee bends, retracing steps, and twirling when walking. Vocal tics may involve various words or sounds (e.g., clicks, grunts, yelps, barks, sniffs, snorts, and coughs). Coprolalia is a complex vocal tic marked by the uttering of obscenities and is present in less than 10% of those with a tic disorder; it is not required for a diagnosis of Tourette disorder. Eye blinking is the most common initial tic.

50-3. C. Patients with TS and those with a tic disorder are at greater risk for developing depressive or anxiety disorders than is found in the general population. Likewise, self-injurious behavior and affective dyscontrol (e.g., anger attacks) are more likely to occur in children with TS, and especially in those with comorbid disorders such as ADHD or OCD. Boys tend to present first with motor or vocal tics, whereas girls tend to present more often with behavioral problems such as OCD symptoms. Patients with tic disorders demonstrate a high incidence of psychiatric comorbidities, with increased rates of ADHD, learning disorders, conduct disorder, oppositional defiant disorder, and OCD. Sleep disorders are also common (e.g., bed wetting, bruxism, insomnia, sleepwalking, and nightmares).

50-4. B. Psychiatric signs and symptoms associated with Wilson disease include abnormal mood states (e.g., lability, irritability, depression, mania, anxiety) and psychosis, including both hallucinations and delusions. Other signs evident on observation or examination include muscular rigidity, gait disturbances, choreoathetoid movements, Kaiser-Fleischer rings, and symptoms suggestive of hepatitis. Patients with Wilson disease may present in early adulthood and symptoms can be difficult to differentiate from schizophreniform or schizophrenic disorders. Feelings of impending doom and increased acute anxiety are usually associated with pheochromocytoma or panic disorder. Wilson disease is an autosomal recessive condition, marked by decreased serum ceruloplasmin (a protein that usually binds copper).

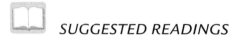 *SUGGESTED READINGS*

Dooley JM. Tic disorders in childhood. *Semin Pediatr.* 2006;13(4):231–242.

Keen-Kim D, Freimer NB. Genetics and epidemiology of Tourette syndrome. *J Child Neurol.* 2006;21(8):665–671.

"He Fell Down the Stairs"

CC/ID: 2-year-old boy who is brought to the walk-in ER for evaluation. His stepfather describes that he slipped on the stairs and hurt his leg, and he is now refusing to walk.

HPI: On exam H.B. is a **quiet, reserved, and passive child.** Though attempts are made to engage him in conversation, he does not appear to cooperate. On physical exam, he presents **with bruises of varying ages on his back and abdomen.** An X-ray of his leg reveals a **femoral fracture.**

THOUGHT QUESTIONS

- Developmentally, what would you expect to find for a 2-year-old boy?
- What is the significance of the findings on his physical exam?
- What is the next step in the management of this case?

DISCUSSION

Between 16 months and 2 years, the average child practices exploration and moving away from the parent or caregiver, followed by then coming back for reassurance and comfort. By 18 months, children are furthering both fine and gross motor development: they can climb up stairs, scribble, and use a spoon. Language also continues to develop, and common objects can be named; at age 2 a child can speak in two-word sentences. Also at 2 years, he or she can jump, and can wash and dry his or her hands. By 3, the child can ride a tricycle, dress with supervision, speak in three- to four-word sentences, and know his or her whole name and some colors. In addition, between 18 months and 3 years, core gender identity is established. (See Table 51-1 for review of social, physical, and language milestones.)

TABLE **51-1** Developmental Milestones (average age attained)

Physical

1 month	Lifts head
6 months	Sits unassisted
7 months	Rolls over
10 months	Crawls
12–15 months	Walks
18 months	Walks up steps
2 years	Jumps in place
3 years	Rides tricycle
4 years	Hops on one foot

Fine Motor

4 months	Grasps object
9 months	Pincer grasp
14 months	Scribbles
18 months	Builds tower of four cubes
2 years	Imitates a vertical line
3 years	Copies a "0"
4 years	Copies a "+"

Social/Personal

1–2 months	Social smile in response to face or voice
7–9 months	Stranger anxiety–shows parental attachment and can differentiate strangers
7–18 months (up to 3 years)	Separation anxiety
12 months	Drinks from a cup
18 months	Uses a spoon, removes a garment
2 years	Puts on clothing, washes, and dries hands
3 years	Dresses with supervision, eats well with utensils
4 years	Dresses without supervision

Language

4–6 months	Babbles
12 months	Speaks first real word
18 months	Names some common objects
2 years	Speaks two-word sentences
3 years	Says first and last name, some colors

The physical exam in this case shows **multiple bruises of varying ages, especially in "hidden" areas of the body** (those usually covered by clothes). Though children often have bruises on their heads, legs, knees, shins, and arms from falls in the home, school, or playground, this child is **bruised in places where bruises are not common (e.g., back, stomach).** In addition, femoral fractures are uncommon. There is significant suspicion that this child has been abused. This child will **need a full skeletal series** to look for any old fractures.

In addition, the child is **speaking only minimally.** It is possible that this child is scared (of the ER, the parental figure's potential reactions, etc.) or has a developmental delay. In either case, this behavior warrants further evaluation.

CASE CONTINUED

The skeletal survey showed a few old posterior rib fractures of various ages. In speaking separately to the stepfather and then the mother, the stories of what happened to the child were quite inconsistent. A review of the ER records shows that the child was seen 2 months ago for a burn and three months before that for head trauma. With this high suspicion for child abuse, Child Protective Services was called. The recommendation for a complete developmental evaluation was made as well.

In evaluating a case of suspected abuse, it is important to **interview each member of the family separately** to better understand the circumstances of the event. Inconsistent or changing stories, or extremely vague or evasive answers may be seen in cases of abuse. It is important to review hospital ER records to see if there are previous instances of suspicious injuries. The most common manifestations of abuse are burns, bruises, cuts, fractures, head trauma, and abdominal injuries.

Approximately 4 million cases of child abuse are reported yearly in the United States. The National Child Abuse and Neglect Data System (NCANDS) reported an estimated 1,400 child fatalities in 2002 (1.98 children per 100,000 children in the general population), though recent studies estimate that 50% to 60% of deaths resulting from abuse or neglect are not recorded. These studies indicate that neglect is the most underrecorded form of fatal maltreatment.

Over 50% of abused children are <5 years old. The NCANDS data for 2002 showed that 41% of child abuse fatalities were in children younger than 1 year, and another 35% were in those between 1 and

4. In 2002, 38% of child abuse fatalities were due to neglect alone; 79% of the perpetrators were one or both parental caregivers. Mothers alone account for 40% of overall abuse (not specifically fatal), fathers alone for 20%, and both together about another 20%. Child abuse is managed on a state level, and the procedures and laws about whom to call differ from state to state. Some states have mandatory reporting of suspected child abuse.

Studies show that victims of childhood violence are more prone to depression, aggression, and affective instability. In longitudinal studies, 74% of adolescents who had been maltreated had at least one significant adjustment problem (e.g., aggression, trouble with the law, running away from home, gang membership, pregnancy [or impregnating someone], clinically significant anxiety or depression), which is almost double the rates of adolescents who have not been abused. The rates of prostitution in women who have been neglected or abused is also much higher, as is substance use. Multiple studies reinforce the fact that childhood trauma and stress increases the risk of depression, anxiety disorders (not limited to PTSD), and suicide attempts. Women with a history of childhood abuse have a risk of depression that is 4 times greater than those without such history. Studies in nonhuman primates suggest that early stressors lead to long-term changes in noradrenergic and serotonergic responsivity. Additionally, a recent study found that people who had experienced child abuse were more refractory to pharmacologic treatment for depression and did better with the combination of psychotherapy and pharmacotherapy.

 QUESTIONS

51-1. While waiting for your attending in the pediatric waiting room, you notice a young child walk away from his mother to look at a toy, quickly run back for a hug, and then go off again to explore further, only to return again. This behavior most typically occurs at what age?
   A. 4 to 6 months
   B. 16 to 36 months
   C. 4 years
   D. 6 years
   E. 9 to 12 months

51-2. A third-year medical student is at her cousin's house babysitting for his 12-month-old child when she is asked about

normal development. Which of the following developmental milestones is most consistent with a 12-month-old girl?
- A. Using a spoon
- B. Copying a "+"
- C. Climbing stairs
- D. Hopping on one foot
- E. Walking

51-3. On a routine exam on a 2-year-old child, which of the following would be of greatest concern regarding child abuse?
- A. Bruises of various ages on shins
- B. Bruises on forehead
- C. Healing burns on back
- D. Consistent explanations by family members
- E. Good compliance with preventative pediatric care

51-4. A 32-year-old woman has sustained a history of childhood abuse by an uncle. She is at increased risk of developing which of the following?
- A. Major depression
- B. PTSD
- C. Presence in an abusive relationship
- D. Depression refractory to medications
- E. All of the above

ANSWERS

51-1. B. This child is walking, and is engaging in a behavior defined by Margaret Mahler as "rapprochement". The fact that the child is walking comfortably suggests that he is likely over a year old. Rapprochement is seen at age 16 to 36 months, and reflects a desire to be separate, grand, and omnipotent, and yet have the mother fulfill wishes and take care of him or her. Behaviorally, the child can appear independent and rejecting of the mother one moment, then clinging and helpless the next. Mahler referred to this as "ambitendency."

51-2. E. Children generally take their first steps around their first birthday. By 18 months, they are usually able to walk up steps and use a spoon. Copying a "+" and hopping on one foot occur around age 4.

51-3. C. A 2-year-old toddler may have lots of falls throughout his or her daily life, depending on a variety of factors, including his gross motor development and his personality. However, bruises on the back or, more significantly, burns are very unlikely to happen in routine play. If the parental figures have consistent stories, and the child can participate and explain what happened (in an older child), the suspicion would be lessened. Noncompliance with pediatric care may add to worries about abuse or neglect.

51-4. E. Childhood abuse clearly increases the risk of developing a number of psychiatric disorders, including mood, anxiety, and personality disorders. Children who are abused are more likely to get into abusive relationships, and are more likely to be refractory to medication.

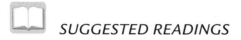

SUGGESTED READINGS

Crume T, DiGuiseppi C, Byers T, et al. Underascertainment of child maltreatment fatalities by death certificates, 1990–1998. *Pediatrics* 2006;(110)2. http://pediatrics.aappublications. org/cgi/reprint/110/2/e18.pdf (PDF 76KB).

National Clearinghouse on Child Abuse and Neglect Information. *Child fatalities resource listing.* 2003. Accessed April 2004 from http://nccanch.acf.hhs.gov/pubs/reslist/rl_dsp.cfm?subjID = 19.

Kini N, Lazoritz S. Evaluation for possible physical or sexual abuse. *Pediatr Clin North Am.* 1998 Feb;45(1):205–219.

Nemeroff CB. Neurobiological consequences of childhood trauma. *J Clin Psychiatry.* 2004;65 (Suppl 1):18–28.

Tenney-Soeiro R, Wilson C. An update on child abuse and neglect. *Curr Opin Pediatr.* 2004 Apr;16(2):233–237.

CASE **52**

"I Can't Get Him to Go to School!"

 CC/ID: 8-year-old boy brought in by his parents because he refuses to go to school.

THOUGHT QUESTION

- ■ Why might a child refuse to go to school?

DISCUSSION

A child may avoid school for many reasons, including wishing to avoid a bully, embarrassment, wanting to avoid teachers or peers (e.g., from enuresis, ADHD causing social difficulties, a learning disability), depression, an organic illness causing difficulties (e.g., hyperthyroidism causing anxiety), separation anxiety, or truancy associated with conduct disorder. A child may also be kept at home (e.g., a mental or physical illness in a parent.)

 CASE CONTINUED

HPI: For the past 6 weeks, since spring break ended, S.R. has **refused to go to school.** During the first week of break, the family had gone camping and shared a tent. After returning home, S.R. came into his parent's bed at night and now refuses to sleep alone. During the second week of break, S.R. followed his mother around everywhere, even to the bank: "It was like having a third arm," she says. He did this preferentially over playing with friends and refused to go to his best friend's sleepover party. He went to school the first few days after break but always found a pretext to go home (e.g., stomachaches, which would resolve on returning home). When his parents insisted that he return to school, he would throw "tantrums" that they "could not bear," and his mother began to ask about the feasibility of home schooling. His pediatrician confirmed he was not ill and suggested they bring S.R. in for a psychiatric evaluation. S.R. admits he has become overwhelmed with the idea that "something will happen to my mom" if he isn't there. He is not depressed, or anhedonic, and has no changes in sleep, appetite, energy, or concentration. He **denies any traumatic event at school,** likes his 3rd grade teacher, participates appropriately in school, and had been doing well academically. However, 4 months ago his grandmother died.

PMHx: None

Meds: None

SHx/FHx: Maternal aunt: panic disorder with agoraphobia. Father: major depressive episode 10 years ago. Mother's mother died suddenly this year, had lived nearby.

DevHx: Unremarkable pregnancy, delivery, milestones.

VS: WNL

PF: Unremarkable, appropriate physical development for age

Labs: WNL

MSE: *General:* Appears his age, **extremely reluctant to have parents leave** the room. *Mood:* "Okay, I guess." *Affect:* constricted, anxious. *Thought process:* goal-directed. *Thought content:* preoccupied with his mother staying within audible distance of him; no perceptual disturbances or delusions, no suicidal or homicidal ideation.

 ## THOUGHT QUESTION

- What is the most likely diagnosis?

 ## DISCUSSION

S.R. meets the criteria for separation anxiety disorder (SAD), characterized by excessive and **developmentally inappropriate anxiety concerning separation** from home or from major attachments—

TABLE 52-1   Criteria for Separation Anxiety Disorder

Excessive distress when away from home or in anticipation of separation
Worry about harm befalling or losing major attachment figures (MAFs)
Not going to sleep if not near a MAF
Refusing school or to be away from a MAF
Fear that an untoward event will lead to separation (e.g., being lost or kidnapped)
Complaints about physical symptoms when separation occurs or is anticipated
Nightmares about separation
Fear of being alone without an MAF

Adapted from American Psychiatric Association. *Task Force on DSM-IV. Diagnostic and statistical manual of mental disorders: DSM-IV.* 4th ed. Washington, DC: American Psychiatric Association, 1994.

TABLE 52-2   School Refusal

Child not going to school	Truant (50%)	May be associated with ODD, CD, or depression
Child remains at home	Being kept at home (10%)	Child physically ill Parent ill Household/work Family or religious holidays Other duties
	Refusing to go to school (25%)	Fears concerning school (e.g., bullying, embarrassment at phys. ed., academic problems) Fears or phobias about going to school (e.g., traveling or types of transport) Symptom of psychiatric disorder (e.g., depression, anxiety, or adjustment disorder Separation anxiety disorder

ODD, oppositional defiant disorder; CD, conduct disorder. Percentages are approximate; ~15% have mixed causes, including truancy and separation anxiety, or psychiatric disorders and separation anxiety.
Adapted from Berg I. School refusal and truancy. *Arch Dis Child.* 1997;76:90–91; Egger HL, Costello EJ, Angold A. School refusal and psychiatric disorders: a community study. *J Am Acad Child Adolesc Psychiatry.* 2003;42(7):797–807.

usually parents. This is evidenced by three or more of the symptoms in Table 52-1. It is accompanied by functional impairment, must last more than 4 weeks, and have an onset before age 18. Basically the child becomes frantically afraid of separation, becomes highly anxious with **symptoms of autonomic arousal** when it happens or is anticipated, and uses various behaviors to avoid it (e.g., tantrums, school refusal). In this child, it is possible that the sudden death of his grandmother precipitated fears of losing his mother, an inference which should be explored. See Table 52-2 for the differential for school refusal.

 QUESTIONS

52-1. At what age is it most common to see normal separation anxiety?
   A. 5 months
   B. 9 months
   C. 18 months
   D. 2 years
   E. 5 years

52-2. Which of the following is correct about separation anxiety as opposed to SAD?
   A. Children may normally experience some symptoms of anxiety on separation until age 3.
   B. Homesickness at the start of camp is an example of separation anxiety disorder.
   C. It is considered abnormal to have fears about leaving home to go to college.
   D. SAD can only be diagnosed after age 6.
   E. Normal separation concerns are often associated with impairment in age-appropriate functioning.

52-3. Which of the following is found in SAD?
   A. The peak age of onset is approximately 3 years old.
   B. Comorbid psychiatric diagnoses are uncommon.
   C. There are increased rates of anxiety disorders in families.
   D. Onset before the age of 7 is a poor prognostic sign.
   E. The prevalence of separation anxiety disorder is approximately 20%.

52-4. Which of the following is correct concerning the treatment of SAD?
   A. Hypnotherapy is the most effective treatment.

B. Randomized placebo controlled trials show nortriptyline to be effective.
C. Family counseling should be used.
D. There is clear longitudinal data suggesting chronicity in 40% of patients.
E. Low-dose antipsychotics are the treatment of choice.

ANSWERS

52-1. B. At about 7 months to 1 year children normally go through a period of separation anxiety and stranger anxiety. This is a normal developmental stage of attachment.

52-2. A. Normal separation anxiety and stranger anxiety may continue in some form until age 3 or 4 years, although the disorder is diagnosable in a child under 4 when there is considerable impairment; there is a specific modifier, "with early onset," for children under 6. Children often have periods of feeling homesick or reluctant to leave home, for periods ranging from the first days of camp to the first days of college. To meet criteria for separation anxiety, this must be a prolonged period (>4 weeks) and cause significant distress or impair functioning.

52-3. C. Increased rates of SAD have been reported in siblings. Also, first-degree relatives of children with SAD have increased rates of anxiety, especially panic disorder and depression. About 40% to 60% of children with SAD have a comorbid psychiatric diagnosis, with the most common being other anxiety disorders and major depression. The prevalence of SAD is 3% to 5%, and the peak age at is 7 to 9 years. The course is variable: the presence of comorbidity, later age at onset, and serious family psychiatric illness may be associated with a greater risk of chronicity. Children with SAD are more likely to have panic disorder later in life.

52-4. C. Family counseling may be of benefit, especially in cases in which family dysfunction complicates the picture. Identifying and treating an anxious parent also helps. The major treatment of SAD is behavioral therapy, in which parents are taught techniques such as graded desensitization and rewards for improvement. There are no good placebo controlled trials evaluating treatment specifically for SAD. However, there was one placebo-controlled study of fluvoxamine used to treat a variety of anxiety disorders in children which reported significant benefits (The

Research Unit on Pediatric Psychopharmacology Anxiety Study Group. Fluvoxamine for the treatment of anxiety disorders in children and adolescents. *N Engl J Med.* 2001;344(17):1279–1285). A variety of other medications have been used, usually in combination with behavioral therapy, and medications include buspirone (5HT$_{1A}$ agonist), SSRIs, or low-dose clonazepam (Klonopin). The long-term effects (therapeutic or otherwise) of various interventions for SAD are not known; in general, longitudinal data are scarce, although there is an approximately 96% remission rate.

 SUGGESTED READINGS

Costello EJ, Mustillo S, Erkanli A, et al. Prevalence and development of psychiatric disorders in childhood and adolescence. *Arch Gen Psychiatry*. 2003;60(8):837–844.

Kearney, C. A., Sims KE, Pursell CR, et al. Separation anxiety disorder in young children: a longitudinal and family analysis. *J Clin Child Adolesc Psychol.* 2003;32(4):593–598.

Berg, I. School refusal and truancy. *Arch Disease Childhood.* 1997; 76(2):90–91.

"My Son Is Always in Trouble at School"

CC/ID: 11-year-old boy brought in by his mother at the recommendation of the school.

HPI: You speak to D.M.'s mother separately, and she tells you that her son has been in detention for most of 5th grade, and the school told her to have him evaluated when he was found with another child's CD player in his bag. The mother tells you that at a recent school function, she was offered condolences about the death of her brother who, in reality, had not died. Apparently D.M. had told his teacher he was unable to complete his project because his uncle had a car accident and died. She hands you a report from school describing his behavior. He has had **many fights** and was **often truant** this year. At home he constantly **argues** with his mother and stepfather, refuses to come inside or put things away, and has **run away** twice for the night. These behaviors started about 2 years ago and have increased in frequency and severity over the past year.

When you see the patient alone, he states that nothing is wrong, and that things are basically fine. When you confront him with the information from the school, he states that he doesn't know how the CD player got into his bag, and that his problems in school stem from other people: "The teacher is mean," and "That kid looked at me funny."

PMHx: None

SHx/FHx: Biological father: Hx of substance abuse, now **incarcerated.** Mother: remarried for 7 years, two other children; stepfather is a salesman and often away for weeks. D.M. was beaten by his biological father in the first 3 years of his life.

DevHx: Unremarkable

PE/Labs: Noncontributory. No evidence of current physical abuse.

MSE: *General:* Appears his age; nonchalant demeanor. *Mood:* "Whatever," though seems angry. *Affect:* constricted, angry. *Thought process:* goal-directed. *Thought content:* withholding, no perceptual disturbances or delusions, not internally preoccupied, no suicidal or homicidal ideation.

 ## THOUGHT QUESTIONS

- What else is important to ask?
- What is your differential diagnosis?

 ## DISCUSSION

At this point the differential diagnosis includes ADHD, oppositional defiant disorder, conduct disorder, major depression, bipolar disorder with "acting out" behaviors, substance abuse, or intermittent explosive disorder. There are a number of aspects that were not covered in the interview that will help differentiate these diagnoses, including **substance use, cruelty to animals or people, destruction of property or fire setting, using a weapon,** mood symptoms, restlessness, hyperactivity, difficulties with attention and concentration, and intelligence.

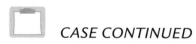 ## CASE CONTINUED

In further discussion with the school, the mother, and the patient, there is no evidence of depressed mood or symptoms of mania. D.M. does not have symptoms of ADHD. He has tried alcohol and marijuana, but is not a habitual user. He once set fire to a neighbor's shed, and has bullied younger children. He has no legal actions pending. He is able to perform adequately on assignments.

 ## THOUGHT QUESTION

- With this further information, what is the most likely diagnosis?

DISCUSSION

Oppositional defiant disorder (ODD) is diagnosed by the presence of argumentativeness, noncompliance with rules, and negativism, but without physical aggression, destruction of property, or cruelty. **ODD may develop into conduct disorder (CD), which is a persistent pattern in which the basic rights of others or major age-appropriate norms or rules are violated.** This includes aggression to people or animals (e.g., bullying, initiating fights, using a weapon, stealing while confronting a victim, forcing sexual activity), destruction of property (e.g., fire setting), deceitfulness or theft (e.g., lying to obtain goods or to avoid obligations, breaking into a house or car, stealing nontrivial items), and serious violations of rules (e.g., running away overnight at least twice, truancy).

In ADHD there may be disinhibition, like blurting out answers. ADHD may also be comorbid with CD or ODD. Major depression may be associated with acting out, and bipolar disorder with impulsive violation of rules and aggression. Substance abuse may have associated irritability, disinhibition, and antisocial behaviors related to obtaining or using the substance, and it is often comorbid with CD. Intermittent explosive disorder is an impulse control disorder in which patients have unprovoked outbursts, but besides unplanned aggression, patients do not engage in violations of rules, theft, or running away. D.M. does not meet criteria for any of these latter disorders. Thus, CD is the most likely diagnosis.

QUESTIONS

53-1. Which of the following is a primary treatment for conduct disorder?
- A. Individual psychodynamic psychotherapy for 6- to 12-year-old children
- B. Home schooling to avoid negative peer interactions
- C. Electroconvulsive therapy
- D. Family therapy and behavioral skills training
- E. Always removing the child from the home

53-2. Which of the following is correct concerning the epidemiology of ODD and CD?
- A. 90% of children with CD will have antisocial PD as adults.

   B. Isolated antisocial behaviors may occur in up to 20% of
       youth in the United States.
   C. The M:F ratio is 1:1.
   D. Peak age of onset is approximately 16 to 20 years.
   E. ODD or CD is present in 40% to 70% of children with
       ADHD.

53-3. Which of the following is a risk factor for CD?
   A. Genetic vulnerability
   B. Physical abuse
   C. Neglectful parenting
   D. Poverty
   E. All of the above

53-4. A common comorbid disorder with CD or ODD is
   A. Obsessive-compulsive disorder
   B. Major depression
   C. Anorexia nervosa
   D. Schizophrenia
   E. Wilson disease

ANSWERS

53-1. D. Therapy should occur within a multisystem-based
approach that includes family, school, legal, and substance abuse
counseling, as well as skills management targeting anger management and conflict resolution. Behavioral techniques taught to the
family and social skills training for the patient are helpful. Individual therapy has not been shown to be helpful as the primary
method of treatment in 6- to 12-year-old children; however, it can
be helpful in adolescents. Residential treatment with clear behavioral plans and special school environments can be helpful, especially if the home environment is not safe, and early intervention is
better. Psychometric testing (e.g., IQ testing) can help clarify level
of intellectual functioning, the presence of any learning disabilities,
and may offer insights into personality structure or other psychiatric issues. Pharmacotherapy can be used to address comorbid
diagnoses and may help in addressing impulsive aggression. Medications are used more frequently in adolescent populations.

53-2. E. In ADHD, the M:F ratio is approximately 4:1. Data
from several epidemiological studies indicate that ODD and CD are
present in 40% to 70% of children with ADHD. About 40% of children with CD will grow up to be adults with antisocial PD. Isolated

antisocial behaviors (e.g., shoplifting, experimentation with alcohol or marijuana) are common, and may occur in up to 80% of youth in the United States. To make a diagnosis of conduct disorder there must be a persistent history and at least three of the behaviors described in the discussion. The peak age of onset is late childhood or early adolescence. There are two subtypes: onset before and onset after 10 years old. Earlier onset may have a worse prognosis.

53-3. E. All of the above. Genetic vulnerability has been supported in adoption studies. "Difficult temperament" may engender increased parental anger and frustration and lead to abuse, or it may directly be associated with later behavioral problems. There are also studies on the biological consequences of childhood abuse: decreased hippocampal volume, altered autonomic reactivity, and maladaptive attachment behaviors, especially with extended and severe abuse. Parental substance abuse, marital discord, poverty, community violence, and abusive and neglectful parenting are all risk factors.

53-4. B. Schizophrenia is not a common comorbid diagnosis. ADHD, substance abuse, and mood and anxiety disorders are seen with regularity. Major depression is the most common.

SUGGESTED READINGS

Burke JD, Loeber R, Birmaher B. Oppositional defiant disorder and conduct disorder: a review of the past 10 years, part II. *J Am Acad Child Adolesc Psychiatry*. 2002;41(11):1275–1293.

Costello EJ, Mustillo S, Erkanli A, et al. Prevalence and development of psychiatric disorders in childhood and adolescence. *Arch Gen Psychiatry*. 2003;60(8):837–844.

Ruths S, Steiner H. Psychopharmacologic treatment of aggression in children and adolescents. *Pediatr Ann*. 2004;33(5):318–327.

van Manen TG, Prins PJ, et al. Reducing aggressive behavior in boys with a social cognitive group treatment: results of a randomized, controlled trial. *J Am Acad Child Adolesc Psychiatry*. 2004;43(12):1478–1487.

"I'm Stressed"

CC/ID: TS is an 18-year-old single white female, freshman in college, who comes to the student health service for "stress."

HPI: She complains of feeling "out of control" since starting college. She denies depressed mood, anhedonia, poor sleep, energy, concentration, or appetite, but says she **doesn't like the way she looks.** She was a cheerleader in high school, was weighed weekly, and maintained her weight closely. As the squad competed nationally, the pressure to be **"thin and perfect"** was strong. In 10th grade someone told her about vomiting to avoid gaining weight. She has **binged and purged** ever since, and has felt "bad" and "guilty," but has not sought help. She has recently gained 7 lb and feels "enormous." At college, she has found the academics harder and social **pressures** greater than in high school. She eats small amounts at meals to try to control weight, but then "raids" the local 24-hour store at night for snacks, which she secretly eats then **vomits.** She does this more than 4 nights a week. A typical binge includes a bag of cookies, potato chips, and a pint of ice cream. She denies using ipecac, laxatives, or diuretics.

PMHx: None

PPHx: As above. No history of noneating-related impulsive or self-injurious behavior.

SHx/FHx: Alcohol and explosive rages in her father. Her mother is "nice," but unable to stand up to him. In her family food is important, and she feels expected to be thin. She has had a few brief relationships with men who have cheated on her; none of these has progressed past an early dating stage.

THOUGHT QUESTIONS

- What might you look for on physical examination?
- What laboratory abnormalities do you expect?

DISCUSSION

Stigmata from bulimia include abrasions or **calluses on the knuckles** and backs of the hands from self-induced vomiting (Russell sign), **dental caries** or erosion from stomach acid, and **parotid enlargement** resulting in a "chipmunk" appearance. Bingeing can cause gastric dilatation and, rarely, rupture. Vomiting may cause **esophagitis,** Mallory-Weiss tears, and rarely esophageal rupture. Ipecac abuse may cause cardiomyopathy. Vomiting can cause hypochloremic metabolic alkalosis from the loss of HCl from gastric fluid. Potassium is lost through emesis, laxative, or diuretic abuse, but most is lost from increased renal excretion because of **metabolic alkalosis. Hypokalemia** leads to skeletal and smooth muscle weakness and to cardiac conduction abnormalities, arrhythmia, and cardiac arrest. Chronic metabolic alkalosis can be associated with hypokalemic **nephropathy** and renal failure.

CASE CONTINUED

VS: BP 120/70, HR 60; weight: 135 lb, height 5'5"

PE: *General:* No acute distress. *HEENT:* bilateral parotid enlargement, dentition fair. *CV:* RR&R, no murmurs.

MSE: *General:* Eye contact good; intense demeanor. *Speech:* normal rate and tone. *Mood:* "Okay," but with clear frustration. *Affect:* reactive, full range. *Thought process:* goal-directed. *Thought content:* preoccupied with being liked, no hallucinations, no suicidal or homicidal ideation. *Insight:* fair. *Judgment:* fair.

Labs: ECG: WNL

$$4.4 \ \frac{13.8}{38} \ 140 \qquad \frac{134 \ | \ 100 \ | \ 12}{3.1 \ | \ 22 \ | \ 1} \ 80$$

THOUGHT QUESTIONS

- How would you proceed from here?
- Does she need to be admitted to the hospital?
- What types of treatments are known to be helpful?

🗩 DISCUSSION

This patient is not medically unstable. Her slightly low potassium can be replaced orally and monitored as an outpatient. Hospitalization is for medical instability or failure to respond to outpatient treatment, and may provide the structure needed to break the binge/purge cycle. On inpatient eating disorder units, food intake is closely monitored, as is bathroom use, to prevent purging.

Cognitive behavioral therapy (CBT) is the mainstay of treatment. It challenges cognitive distortions and overvalued ideas that lead to the binge/purge cycle, such as body image distortions and rituals ("If I eat one bite of pie I must exercise for 50 minutes," or "I'm worthless unless I'm thin"). It offers alternatives in addressing impulses (e.g., wait 5 minutes before purging and write down how you feel). Information is given about nutrition, meal planning, and medical consequences. Medications are also used in treating bulimia and comorbid disorders. **SSRIs** are used in normal-weight bulimics to help with impulsivity and binge/purge behaviors. **Naltrexone** has been used in severe bulimics who cannot stop purging, but must be used with caution because of liver toxicity. **Buproprion should be avoided** in bulimia, as it has been associated with seizures, as should lithium because rapid shifts in fluid balance can cause fluctuation of lithium levels and toxicity (Table 54-1).

TABLE 54-1   Review of Selective Serotonin Reuptake Inhibitors

General	■ Block the reuptake of serotonin, and minimally that of other neurotransmitters
	■ Do not use within 2 weeks of an MAOI and do not start an MAOI within 2 weeks of SSRI treatment (5 weeks for fluoxetine); note that the antibiotic linezolid has MAOI-like properties
	■ Common side effects generally include **decreased libido, abnormal or delayed ejaculation, impotence**, anorexia, constipation, headache, **nausea, anxiety**, insomnia, and easy bruising
	■ Rare but more serious side effects include increased suicidal ideation and suicide (particularly in children and adolescents), hyponatremia, seizures, and mania or hypomania
	■ Doses are generally the same for anxiety and depression, except for OCD which requires a higher dose and longer duration for effect to begin
	■ Doses should be lowered in debilitated or geriatric patients, or in those with liver or renal impairment

(Continued)

TABLE 54-1   Review of Selective Serotonin Reuptake Inhibitors (*continued*)

	■ Check for possible drug interactions (N.B. **p450 system**) ■ Uses below reflect FDA approved uses only, though in theory, they should be interchangeable
Fluoxetine (Prozac)	Bulimia, depression, OCD, panic disorder, and premenstrual dysphoric disorder (PMDD) **Longest half-life of the SSRIs;** most activating/energizing
Paroxetine (Paxil)	Depression, OCD, panic disorder, social anxiety disorder, and generalized anxiety disorder **The shortest half-life of the SSRIs,** and therefore the worst withdrawal phenomena (e.g., dysphoria, flu-like feelings, myalgias and arthralgias, electric-shock-like sensations, disorientation); more anticholinergic than other SSRIs, and possibly more sedating
Sertraline (Zoloft)	Depression, OCD, panic disorder, PTSD, PMDD, and social anxiety disorder
Fluvoxamine (Luvox)	OCD. **Check interactions,** N.B. theophylline and warfarin
Citalopram (Celexa)	Depression
Escitalopram (Lexapro)	Depression and generalized anxiety

QUESTIONS

54-1. Which of the following is a criterion for diagnosing bulimia?
A. Being <75% of ideal body weight
B. Strict control over food consumption
C. Amenorrhea
D. Episodes of binge eating followed by guilt or shame
E. Lack of preoccupation with weight

54-2. Which of the following is correct in bulimia nervosa?
A. The peak age of onset is 10 years.
B. Mortality is >50%.
C. 80% will have chronic symptoms at 5 years.
D. The relapse rate is ~10%.
E. The M:F ratio is 1:10

54-3. Which of the following is commonly postulated in understanding bulimic behaviors?
A. Bingeing is noradrenergically mediated and related to the intrinsic response to starvation.

    B. Purging is a response to inadequate parental discipline.
    C. Purging is a self-injurious or punishing behavior.
    D. Bingeing is an inappropriate response to hunger.
    E. Binging represents direct fulfillment of unrequited
       oedipal urges.

54-4. Which of these comorbid psychiatric disorders is common in bulimia?
    A. Borderline personality disorder
    B. Avoidant personality disorder
    C. Schizotypal personality disorder
    D. Narcissistic personality disorder
    E. Obsessive-compulsive personality disorder

ANSWERS

54-1. D. Bulimics are usually normal or slightly overweight, and are not usually amenorrheic. Binges typically last ~1 hour and are very caloric. Compensatory measures after bingeing include vomiting, laxatives, periods of starvation, use of diuretics, thyroid preparations, etc. Patients often describe a sense of losing control. Episodes are often followed by guilt, shame, or depression. Bulimics who do not purge but use starvation or exercise belong to the nonpurging subtype. Of note, the weight criterion for anorexia differentiates bulimia from anorexia of the binge/purge subtype.

54-2. E. Bulimia was only rigorously defined in 1980, so there are few long-term studies. The M:F ratio is 1:10. The prevalence is approximately 1% to 3% of adolescent and adult women in the United States and Europe. The onset is usually around 18 years old. After 5 to 10 years, 50% have full recovery, 20% continue to meet criteria for bulimia, and 33% of recovered bulimics relapse within 4 years. The mortality rate is approximately 3%. Personality disorders with impulse control problems are associated with a poorer prognosis.

54-3. C. Bingeing has been postulated as an attempt to fill a sense of emptiness and provide self-soothing and self-nurturing. Purging may be both to try to avoid weight gain and as part of a pattern of self-injurious or punishing behavior after giving in to a binge. Unexpressed anger or other strong or intolerable emotions often trigger binge/purge episodes.

54-4. A. It is always important to assess for comorbid psychiatric illness. Major depression coexists in 35% to 70% of patients, substance abuse in 15% to 30%, and axis II disorders, particularly borderline PD, in 25% to 75%. Other problems that may be associated with bulimia or the comorbid disorders include chaotic lives and relationships, impulsive or self-injurious behaviors, anxiety, and compulsivity. Also 25% may steal compulsively, especially food.

 ## SUGGESTED READINGS

Bacaltchuk J, Hay P. Antidepressants versus placebo for people with bulimia nervosa. *Cochrane Database Syst Rev.* 2004;4:CD003391.

Hay PJ, J Bacaltchuk J, Stefano S. Psychotherapy for bulimia nervosa and binging. *Cochrane Database Syst Rev.* 2004;3:CD000562.

"Everything's Fine"

 CC/ID: "The student health nurse made this appointment. Everything is under control."

HPI: A.M. is a 24-year-old, **5'5"**, first-year medical student, who says the nurse told her to come in "because of my history." As a college freshman she felt "out of control," dieted and lost weight to **75 lb**, and was hospitalized for 3 weeks. Afterward she was able to stay at 97 lb, but has never attained her "target weight" of 120 lb. Now her weight "may have slipped." She states, "I've read the books—when I'm overwhelmed, controlling my eating boosts my self-esteem." She has some difficulty concentrating, but completes her work. She sleeps "fine" at 5 hours a night. "I shouldn't need more—it gives me a chance to exercise." She exercises 2 to 3 hours a day.

PMHx: None

PPHx: As above

SHx: When she was 18 years old, her parents divorced. Father works in theater; one sister is a lawyer, the other a professional tennis player.

THOUGHT QUESTIONS

- What might you expect to see on physical examination?
- What laboratory abnormalities are seen in low weight individuals? Why?
- What other questions are crucial to ask?

CASE CONTINUED

VS: **BP 90/50, HR 45; weight 78 lb, height 5'5"**

PE: *Gen:* cachectic, in no acute distress, dressed in multiple layers of clothing. *HEENT:* temporal wasting, trace facial lanugo. *CV:*

mid-systolic click, bradycardia, and regular. *Abdomen:* scaphoid. *Ext:* dry cracked skin, no lanugo.

Labs: See figure

$$2.4 \quad \dfrac{11.8}{32} \quad 110 \qquad \dfrac{134 \mid 105 \mid 14}{3.1 \mid 20 \mid 1} \quad 55$$

MSE: Well-related, but slightly withdrawn. *Mood:* "Okay," but upon greater evaluation describes annoyance. *Affect:* slightly blunted, neutral. *Thought process:* goal-directed. *Thought content:* slightly guarded but does betray some idiosyncratic thoughts regarding food; no hallucinations, delusions, or suicidality. *Insight:* fair. *Judgment:* poor.

THOUGHT QUESTION

■ What else is important to be asked about?

DISCUSSION

It is important to ask questions about menstrual history and whether she binges or purges. This is important information diagnostically and for risk assessment. It is also important to ask about eating rituals and to look for false beliefs that can be addressed in treatment.

Amenorrhea and impotence (in males) are criteria for anorexia nervosa. Amenorrhea is associated with abnormal patterns of LH secretion and very low estradiol. At about 90% of ideal weight, menstruation may return, but the timing varies. This patient is approximately 65% of her minimum ideal weight. **Some lab abnormalities are associated with starvation:** T3 may decline by 50% because of reduced T4 to T3 conversion and increased inactive rT3; peripheral glucose may be low; cholesterol may be high due to decreased degradation and clearance. These changes are adaptive in starvation, but may perpetuate the disease and behaviors of anorexia nervosa. Hematologic changes include leukopenia, mild anemia, and hypoplastic marrow; these changes are reversible with weight gain. Lanugo, fine hair seen in sustained starvation, begins on the face and progresses to the extremities. Patients may have functional mitral valve prolapse when loss of cardiac muscle causes "floppy" valves. Finally, cerebro-cortial shrinkage occurs at extreme and persistent starvation, and may not be reversible. **Other lab abnormalities may reflect associated behaviors (e.g., vomiting or laxatives).**

The differential diagnosis includes major depression with loss of appetite, schizophrenia with delusional avoidance of food, and chronic medical illnesses such as Crohn's disease, Addison's disease, or hyperthyroidism. This patient does not meet criteria for these disorders.

 ## CASE CONTINUED

She has no binging or purging. She has not menstruated since age 18. Eating rituals include mincing food and a restricted diet (apples, bagels, and carrots). She refuses hospitalization, stating "I can change my diet and gain."

 ## THOUGHT QUESTIONS

- Would you hospitalize her?
- How would you treat her?

 ## DISCUSSION

Because of her severe medical complications (bradycardia, hypotension, ECG changes), she needs hospitalization. She could die from an arrhythmia, and may have complications of re-feeding including CHF. CBT focuses on cognitive distortions, such as body image distortion, magical thinking (pale foods have fewer calories), rituals (the fork cannot touch my lips), food restrictions, and overvalued ideas. It also addresses medical consequences like possible osteoporosis, infertility, and increased perinatal mortality in women who are able to conceive. Treatment of comorbid disorders (e.g., OCD or depression) is important. Cyproheptadine has been used in nonpurging anorexics that have difficulty gaining weight and are anxious and depressed.

 ## QUESTIONS

55-1. Which of the following is a major criterion for diagnosing anorexia nervosa?

    A. Excessive exercise
    B. Amenorrhea
    C. Insight into the seriousness of her condition
    D. Refusal to maintain weight above 65% of ideal
    E. Use of compensatory measures such as laxatives

55-2. Which of the following is true about the epidemiology of anorexia nervosa?
    A. It occurs in 5% of adolescent girls.
    B. The M:F ratio is ~1:10.
    C. The peak age of onset is 20 to 25 years.
    D. 25% have amenorrhea.
    E. 73% think they have a problem and seek help.

55-3. Which of the following is correct about the prognosis of anorexia nervosa?
    A. 15% will have a full recovery.
    B. Mortality is ~50%.
    C. Purging is a good prognostic sign.
    D. Most anorexics are very poorly motivated for treatment.
    E. Onset over age 25 is a good prognostic sign.

55-4. Which of the following is correct about the psychology of anorexia?
    A. In Western cultures, being overweight is associated with success.
    B. Control of eating is fundamentally an impulsive gesture.
    C. Anorexia may represent a way to deal with the sexual tensions of puberty.
    D. Anorexics are often nonconformists.
    E. Anorexics are rarely perfectionist and rigid.

ANSWERS

55-1. B. Although anorexics may engage in excessive exercise, it is not a diagnostic criterion. Major criteria for this illness include refusal to maintain body weight at or above 85% of ideal, intense fear of gaining weight although underweight, disturbance of body image or denial of severity of illness, and amenorrhea. There is a subpopulation of anorexic patients who engage in binge/purge behaviors. They are differentiated from bulimics by meeting weight criteria for anorexia.

55-2. B. The M:F ratio is approximately 1:10. What is known about this illness is based on people who are in treatment, and thus may not represent the general population. It may be biased toward those with more severe illness, because most patients with eating disorders have poor insight into their illness and do not seek help voluntarily. The usual age of onset is 14 to 15 years, although there are two peaks, one in early adolescence and one in late adolescence (though the range is 9 to 50+ years). The lifetime prevalence rate is approximately 0.55% of adolescent girls in the United States. Amenorrhea is one of the diagnostic criteria.

55-3. D. Most anorexics have poor insight and are not motivated to come to treatment. Ten-year outcome studies show 25% have complete recovery, 50% have marked improvement with good functioning, 7% die, and 18% function poorly and are chronically underweight. Studies have shown mortality rates as high as 20% over 20 to 30 years. Good prognostic factors in anorexia include onset under age 18 years, no hospitalizations, and no purging.

55-4. C. Anorexia may be associated with tension generated by the physical and social changes in puberty. Control of eating may increase self-esteem and self-efficacy, given a perceived global sense of ineffectiveness. Characteristics of anorexics include obsessional and inflexible thinking, social introversion, perfectionism, insecurity, regimentation, minimization of affect, and excessive conformance. They may also deny weakness and hunger. Anorexia is rare in non-Western developing countries, but with immigration the prevalence normalizes. In Western cultures, thinness may be equated with achievement and success. Family characteristics may include emphasis on appearance, and appearance equated with success. Of note, while anorexia is associated with obsessionality, rigidity, and minimization of affect, bulimia tends to be associated with impulsivity, acting out, and labile affect.

SUGGESTED READINGS

Steinhausen HC. The outcome of anorexia nervosa in the 20th century. *Am J Psychiatry*. 2002;159(8):1284–1293.

Stice E. Risk and maintenance factors for eating pathology: a meta-analytic review. *Psychol Bull*. 2002;128(5):825–848.

Treasure J, Schmidt U. Anorexia nervosa. *Clin Evid*. 2004;(11): 1192–1203.

Currin L, Schmidt U, Treasure J, et al. Time trends in eating disorder incidence. *Br J Psychiatry*. 2005;186:132–135.

CASE 56

"He Makes in His Pants"

CC/ID: 6-year-old boy who has been referred to you by his pediatrician for evaluation of his soiling problem.

HPI: George has **never achieved complete control of his bowels** and soils himself frequently. This is usually manifest by a small amount of **semi-liquid stool, which is poorly formed.** His parents started toilet training him at the age of 2 years, and he gained control of his bladder relatively easily. However, they have become increasingly frustrated with his soiling and report that punishing him does not seem to make any difference. His mother describes that he **seems to hold his stool for as long as possible,** and then it causes him distress when he finally goes. She says she is at the end of her tether with him. He has a healthy appetite and no other complaints. When you ask him about this problem, he tells you that he does not like to "do number two's." He does not hide the feces in inappropriate places.

PMHx: None

Meds: None

Allergies: NKDA

PPHx: None

SHx: George is the eldest of three, with a 4-year-old brother and a 2-year-old sister. He gets on well with his siblings. His brother achieved control of his bowels after a relatively short period. He attends school and seems to be doing all right, though his teacher reports that his soiling is sometimes a problem, and the other children sometimes make fun of him and call him names.

FHx: Asthma. No history of enuresis or encopresis in any family member.

DevHx: George was born by C-section due to a difficult labor and weighed 10 lb. He reached all other developmental milestones at the appropriate ages.

THOUGHT QUESTIONS

- What possible causes of this problem need to be considered?
- What investigations should you consider?
- How would you treat this child?

DISCUSSION

Encopresis is defined as the repeated involuntary or intentional passage of feces in inappropriate places at least once a month for at least 3 months in a child who is chronologically or mentally aged at least 4 years. It is not caused by a substance (e.g., laxatives), or a medical condition other than constipation. It occurs in about 1% of children aged 5 years and is significantly more common in boys than girls. Studies have reported prevalence rates of 1.3% of boys and 0.3% of girls aged 10 to 12 years.

As with enuresis, it may be primary (meaning the patient has never attained bowel control) or secondary (meaning that the patient once had bowel control and now has lost it). Studies have revealed that the primary type is more likely to be associated with developmental delays and enuresis. The secondary type may be associated with psychosocial stressors and conduct disorder. It is further divided into two clinical subtypes, those with constipation and overflow incontinence (retentive), and those without (nonretentive). In the retentive type, the feces are usually soft, poorly formed with continuous leakage, and small amounts are passed in the toilet. This type usually responds to treatment of the constipation. Intentional soiling can occur in children who have bowel control but choose to excrete for psychological reasons; it may be associated with CD or ODD. **The majority of children with involuntary soiling have a retentive overflow type, but it may be caused by diarrhea or anxiety.** Physical exam should evaluate the child's general health (signs of malnutrition/wasting), thyroid function, neurological function of the lower limbs (neuromuscular disorders), abdomen (retained stools), and perianal areas (fissures, ulcers, rashes). Physiologic investigations include anal manometry (may reveal abnormal expulsion dynamics) and electromyogram (EMG). These should probably be reserved for those who have failed usual treatments or when there is a high index of suspicion of an organic cause. They may require referral to a specialist center.

A plain X-ray of the abdomen may help in diagnosis of the retentive subtype. Psychological testing may be appropriate in patients with behavioral problems. There is no reported significant association between encopresis and child abuse.

CASE CONTINUED

It seems that George's soiling causes significant distress to the family. Unfortunately, punitive attitudes can lead to an element of oppositional behavior manifested by the child further holding stool. After discussing the case with your pediatric colleague, he decides to start a regimen of regular stool softeners following an initial catharsis (necessary to ensure the bowel is empty). If stool softeners fail, then laxatives should be prescribed. You instruct the parents on how to follow a program of **behavioral modification** with success positively reinforced with small rewards. The family and child are educated about bowel functioning, which helps relieve their levels of anxiety. You encourage his intake of fresh (if possible raw) fruits, vegetables, water, fruit juices, and high fiber cereals. When they return for a followup visit 6 months later, George has mastered normal bowel habits without further episodes of soiling.

QUESTIONS

56-1. Which of the following is in the differential diagnosis of encopresis?
  A. Hirschsprung disease
  B. Pyloric stenosis
  C. Meckel diverticulum
  D. Enuresis
  E. Depression

56-2. Which of the following is accurate concerning encopresis?
  A. It is always associated with a behavioral disturbance.
  B. Treatment is not usually successful.
  C. It may be associated with abnormal expulsion dynamics.
  D. It is always related to psychological causes.
  E. An initial catharsis is rarely needed.

56-3. Which of the following is correct concerning the possible psychological causes of encopresis?
  A. It is usually related to childhood sexual abuse.
  B. These causes may not predict treatment outcome.

C. They may play a more important role in the primary type.
D. They include developmental delay.
E. Early and punitive bowel training is associated.

56-4. Which of the following is correct concerning the treatment of encopresis?
A. Treatment rarely involves education.
B. Treatments have been reported to be successful in almost 30% of children.
C. Psychological interventions are rarely needed.
D. Imipramine is a rarely first-line treatment for this disorder.
E. Operant conditioning involves the bell and pad technique.

ANSWERS

56-1. A. Medical causes of encopresis include Crohn disease, Hirschsprung disease, other smooth muscle disorders (e.g., congenital amyotonia, cerebral palsy, and infectious polyneuritis), hypothyroidism, spinal cord lesions, malnutrition, and stenosis of the rectum or anus. These should be ruled out if there is a suspicion of an organic cause and referral may need to be made to a specialist pediatric center. Older children may have encopresis due to prolonged gastroenteritis or lactose deficiency. Children with attention deficit or impulse-control disorders may have soiling episodes due to inattention.

56-2. C. Studies have shown that a significant percentage of children with retentive encopresis have difficulty relaxing their anal sphincters. This disorder is not invariably associated with behavioral disturbance; there are a significant number of children who have not gained adequate control of their sphincters or have difficulty recognizing the need to defecate in time. An initial catharsis using an enema or stool softeners is usually needed to empty the bowel completely. Of note, there is little if any significant relationship with enuresis.

56-3. E. Early and harsh methods of bowel training and developmental delay may be associated with encopresis. There is not a significant causal relationship reported between sexual abuse and encopresis. Although physiological variables were found to relate to outcome, psychological factors were not. Psychological factors may play a more important role in the secondary type (onset after a period of control) of encopresis.

56-4. D. There are some case reports of imipramine being effective in encopresis, but the mechanism of action is unclear, and it should probably be reserved for those who have failed the conventional methods. Treatment involves a combination of education, behavior modification, and physiologic methods involving an initial catharsis and regular use of stool softeners or laxatives. These methods have been shown to be highly successful in almost 80% of children. Maturation may contribute to spontaneous remission of symptoms. The inability to defecate a rectal balloon is associated with poorer treatment outcome. Psychological interventions are needed for those children with behavioral problems, intentional soiling, or those with contributing psychodynamic factors. Operant behavior modification techniques reward the desired behavior (defecating in the toilet) with praise or a star chart. Treatment usually takes about 6 months and may need regular encouragement from the physician.

SUGGESTED READINGS

Joinson C, Heron J, von Gontard A. Psychological problems in children with daytime wetting. *Pediatrics* 2006;118 (5):1985–1993.

Loening-Baucke V. Encopresis and soiling. *Pediatr Clin North Am.* 1996;43(1):279–298.

Mikkelsen EJ. Enuresis and encopresis: Ten years of progress. *J Am Acad Child Adolesc Psychiatry.* 2001; 40:1146.

CASE 57

"He Keeps Wetting the Bed"

CC/ID: 8-year-old boy who has been brought to the outpatient clinic. He has been wetting his bed since he was taken out of diapers at $2^1/_2$ years of age.

HPI: This has been happening about **two nights per week.** Peter is afraid to stay over at a friend's house and does not want to go away to camp this summer. Peter has never been completely continent for any period more than a few weeks. His parents had tried restricting fluids before bedtime and toileting him during the night but with limited success. His parents are now more concerned.

PMHx: None

PPHx: None

SHx: Peter is the youngest of four children, the eldest of which is 12. He started school at age 5 and has been doing well. He is a friendly child and likes to attend social events with his friends. He gets on well with his siblings and is generally well liked and popular. Peter's father works as an insurance broker, and his mother is a homemaker. The parents denied any significant financial or social difficulties.

FHx: His father had some difficulties with bedwetting himself intermittently until the age of 9.

DevHx: Peter was born by normal delivery, weighed 8 lb, and reached the other normal developmental milestones at the appropriate ages.

Labs: UA normal

THOUGHT QUESTIONS

- What do you think is happening in this boy?
- What would be significant to ask about in his history?
- What treatments are available for this disorder?

DISCUSSION

The diagnosis of enuresis is made when there is repeated void-ing of urine into clothing or bedding at least twice a week for a period of 3 consecutive months in a child whose chronological or mental age is at least 5 years. It can cause significant distress or interfere with social or academic functioning. It is not due to the effects of any substance or medical condition. It may be **nocturnal or diurnal** (daytime). In the primary type, the child has never attained complete bladder control for longer than 1 year. The sec-ondary type begins after a period of successful control (approxi-mately 1 year), and it begins commonly between the ages of 5 and 8 years. **Like encopresis, it is due to a combination and interac-tion of physiological and psychological factors.** Daytime and sec-ondary types are more likely to be related to stress and behavioral problems and tend to occur between 5 and 7 years and again at adolescence. The correlation with psychological disturbance appears to increase with age. The majority of children do not wet on an intentional basis. Those who do so may have an ODD or even psychosis. Sleep studies have revealed that enuretic episodes tend to occur during delta sleep, but can occur during all phases.

The differential diagnosis includes **urinary tract infections— particularly in girls,** who are more susceptible—so a urinalysis should be performed. Organic causes may need to be ruled out and may need a specialist referral. The maximum amount of urine a child should be able to hold should be equivalent to their age plus 2 in ounces; lesser amounts suggest a small bladder capacity. Inves-tigate the child's developmental history and see if there are any sig-nificant stressors related to past or current events. Any behavioral disturbances should be treated.

Treatment involves a combination of pharmacologic agents and behavioral techniques. If there has been a significant event such as death or divorce of a parent, then psychotherapy (individual or family) would be appropriate. Initial interventions include fluid restriction for 2 hours before bed, toileting at night (majority of urine is produced in the first third of the night), and the use of star charts to document successes with the child's receiving the reward in the morning. Criticism should be avoided. The bell and pad method involves the child's sleeping on a special pad attached to a bell. When the child voids, the bell rings, waking him or her. The parent toilets the child and then resets the system. With conditioning, the child learns to wake before the bell. This is generally successful in two-thirds of cases, but it may take up to 2 months and parents should persist. The bell and pad is usually used when more simple behavioral methods have failed and works best when the child can understand the concept (e.g., at about 8 years of age). About one-third may relapse after 1 year, and the intervention should be restarted. Spontaneous remission may occur with continued maturation.

CASE CONTINUED

Peter was started on a program with the bell and pad combined with star charts and positive reinforcement. After 2 weeks, there was notable improvement; by 10 weeks, he was no longer enuretic.

QUESTIONS

57-1. Which of the following is correct about enuresis?
   A. It is defined as the voluntary voiding of urine.
   B. Few children have nocturnal episodes only.
   C. It is present in approximately 2% of boys aged 18 years.
   D. Incidence rates are lower for girls.
   E. Boys more commonly suffer from urinary tract infections.

57-2. Which of the following is correct concerning enuresis?
   A. The vast majority do not wet on an intentional basis.
   B. Psychological factors are not important in the secondary type.
   C. There is a higher incidence in higher socioeconomic groups.
   D. It is not associated with developmental delay.
   E. Those associated with behavioral disturbance tend to have normal bladder function.

57-3. Which of the following is correct considering the etiology of enuresis?
    A. It has not been reported to occur in family members of the proband.
    B. Concordance rates are equal for monozygotic and dizygotic twins.
    C. Bladder infection should be ruled out.
    D. Obstructive lesions may be found in approximately 20% of sufferers.
    E. It is associated with smaller families. -

57-4. Which of the following is accurate about the medical treatment of enuresis?
    A. Medical interventions include imipramine or desmopressin (DDAVP) only.
    B. Monthly ECGs are recommended for those taking imipramine.
    C. Imipramine is continued indefinitely.
    D. DDAVP may be used in those who have failed other methods.
    E. Side effects of imipramine include nasal congestion, nosebleeds, headaches, and mild abdominal pain.

ANSWERS

57-1. D. Enuresis is less prevalent in girls than in boys, with the male to female ratio being about 2:1. The prevalence of enuresis is relatively high between the ages of 5 and 7, when approximately 15% of boys and 12% of girls are enuretic less than once a week. By 9 to 10 years old, approximately 6% of boys and 3.5% of girls are enuretic less than once a week. By 14 years of age, 1.9% of boys and 1.2% of girls are still enuretic less than once a week. Finally, by 18 years of age, 1% of boys continue to experience enuresis compared to its extreme rarity in girls. Boys may more commonly have a congenital abnormality of the genitourinary tract, but girls are more susceptible to urinary tract infections. The majority of sufferers have nocturnal enuresis only (unlike encopresis); daytime symptoms may suggest an underlying bladder dysfunction. (Evans JH. Evidence based management of nocturnal enuresis. *BMJ.* 2001;323(7322):1167–1169.)

57-2. A. In the vast majority, wetting is involuntary. Intentional wetting may indicate more serious psychological disturbance, such as ODD or psychosis, which should be attended to clinically.

Although most children with enuresis do not have higher rates of psychiatric disorders, children with enuresis tend to have significantly more developmental delay than those without the problem. The correlation between enuresis and psychological disturbance increases with age. Children who are socially disadvantaged, from lower socioeconomic groups, or under psychosocial stress have higher rates of enuresis. It was reported that enuretic children with behavioral disturbance had higher rates of dysfunctional bladders with smaller capacities.

57-3. C. Organic causes such as urinary tract infections (particularly in girls), urinary tract obstruction, bladder calculi, constipation, diabetes (insipidus and mellitus), congenital anomalies of the genitourinary tract, sleep apnea, or a seizure disorder should be ruled out. Obstructive lesions have been reported to occur in only 4% of children with enuresis. Enuresis may recur in families, with up to 75% of children having a first-degree relative with a similar problem; a large study reported that a maternal history of enuresis increases the child's risk by 5.2, and a paternal history increases the risk by 7.1. Twin studies have revealed greater levels of concordance between monozygotic twins (68%) compared to dizygotic twins (36%). Linkage studies have implicated several chromosomes, including chromosome 22. Enuresis has been associated with larger families.

57-4. D. Pharmacotherapies for enuresis may include imipramine or desmopressin (DDAVP). DDAVP has efficacy and relapse rates similar to imipramine and may be used in those who have failed other methods. Its side effects include nasal congestion, nosebleeds, headaches, and mild abdominal pain. There have been reports of hyponatremic seizures with prolonged use, so evening fluid intake should be limited. Parents should be warned to look out for nausea, vomiting, or headache which may the warrant an electrolyte assay. Imipramine is usually given in doses of 25 to 125 mg at night. Many studies have documented its success, though less than that found using alarms or bell systems. Monitor for intolerable anticholinergic side effects. Baseline ECG is recommended, with monitoring for those receiving higher doses (it may cause cardiac arrhythmias and seizures). Imipramine has a narrow therapeutic index, and accidental overdose may be fatal. After the child had been dry for 3 to 6 months, medication is usually tapered and stopped. Other agents under study include SSRIs and indomethacin. Recent work has suggested that oxybutynin may be helpful in those whose nocturnal enuresis is due to bladder instability. The problem usually remits spontaneously, and only a small number continue to suffer from this problem into adulthood.

SUGGESTED READINGS

Butler R, Stenberg A. Treatment of childhood nocturnal enuresis: an examination of clinically relevant principles. *BJU Int.* 2001; 88(6): 563–571.

Butler RJ. Combination therapy for nocturnal enuresis. *Scand J Urol Nephrol.* 2001; 35(5): 364–369.

Mikkelsen EJ. Enuresis and encopresis: ten years of progress. *J Am Acad Child Adolesc Psychiatry.* 2001; 40(10):1146–1158.

Joinson C, Heron J, Butler U, et al. Psychological differences between children with and without soiling problems. *Pediatrics.* 2006;117(5)1575–1584.

"My Son Isn't Talking"

CC/ID: 18-month-old boy brought in by his parents because of a speech delay.

HPI: B.D. is the first child born to his parents. His mother had an uneventful pregnancy and delivery. They report that he has been "easy" and "quiet," and only gets upset when they don't remove the tags on his clothes or when the neighbor mows his lawn. B.D.'s parents are concerned about his **not yet talking,** but his paternal great-grandmother said that all the boys in the family talked late, so not to worry. Otherwise, they thought that everything was fine until they went to a playgroup and noticed that his **behavior was quite different from other kids his age. He spends hours sitting by himself, rocking, spinning** the wheels on a toy car, or staring at his hands. He **does not interact with the other children,** nor does he seem to relate to the teachers. He neither speaks nor actively indicates his wants. He does seem to be somewhat upset when his parents leave.

PMHx: None

PSHx: None

Meds: None

FHx: Language delay as above.

DevHx: Physical milestones (rolling over, sitting up, walking) WNL.

VS: WNL

PE: Unremarkable

Labs: Chemistries, LFTs, ammonia, CBC, lead screen, sleep-deprived EEG: all WNL.

MSE: Appears his age; some odd facial expressions and grimacing, and poor eye contact. *Behavior:* spins a tennis ball, not responsive to interview, does not smile or react to you.

THOUGHT QUESTIONS

- What is in the differential diagnosis?
- What is the prognosis and treatment?

DISCUSSION

Two clinically striking elements in B.D.'s case are his lack of interpersonal relatedness and his significant language delay. The differential diagnosis includes visual or hearing impairment, Rett syndrome, Asperger syndrome, childhood disintegrative disorder (CDD), toxic and metabolic conditions (e.g., lead or inborn errors of metabolism), and autistic disorder. The central characteristics of all **autism spectrum** disorders include

- **Deficits in social interactions**
- **Deficits in communication**
- **Repetitive behaviors and restricted or stereotyped interests**

all of which are present **before 3 years of age.**

An impairment in social interaction is usually the most characteristic deficit in autism and often presents itself as the inability to form relationships and to reciprocate. Examples include a lack of eye contact and facial expression; patients are incapable of reading social cues or perceiving others' moods. Of note, until about 18 months old, autistic children may have reached normal developmental milestones. About half of autistic children are nonverbal, but this seems to be decreasing with early intervention programs. If verbal, autistic persons still have significant difficulty in social or reciprocal communication. Autistic patients may vocalize monologues about restricted topics, immune to the interests of others in their environments. Restrictive or repetitive behaviors may include repetitive motor behaviors such as arm flapping, rocking, and spinning, or higher level repetitive behaviors, such as restricted and all-encompassing interests (e.g., minerals, dates, swords). Rigid routines and rituals are also common.

Asperge syndrome is defined by significant social deficits and repetitive behaviors and interests, in the absence of language or cognitive delay. **Rett syndrome** is a disorder that occurs almost exclusively in girls, aged 5 to 48 months (although there have been rare documented cases in males). These patients have decreased head growth, loss of purposeful hand movements, stereotyped hand wringing, gait apraxia, and loss of previously developed language skills. **Childhood disintegrative disorder (CDD)** is a rare condition in which development is normal at least through age 2, followed by a regression in language, social interaction, and motor abilities. Although child abuse and neglect can cause psychological abnormalities, language delay, and poor social skills in a toddler, the theory that autism is caused by "bad parenting" has not been shown to have validity. **Hearing dysfunction** leading to language delay must always be ruled out.

In completing the workup, it is important to order a **thorough developmental assessment.** This provides a baseline, and if indicated can help steer the child toward appropriate early intervention programs. Some children, especially those who develop some language skills, may grow up to live self-sufficient, albeit marginalized and isolated, lives in the community, frequently living in structured environments. For individuals with more severe autism, chronic placement is usual. **Better prognosis is associated with higher intelligence, functional speech, and less bizarre symptoms and behaviors. Autism is often accompanied by behavioral outbursts, agitation, and self-injurious behaviors which, along with seizures, become more common with advancing age.** Autism researchers have felt that there is a window of opportunity to intervene in early childhood, in order to possibly modify the ultimate outcome. Encouraging data first arose in the 1980s when it was reported that 50% of patients in an intensive early intervention program were in regular classrooms by elementary school. Currently there are several types of early intervention programs in use. In general, treatment consists of special schools that can focus on behavioral interventions, language skills, social skills, and other discrete skill acquisitions. Teaching parents behavioral management techniques may be very helpful in managing these complex children.

CASE CONTINUED

B.D. underwent a full assessment, including audiometry, which confirmed the diagnosis of autistic disorder. He then began a comprehensive early intervention program, which included speech, language, and socialization training.

QUESTIONS

58-1. Which of the following is found in autistic disorder?
   A. It is more common in girls than boys.
   B. There is no evidence of a genetic contribution.
   C. Most children with autistic disorder have a special talent (i.e., savants).
   D. 75% are mentally retarded.
   E. Verbal IQ is usually better than performance IQ.

58-2. Which of the following is correct regarding language impairment in autism?
   A. Approximately 80% of autistic patients have functional speech.
   B. Pressured speech is common.
   C. Echolalia is rare.
   D. Speech tends to be repetitive and stereotyped.
   E. Loosening of associations is characteristic.

58-3. Which of the following is true about behavior in autistic individuals?
   A. They prefer variations in routine.
   B. They may be very sensitive to specific sounds which may lead to acting-out behaviors.
   C. They often enjoy imaginative play with dolls or figures.
   D. A typical example of repetitive play in a 4 year old would be playing a game of solitaire.
   E. Self-injurious behaviors are more common in Asperger syndrome than in autism.

58-4. Which statement about autism and its relation to other neurological disorders is correct?
   A. It is commonly comorbid with late-life Parkinson disease.
   B. There is no increased incidence of seizure disorders.
   C. It is commonly comorbid with Wilson disease.
   D. It is commonly seen in fragile X syndrome.
   E. Hemiballismus is a common complication.

ANSWERS

58-1. **D.** Approximately 75% of children with autistic disorder are mentally retarded (defined as having a full-scale IQ of less than 70 to 75). IQ is one of the most important predictors of course and outcome. Autistic disorder is four times more prevalent in boys than in girls, with an overall prevalence of 0.04 to 0.5%. Only a small number of autistic individuals are savants (10%) and have phenomenal abilities such as calendar calculation or memory. Autism has high concordance in monozygotic twins and an increased prevalence in siblings, suggesting a genetic component.

58-2. D. In keeping with the repetitiveness of their interests and behaviors, autistic individuals' speech also tends to be repetitious and stereotyped, and frequently includes echolalia and neologisms. It is estimated that only about half of autistic children develop functional speech, with a characteristic delay in the development of speech, deviancy in speech patterns, and a lack of social aspects to their speech. Pressured speech is usually seen in mania, and loosening of associations in schizophrenia.

58-3. B. Autistic individuals may be unusually sensitive to specific sounds and may react with acting-out behaviors. Additionally, they often have difficulty with new experiences. Autistic children usually prefer playing with objects like spinning plates or tops rather than imaginative play with dolls, which requires a social sense, characteristically lacking in autism. They often perform repetitive, stereotyped motor acts. Some engage in self-injurious behaviors, including biting themselves or banging their heads.

58-4. D. Autism can be associated with various neurological diseases, including tuberous sclerosis, seizure disorders (25% will have seizures by adolescence), and fragile X syndrome (the most common hereditary cause of mental retardation). Autism may also be associated with in utero exposure to maternal rubella. Wilson's disease is an autosomal recessive disorder in which copper accumulates because of a mutation in the copper transport gene, causing liver, basal ganglia, and other organ damage. It is characterized by a large amplitude tremor, parkinsonian symptoms, and nonspecific psychiatric symptoms, but not autism. It usually presents in the teenage years. Hemiballismus is a rare movement disorder in which the limbs of one side (arms more than legs) are flung about involuntarily. It is caused by lesions in the contralateral subthalamic nuclei and has a variety of infectious, vascular, traumatic, and autoimmune causes.

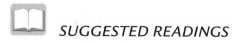 *SUGGESTED READINGS*

Constantino JN. Todd RD. Autistic traits in the general population: a twin study. *Arch Gen Psychiatry.* 2003;60(5):524–530.

Hollander E, Phillips AT, Yeh C. Targeted treatments for symptom domains in child and adolescent autism. *Lancet.* 2003;362(9385):732–734.

Muhle R, Trentacoste SV, Rapin I. The genetics of autism. *Pediatrics.* 2004;113(5):e472–486.

Shea S, Turgay A, Carroll A, et al. Risperidone in the treatment of disruptive behavioral symptoms in children with autistic and other pervasive developmental disorders. *Pediatrics.* 2004;114(5):e634–e641.

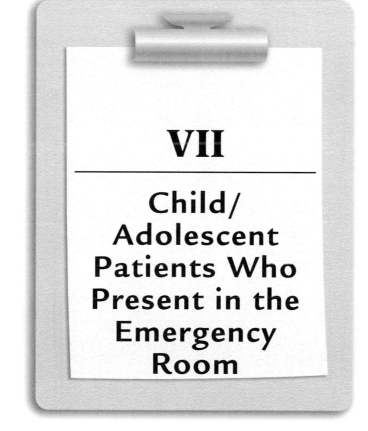

VII

Child/ Adolescent Patients Who Present in the Emergency Room

CASE 59

"I Didn't Meant to Do It"

 CC/ID: 16-year-old Asian female whom you have been asked to evaluate in the ED. She was brought in after taking an overdose of acetaminophen.

HPI: Ms. S. took approximately 20 acetaminophen tablets the prior evening after an argument with her parents over whether she would be able to attend a school friend's party that upcoming weekend. Following the argument, she went upstairs to her room, took the tablets, and went to sleep. She woke her parents early in the morning, explained her actions, and they called an ambulance.

 THOUGHT QUESTIONS

- What are your primary concerns in this situation?
- What should you look for in her history?

DISCUSSION

Medical issues: In the overdose of any pharmaceutical agent, acetaminophen accounts for the most hospitalizations. Many of those who overdose with acetaminophen do not understand the lethality involved and do not seek treatment until it is too late. Most gastrointestinal absorption of acetaminophen occurs within 2 hours of ingestion, even after overdose. The medical management of her overdose is most important. She may be at risk of serious and **fatal hepatotoxicity** (hepatic metabolism accounts for 90% of the elimination of absorbed drug) as well as nephrotoxicity. Acetaminophen is oxidized in the liver to form toxic *N*-acetyl-*p*-benzoquinonemine (NAPQI), which is then conjugated with glutathione to form nontoxic compounds. Hepatocytes are damaged when the amount of NAPQI exceeds the supply of glutathione. Those treated within 10 to

16 hours after ingestion have a significantly lower risk of hepato-toxicity. Treatment modalities are described below.

The early (less than 24 hours) signs of toxicity may be nonspecific, with lethargy, pallor, diaphoresis, anorexia, nausea, and vomiting (Table 59-1); metabolic acidosis and coma are rare presentations of overdose. **After 24 hours, acute symptoms may subside, but increases in AST, ALT, bilirubin, prothrombin time, abdominal pain, liver tenderness, and oliguria may develop. After 48 hours, hepatotoxicity can lead to acute liver failure, coagulopathy (treat with vitamin K or fresh frozen plasma), and AST levels in the thousands.** If the patient avoids hepatic failure, the laboratory abnormalities may return to normal within 2 weeks. For those who require transplant, psychiatric consultation should be arranged before encephalopathy develops.

Approach: Initial contact with the patient should **focus on developing rapport.** The complete psychiatric evaluation may be interrupted by medical needs, but it is of vital importance to ascertain whether the patient is still feeling suicidal and whether there is a need for more intensive monitoring and precautions, such as one-to-one observations.

History: **Was this a planned suicide attempt or an impulsive act?** Did she make any preparations, such as a suicide note, a will, or saying goodbye to anyone? Was she alone at the time? How was her

TABLE 59-1   Liver Damage Induced by Acetaminophen

Stages of Liver Damage	Signs and Symptoms
Stage 1: No injury	Usually within 24 hours: **nonspecific symptoms** such as nausea, vomiting, malaise, or sweating; may be asymptomatic
Stage 2: Damage begins	Usually 24 hours after ingestion: nausea, vomiting, tenderness or pain in the epigastrium or right upper quadrant
Stage 3: Maximum damage	Usually 3 to 4 days after ingestion. Symptoms and signs depend on the amount of damage that occurred. Fulminant hepatic failure may be evident with coagulopathy, encephalopathy, or coma. Hypoglycemia or metabolic acidosis may be seen. Renal failure may progress alongside hepatic injury. Death may be caused by infection, hemorrhage, multiorgan failure, respiratory failure, or cerebral edema.
Stage 4: Recovery	Hepatic enzymes may return to baseline by day 7; eventually the liver regenerates.

mood at that time? Did she think anyone would find her? Was she aware of the potential toxicity of acetaminophen? What was her intent? What did she think would happen? How does she feel being alive now (i.e., that she did not die)? How did she think her family and friends would react? Has she ever tried to harm herself in the past? If yes, examine those experiences in detail. Is there a family history of suicide, mood disorders, or alcoholism? Does she know anyone who has attempted to or succeeded in killing him or herself? Are there current stressors in her life? **What social and psychological support does she have? What coping mechanisms does she use** to deal with stressors or problems? Are there underlying physical or psychiatric illnesses? Does she have any problems with alcohol or substance use? What are her premorbid personality traits? Finally, as suicide is arguably the most severe and feared outcome of a psychiatric illness, it behooves the clinician to go through, in detail, the 24 hours leading up to the suicide attempt; the action, even if impulsive, usually does not come out of nowhere, but is precipitated by some stressful occurrence, usually idiosyncratic to the patient. The history should help resolve the cause, with an eye to its future prevention.

Mental status: A comprehensive mental state examination should be performed. If a serious psychiatric disorder is diagnosed or if there is continued risk of a further suicide attempt, she should be admitted to a psychiatry unit. In this case, if concern exists, the threshold for admission should be rather low, given this patient's not telling her parents after the overdose of acetaminophen.

TREATMENT OF ACETAMINOPHEN OVERDOSE

- May induce emesis (with ipecac), gastric lavage (rarely used, as drug is rapidly absorbed), or activated charcoal if the overdose was taken within 4 hours, and *N*-acetylcysteine therapy if within 8 hours of ingestion.

- *N*-acetylcysteine (Mucomyst) provides cysteine for increased glutathione synthesis to conjugate and detoxify the excess buildup of the toxic metabolite (NAPQI). Possible side effects include rash.

- There may be no evidence of liver damage until 24 to 48 hours after ingestion. Detectable levels of the drug can fall rapidly, so patients need intensive monitoring with serial drug and enzyme levels.

- The risk of hepatotoxicity after acute ingestion is calculated by comparing levels to a treatment nomogram. Extended release preparations should be acknowledged and are treated in a similar manner, though with a different time course. Levels between 150 and 200 μg/mL indicate possible toxicity; those above 200 μg/mL are associated with probable toxicity.

CASE CONTINUED

Upon examination she states that she was angry with her parents and had "no idea" that this would land her in the hospital. She tearfully tells you that she does not wish to die and regrets this impulsive action. She has no significant past medical, psychiatric, or family history, and she denies any additional history of deliberate self-harm.

MSE: *Affect/Mood:* states she is euthymic but embarrassed, manifests tearfulness and anxious affect. *Thought process:* no evidence of thought disorder. *Thought content:* she is hopeful about her future and regrets the attempt; no evidence of psychosis, suicidal, or homicidal ideation. *Cognitive function/insight:* intact.

She is admitted to the medical service as an inpatient for 5 days until her liver enzymes return to normal. During this time, you are able to perform brief dynamic psychotherapy, and she does well. Possible sources of external and internal support for the patient are identified to help her cope with future stressors. She is discharged to the care of her family, with a followup evaluation scheduled.

QUESTIONS

59-1. Which of the following is accurate about acetaminophen overdose?
- A. Decreased risk of toxicity is found in chronic alcoholics and those taking medications that induce the P450 isoenzymes system.
- B. Acetylcysteine is used to replace hepatic glutamate.
- C. Adolescents frequently underestimate the possible danger of this medication.
- D. It is an uncommon cause of acute liver failure.
- E. Ibuprofen has no hepatotoxicity.

59-2. Increased risk of completed suicide is associated with which of the following?
- A. Social isolation
- B. Epilepsy
- C. Antisocial personality disorder

D. Multiple sclerosis
E. All of the above

59-3. Features of the mental status that are associated with increased risk of suicide include
A. Feelings of hopelessness and pessimism
B. Delusions of poverty or control
C. Agitation
D. Depression
E. All of the above

59-4. Suicide rates
A. Decrease with increasing age
B. Are higher in urban than rural areas
C. Are higher among non-Whites in the United States
D. Are lower in immigrants compared with their country of origin
E. Are higher in Asians than African Americans in the United States

ANSWERS

59-1. C. Adolescents often underestimate the danger of acetaminophen overdose, and it is a common cause of drug-induced acute liver failure. There is increased risk of toxicity in patients with alcohol dependence, malnourishment, and in those taking medications that induce P450 isoenzymes (e.g., isoniazid, some anticonvulsants). However, acute ingestion of alcohol may protect from toxicity by competing for P450 enzymes. Acetylcysteine is used to replace hepatic glutathione, which is used to conjugate and detoxify the toxic metabolites of acetaminophen. N-acetylcysteine may improve survival even in acetaminophen-induced hepatic failure, long after the acetaminophen has been metabolized. Patients with serious coagulopathy, encephalopathy, and refractory metabolic acidosis require urgent referral to a transplant center. All adolescents and pediatric patients should be admitted, observed, and treated for at least 48 hours postingestion. Ibuprofen is, in itself, hepatotoxic in overdose, though not to the same predictable extent as acetaminophen.

59-2. E. Increased risk of completed suicide is associated with social isolation, divorced/widowed, male gender, epilepsy, AIDS, head injury, Huntington's chorea, multiple sclerosis, antisocial personality disorder, and insomnia. Older Caucasian and younger

African-American males (25 to 34 years old) have higher rates of suicide than their counterparts. There is a disproportionately high rate of suicide among younger Native Americans/Alaskans. However, in all age groups, Caucasians commit suicide twice as often as do African-Americans or Hispanics. Females have more attempts (3:1), but males have greater rates of completion (4:1), as they tend to use more lethal means. Stressors that may precipitate suicide in young people include separation, rejection, unemployment, and legal problems. In interview and evaluation, problems surrounding and precipitating the suicide attempt should be explored, as well as alternative solutions that the patient had envisioned. Approximately 1% of those who attempt suicide will succeed in the following year. Increased risk is associated with a previous suicide attempt or attempts, previous psychiatric treatment, living alone, a history of trauma or abuse, impulsive tendencies, and alcohol abuse or/dependence. One percent of Americans die by suicide, and it is the eighth leading cause of death in the United States. Adolescent rates have tripled since the 1950s. Knowledge about risk factors should inform the physician's thorough assessment.

59-3. **E.** Feelings of hopelessness and pessimism, delusions of poverty or control, agitation, and command auditory hallucinations are all features that are associated with increased risk of suicide. The majority of suicide victims suffer from depression at the time of death, but the degree of hopelessness may be more predictive than the level of depression. Other causes of increased risk include a history of anorexia nervosa, incest or child abuse, depression with severe anxiety/panic attacks, and a previous attempt.

59-4. **B.** Suicide rates are higher in urban than in rural areas. Rates increase with increasing age; the peak for males is after age 45 and for females after age 55. Elderly persons attempt suicide less often than younger ones but are more often successful, and they account for 25% of all suicides. The rate of suicide among those over 75 years is more than 3 times that of the young. The rate for Whites is higher (nearly twice the rate) than for non-Whites. Among non-Whites the rates for African-Americans is higher than that for Asian-Americans. Rates are increased among immigrants in a new country when compared to their peers back in their country of origin and to nonimmigrants in their new country. The most common methods for men include firearms and hanging, while women tend to overdose on medications. The 6 months following a psychiatric hospitalization is a high-risk period.

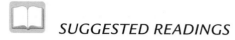

SUGGESTED READINGS

James LP, Wells E, Beard RH, et al. Predictors of outcome after acetaminophen poisoning in children and adolescents. *J Pediatr.* 2002;140(5): 522–526.

Stovall J, Domino FJ. Approaching the suicidal patient. *Am Fam Physician.* 2003;68(9):1814–1818.

"He Is Not Making Any Sense"

CC/ID: 13-year-old boy who is brought to the ED by his neighbor, who found him lying on the ground appearing to be drunk with a **plastic bag filled with glue** beside him.

HPI: Kevin's neighbor found him about 30 minutes ago, **barely responsive** and unable to speak clearly. He had contacted the boy's parents who arrived shortly from work. They were extremely shocked and say they had no idea that their son was involved with drugs of any kind.

PMHx: Fractured collarbone at age 8 following a fall from a tree

PPHx: None

SHx: Kevin is the youngest of five boys, the oldest of which is 22. His father works as an electrician, and his mother works as a stenographer at the local courthouse. Though his parents describe him as a "good kid" who has not been a problem, he has been caught truant several times at school.

FHx: Paternal uncle has problems with alcohol.

VS: Afebrile, BP 110/70, HR 65, RR 12

PE: *HEENT:* eyes closed, PERRLA, **nystagmus bilaterally**; perioral red rash. *CV:* RR&R, no murmurs. *Lungs:* clear to auscultation and percussion. *Abdomen:* soft, nontender, normal bowel sounds. *Neuro:* **reflexes sluggish; ataxic** and unable to stand unaided; **incoordinated** and unable to perform either finger-to-nose or heel-to-shin tests; **mild bilateral tremor** in both upper limbs.

Labs: Noncontrast head CT: WNL. CBC and SMA7: WNL.

MSE: *General:* Kevin appears younger than his stated age, with a small frame. There are remnants of glue on his clothing, and the **odor of solvents** is quite strong. *Speech and behavior:* He is

drowsy and his speech is **slurred.** *Affect:* restricted and appears confused. *Mood:* "Weird." *Thought process:* slowed but no abnormalities of form. *Thought content and perception:* describes seeing "special lights and colors everywhere" and that his body feels smaller; denies auditory hallucinations; denies suicidal and homicidal ideations. *Cognitive function:* oriented to person and place but not time; immediate and short-term recall are impaired. *Insight:* limited.

THOUGHT QUESTIONS

- What is your differential diagnosis?
- How would you treat this young man?
- What are your concerns about his prognosis?

DISCUSSION

Although it appears that Kevin is suffering from the effects of acute inhalant intoxication, other substances such as alcohol should be considered, and it is also important to look for signs of a head injury. Symptoms of acute inhalant intoxication include initial euphoria, dizziness, lethargy, slurred speech, incoordination, hypotonic reflexes, ataxia, tremor, nystagmus, diplopia, and stupor or coma; a perioral rash is commonly seen. Chronic use may be associated with inattention, uncoordination, disorientation, and cognitive impairment. In addition to their psychoactive properties, inhalants can also cause aspiration, suffocation, respiratory depression, or cardiac arrhythmias, which may be fatal. Delirium, psychosis, cognitive impairment, mood and anxiety disorders, as well as dependence with withdrawal symptoms may occur (Table 60-1). Polysubstance abuse is common in inhalant abusers. Those with conduct disorders may develop antisocial personalities and serious alcohol and substance abuse or dependence. Use during pregnancy can lead to infant growth retardation, dysmorphic facial features, and perinatal death. Tolerance and dependence can occur with toluene, found in some glues and cements. Gasoline may cause euphoria, violent excitement, and coma or death. Volatile nitrites, found in deodorizers, can cause headache, flushing, severe hypotension, syncope, ECG abnormalities, and bronchial irritation. Treatment is generally supportive, monitoring for any arrhythmias and breathing or circulatory difficulties.

TABLE **60-1**   Signs and Symptoms of Inhalant Intoxication

Cardiovascular	Arrhythmias, hypotension, sudden death
Chemistry	Metabolic acidosis, hypokalemia, hypercalcemia, hyperphosphatemia
Gastrointestinal	Nausea, vomiting, pain, hematemesis
Neurological	Ataxia, intoxication (without alcohol), nystagmus, poor coordination, headache, hallucinations, lethargy, agitation, seizures, respiratory depression, coma, peripheral neuropathy
Pulmonary	Wheezing, rhonchi

It has been reported that approximately 20% of American 8th graders have used inhalants. Most try them once or a few times and then stop. However, a small proportion may progress to more frequent and chronic use, in addition to using alcohol and other illicit drugs. Inhalant abuse is thought to be more common in poor and inland areas.

     CASE CONTINUED

After a few hours, Kevin's mental status returns to normal. He reveals that he had used inhalants twice before with some older boys from school, but that he has never taken alcohol or other substances. Both he and his parents are educated about the possible effects of solvent abuse and referred for a combination of individual and family therapy. Fortunately, there was no evidence of long-term sequelae or relapse at the followup visit.

     QUESTIONS

60-1. Which of the following is accurate concerning solvent abuse?
   A. It may contribute to 1% of drug-related deaths in the United States.
   B. A survey of high school seniors revealed that 18% use inhalants regularly.
   C. It has been suggested that most users will use inhalants a few times then stop.
   D. Inhalants cause few drug-related emergencies.
   E. There are substantial ethnic differences in inhalant abuse in the United States.

60-2. Which of the following is a complication of chronic abuse of solvents?
A. The development of a dementia syndrome
B. Irreversible cognitive deficits
C. Possible toluene-induced white matter brain changes
D. Association with dependence on alcohol
E. All of the above

60-3. Which of the following is correct concerning the medical complications of chronic inhalant use?
A. Pancreatitis is common.
B. There may be muscle weakness, rhabdomyolysis, and myoglobinuria.
C. Chorea is characteristic.
D. Constipation is common.
E. Severe blood dyscrasias never occur.

60-4. Which of the following is correct concerning psychiatric disorders induced by inhalants?
A. Depression is the least common mood disorder caused by inhalants.
B. Psychotic features generally last a few months.
C. If agitation or psychosis occurs, benzodiazepines may be beneficial.
D. Panic disorders may occur.
E. Depressive symptoms should be initially treated with antidepressants.

ANSWERS

60-1. C. Inhalants cause less than 1% of drug-related emergencies. Of these, about one-fifth occur among 10- to 17-year-olds. Inhalant use seems to be much higher among boys than girls. In the United Kingdom, detailed records reveal that inhalants have become a leading cause of adolescent mortality. The 1991 U.S. National Household survey revealed that approximately 5.6% of the population had used inhalants in the past. No association was found with any particular ethnic grouping, though previous work had found higher rates among Native Americans. Inhalants may include a variety of toxic substances, mostly volatile hydrocarbons (e.g., toluene, trichloroethane, dichloromethane, butane, and gasoline), ketones, anesthetic agents, and alkyl nitrites. These are found in a variety of products, including paint thinners, solvents, propellants in spray cans, and fuels. One should suspect solvent abuse particularly in younger patients who present with unexplained arrthymias, renal tubule acidosis, carbon monoxide poisoning, pancytopenia, methemoglobinemia, or intoxication without evidence of alcohol ingestion.

60-2. E. Dependence on inhalants may lead to long-term irreversible cognitive decline and structural changes in the brain; toluene is a solvent and, as such, can be seen as "dissolving" the "greasy" fat-laden myelin that makes up much white matter in the brain. However, there have been reported cases of some improvement upon cessation of use, but in general the cognitive impairment may continue or worsen, particularly in the context of future relapses. Persons who have used products that contain toluene (e.g., gasoline, adhesives, and paint thinners) for over a year have been reported to manifest abnormalities of behavior, speech, and thinking, with hallucinations and delusions.

60-3. B. There are many possible medical complications from long-term abuse of inhalants and include nausea, vomiting and hematemesis, muscle weakness, rhabdomyolysis, renal dysfunction, hepatotoxicity, pulmonary disorders, anemia, peripheral neuropathy, and reversible cerebellar dysfunction or cerebellar degeneration. Severe blood dyscrasias can occur.

60-4. D. Panic and generalized anxiety are the types of anxiety disorders most frequently seen with inhalants. Depression is the most common type of mood disorder, but antidepressants are rarely needed, as resolution tends to occur with cessation of use. Psychosis or agitation may be treated with haloperidol, but benzodiazepines should not be used, to avoid possible further respiratory compromise.

SUGGESTED READING

Wu LT, Howard MO. Psychiatric disorders in inhalant users: results from the National Epidemiologic Survey on Alcohol and related conditions. *Drug Alcohol Depend.* 2007 May 11;88(2–3): 146–155.

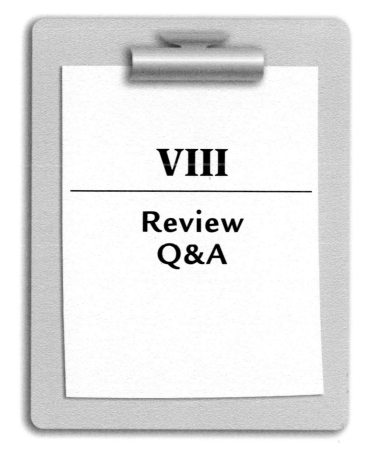

VIII

Review
Q&A

Questions

Questions

1. A 21-year-old college student was just diagnosed with schizophrenia. He and his family are concerned with his returning to school and being able to maintain his grades and ultimately his career plans. The symptoms in schizophrenia responsible for the most functional impairment are

    A. Hallucinations
    B. Delusions
    C. Negative symptoms
    D. Disorganized thinking
    E. Disorganized behavior

2. Mr. P. comes in to the ER intoxicated, and the resident learns he has a long history of alcohol and drug abuse. If he were to have a personality disorder, which would be most likely?

    A. Dependent
    B. Antisocial
    C. Schizoid
    D. Paranoid
    E. Schizotypal

3. A 37-year-old woman with a 15-year history of an idiopathic seizure disorder presents with atypical seizures which, after 24-hour EEG monitoring, are diagnosed as pseudoseizures. Pseudoseizures are diagnosed as which of the following?

    A. Somatization disorder
    B. Hypochondriasis
    C. Conversion disorder
    D. Hysteria
    E. Pseudoneurologica fantastica

4. A 58-year-old successful female internist finally presents to the psychiatrist at the request of her daughter, a medical student, for evaluation of her anxiety. She is constantly preoccupied about how she is doing in her career, the health of her patients, her daughter's happiness in school, and her retirement in ~10 years (bills, etc). She smiles throughout the examination and, despite her concerns, tells the

409

psychiatrist that everything is wonderful as long as she keeps vigilant about these issues. She explains her poor sleep and muscular tension as secondary to her needing to keep on top of things. She refuses medication for what she considers an adaptive response to life's stresses. What would be the best option to recommend for her care?

A. Treatment over objection, with medications
B. There is no treatment for her condition other than pharmacotherapy
C. She does not require treatment because, as she puts it, her preoccupations are adaptive
D. Cognitive-behavioral therapy
E. Family therapy

5. A 35-year-old man was brought in by police after he attempted to assault an officer and is currently restrained to a stretcher in the emergency room. He is belligerent and is trying to free himself from the restraints. He will not talk to you, but you are able to perform a brief exam which is notable for hypertension, tachycardia, vertical nystagmus with normal size light-reactive pupils, and muscular rigidity. He seems not to notice the gaping wound in his side that resulted from his falling onto a sharp pole during the struggle. The time course of intoxication with this compound is on the order of

A. 30 minutes to 3 hours
B. 6 hours to 3 days
C. 6 to 10 hours
D. 2 to 3 hours
E. Chronic

6. Upon interview, a patient in a psychiatric hospital gushes over the qualities of her intern psychiatrist, much to this new doctor's pleasure. However, the nurses note that this patient has been a holy terror and want her discharged off the unit as soon as possible. A rift among the staff occurs, and neither can see the other's perspective. This is an example of the patient's use of

A. Splitting
B. Projective identification
C. Reaction formation
D. Identity diffusion
E. Multiple personalities

7. A 72-year-old woman's husband died 3 months ago. She comes in for her yearly physical exam, and describes depressed mood, tearfulness, and states that at times she thinks she hears her husband's voice. On exam she is appropriately dressed and groomed, has good eye contact, and is tearful in the interview when discussing her husband's death. She is not suicidal. What is the most likely diagnosis?

A. Major depression
B. Schizophrenia
C. Normal bereavement
D. Brief psychotic disorder
E. Complicated grief reaction

8. Mr. R. has been taking an SSRI for the past 9 months. He has run out of medications. Which of the following antidepressants has the least likelihood for inducing withdrawal phenomena?
A. Paroxetine
B. Venlafaxine
C. Sertraline
D. Fluoxetine
E. Citalopram

9. A 65-year-old attorney is spending time with his family and his 18-month-old granddaughter. When the child is given to him, he holds her at arms' length, obviously uncomfortable, and at dinner when she is crying, he snaps, "Act like a young lady." He prides himself on his accounting skills and the fact that he has never made a mistake on any forms. When confronted with clients who contest wills by their family members, he advises, "You should relate to your family more," without explaining further. He is stubborn and cold, but not mean. His symptoms are most characteristic of what disorder?
A. Narcissistic personality disorder
B. Obsessive-compulsive personality disorder
C. Intermittent explosive disorder
D. Obsessive-compulsive disorder
E. Schizotypal personality disorder

10. Ms. R. is a 35-year-old woman with schizophrenia who was recently admitted for a suicide attempt, having taken an overdose of her prescribed medications. The percentage of patients with schizophrenia who attempt and who complete suicide, respectively, is approximately
A. 5%, 1%
B. 10%, 5%
C. 25%, 1%
D. 40%, 1%
E. 40%, 10%

11. A 7-year-old boy presents after a year of a variety of physical and vocal tics including shrugging, neck movements, blinking and grunting. He has no other underlying medical problems and is taking no medications. Which of the following medications has been shown to be most efficacious in the treatment of this disorder?

A. Propranolol
B. Carbamazepine
C. Haloperidol
D. Sertraline
E. Lorazepam

12. A 69-year-old man is brought to the walk-in area of the ER by his nephew who notes that he has been more confused and tired over the past 4 to 6 weeks, with more difficulty with memory. The patient complains of a headache that has recently worsened and notes that he has been somewhat nauseous and thought he had a "bug." His PMH is significant for a history of pancreatitis, and one admission for alcohol detox "a few years ago." He denies drinking in the last month or so and denies any history of head trauma. On exam he is noted to have mild weakness, hyperreflexia, and a positive Babinski sign on the right. Which of the following is the most likely cause of his symptoms?
A. Bacteria
B. Blood
C. Prion
D. Fungus
E. Plaques and tangles

13. A medical student comes to your office after interviewing a 23-year-old woman with a recent diagnosis of schizophrenia. The student wants to understand the usual clinical course of schizophrenia. You say that it is best characterized by
A. Discrete exacerbations and complete remissions
B. A steady level of deterioration
C. Maintenance of functional status despite a near-constant presence of symptoms
D. Progressive functional decline with acute exacerbations and partial remissions
E. Clinical stability after the first psychotic episode

14. Mr. H. is a 45-year-old criminal with a diagnosis of antisocial personality disorder. What is the primary behavioral pathology of patients with this diagnosis?
A. Mistrust of the motives of others
B. Social anxiety
C. Overly deliberate planning
D. Disregard and violation of the rights of others
E. Constricted affect

15. A 28-year-old woman with Crohn disease presents to a psychiatrist complaining of 3 weeks of apathy and food losing its taste. Additionally, she reports having difficulty sleeping due to thinking of all the things she has to do over the next few months, and she expresses concerns that she is to blame for most of the current problems she is experiencing at work. She has not contemplated suicide, but she does manifest hopelessness and feels "blue." Before initiating psychopharmacologic treatment, it is most important to assess which of the following?

    A. Family history of depression
    B. History of manic symptoms
    C. Social support structure
    D. Whether her problems at work are in fact her fault
    E. Taste testing

16. An 11-year-old boy is referred for "behavioral problems." He was caught stealing items from his classmates, "talks back" to his teachers and mother, and initiates physical fights with kids at school. He has also been truant at least once or twice per week for the last 6 months, and he ran away for 2 nights last week because he didn't like being told to do his chores in the home. He tells you that none of these things were his fault, and there are people talking to him in his head telling him to do these things. He does not appear to be responding to internal stimuli. What is the most likely diagnosis for this boy?

    A. Oppositional defiant disorder
    B. Conduct disorder
    C. Normal development
    D. Schizophreniform disorder
    E. Antisocial personality disorder

17. When interviewing a manic patient, you cannot get a word in edgewise, and you notice that when you try to interrupt her, she becomes irritable and combative. The appropriate conduct at this point is to

    A. Let her continue her story, hoping that you will be able to glean some history
    B. Keep trying to interrupt her, but when she gets louder, fall back
    C. Reflect to her that she seems to have a lot to say, but there are some specific questions you need to ask to complete your evaluation
    D. Terminate the interview
    E. Give her a dose of haloperidol and lorazepam because the interview is fruitless anyway

18. A 26-year-old theater major is in her last year of training. She has an impressive résumé but has developed a reputation among her colleagues as someone they try to avoid. She attempts to insert herself into every conversation, much to the dismay of others. She especially enjoys gaining the attention of men by wearing high heels, short skirts, and excessive make-up to school. She believes that each friend she has is "the best," but has a difficult time describing that person's attributes in any detail. She denies any deliberate self-harm or identity disturbance. She presents for treatment of periods of depression lasting a few days. What is the ideal treatment of this patient?

    A. Dialectical behavioral therapy
    B. SSRI
    C. Mood stabilizer
    D. No treatment is required
    E. Psychodynamic psychotherapy

19. While riding the subway, a successful 29-year-old man experiences intense and vivid mental images of stabbing the elderly woman across from him in the eye with his pen. Though recognizing that he would never act on such thoughts, he becomes visibly anxious and turns away from her. This symptom is an example of a(n)

    A. Intrusive image
    B. Delusion
    C. Visual hallucination
    D. Thought insertion
    E. Dissociative experience

20. A 30-year-old man presents to a psychiatrist with symptoms of irritability, late insomnia, diurnal mood variation, poor appetite, and low sex drive. He is treated with a medication. What is the likelihood of his responding to initial treatment?

    A. 25%
    B. 50%
    C. 65%
    D. 80%
    E. 100%

21. A 28-year-old woman PhD student who is being treated with a mood stabilizer for bipolar disorder complains about being an "addictive person." Between sessions, she calls you complaining about her "cravings" for cigarettes and nicotine gum. She also intermittently abuses cocaine and recently had a 3-day binge of cocaine, marijuana, hallucinogens, and "NoDoze" (caffeine pills). She says that buproprion has decreased her nicotine cravings in the past and denies that it ever made her manic. She requests to restart on buproprion in combination with her mood-stabilizer as soon as possible. What should you do first?

A. Restart her on buproprion and monitor her closely for emergence of any symptoms of mania.

B. Clarify what other approaches she has taken to stop smoking in the past, why they did not work, and what exactly her goals would be with this new approach.

C. Whatever you do, do not give her an antidepressant. Given the risk of mania, smoking cessation is not an indication to use an antidepressant in a patient with bipolar disorder.

D. Offer her the nicotine patch and refer her to a cognitive-behavioral therapist for motivational therapy for substance abuse.

E. Try another antidepressant with a less-likely risk of inducing mania.

22. A patient presents with symptoms suggestive of a major depressive disorder. Her history reveals a mother who suffers from bipolar disorder. The likelihood that this patient will develop a bipolar (i.e., not unipolar) disorder is

A. 1% to 10%

B. 30% to 50%

C. >75%

D. This has not been studied.

E. By definition she can only have a unipolar disorder because she first experienced depressive symptoms.

23. A 17-year-old girl has developed ritualistic behavior, marked by repeated jiggling of the toilet handle, turning lights on and off, repeating under her breath words she has just said, and constantly counting her steps. She is prescribed a medication. What is the most likely course of her illness?

A. Chronic remission if her symptoms remit with this medication

B. Chronic course not affected by the presence of medication

C. Chronic course with partial amelioration by medication

D. Episodic course with periods of remission

E. Progressive and deteriorating course

24. A 70-year-old man presents with 2 months of apathy and depressed mood worse in the morning, initial insomnia, poor appetite, and a conviction that he cannot eat due to the rotting away of his internal organs. He has lost 20 pounds in the last month. He feels that he is receiving a deserved punishment for not being as available to his children and spouse as he should have been. Medical workup has been negative. Which of the following is an appropriate regimen for his treatment?

    A. Tricyclic antidepressant
    B. Monoamine oxidase inhibitor
    C. SSRI
    D. Electroconvulsive therapy
    E. Antipsychotic medication

25. A 25-year-old woman is embarrassed in stating that she feels she must keep rereading the directions on a box of macaroni and cheese or her beloved grandmother will die. This is an example of

    A. An obsession
    B. A compulsion
    C. A delusion
    D. An overvalued idea
    E. Loss of ego boundaries

26. A 24-year-old woman is depressed and anhedonic, with passive suicidal ideations. Upon taking a history you discover that 3 to 4 times per week for the last year, she has been bingeing and vomiting. In considering an antidepressant for her, which of the following is the correct pairing?

    A. Paroxetine—long half life—should be avoided
    B. Buproprion—risk of seizures—should be avoided
    C. Fluoxetine—short half life—good choice
    D. MAOI—multiple dietary restrictions—good choice
    E. Tricyclic antidepressant—safe in overdose–good choice

27. A 42-year-old disheveled man is in the psychiatric emergency room, tremulous and pacing. His blood pressure is 180/100, and his pulse is 120. He looks anxious and tries to cooperate with the interview but is not making any sense. He keeps looking around and commenting on the little people on the bed rails. What is the correct treatment for this patient?

    A. Nothing; he will "re-compensate" with time
    B. IM lorazepam, IM thiamine, and admission to a
       psychiatric inpatient unit
    C. IV lorazepam, IV thiamine, and admission
       to a medical unit
    D. Naltrexone
    E. Haloperidol

28. A 35-year-old executive has a fixed daily routine, much to the dismay of his wife. She notes that at work he must do things perfectly, and she is frustrated with his long hours despite the fact that he has risen to the top of his company and is liked a great deal. He is aware of his rigidity and conscientiousness and describes his habits as necessary to make a good living. On the weekends he is relatively able to relax and spend time with his family and friends. During the week he eats and goes to sleep without difficulty. After multiple arguments with her and at her request, he presents to the psychiatrist for "treatment of his obsessive-compulsive disorder at work." What is likely to be the best treatment?

  A. SSRI
  B. Exposure and response prevention
  C. Flooding
  D. Systematic desensitization
  E. Couples therapy

29. Mr. G. is a 19-year-old male who was just admitted to a psychiatric unit with a diagnosis of schizophreniform disorder. The resident is taking a detailed history from the family about his premorbid symptoms and functioning. The prodromal phase of schizophrenia commonly includes

  A. Strange ideations
  B. Hallucinations
  C. Delusions
  D. Disorganized speech
  E. Suicidality

30. A 67-year-old woman has just experienced the death of her husband of 30 years. One month later, she presents to a psychiatrist complaining of hearing her husband's voice when she is cooking dinner and frequently thinking she sees him out of the corner of her eye. She finds these experiences disturbing. What is the appropriate treatment for her condition?

  A. Antidepressant medication
  B. Antipsychotic medication
  C. Reassurance and observation
  D. Electroconvulsive therapy
  E. Inpatient hospitalization

31. Ms. O. is diagnosed with major depression. She is a Scientologist and does not want medication or therapy for her illness. She denies suicidal ideation. Given the natural course of major depression, most episodes clear within what length of time?

  A. 2 months
  B. 6 months
  C. 1 year
  D. 5 years
  E. never, without treatment

32. A 35-year-old firefighter has begun to worry incessantly and shows great unease in most contexts and situations. He has been followed in the resident clinic for the past 2 years and is being treated for generalized anxiety disorder; however, his symptoms have not responded to increasing doses of benzodiazepines. On transfer of care, the new resident picking up his case decided to take a more detailed history and was struck by the patient's reporting that these symptoms began a few months after an incident in which his partner was killed by a falling ceiling, and his symptoms are more specific to PTSD than GAD. The initial drug of choice in treating uncomplicated PTSD is
  A. Norepinephrine dopamine reuptake inhibitor
  B. Selective serotonin reuptake inhibitor
  C. Serotonin norepinephrine reuptake inhibitor
  D. Tricyclic antidepressant
  E. Antipsychotic

33. A 40-year-old agitated and violent man arrives in the psychiatric emergency room and rushes at the security guards. He yells that he has lawsuits pending at 20 other hospitals and that he should be released immediately or he will sue. He also states that he owns 10 successful businesses and was planning to run for governor. Per the family, the patient has had increased energy, started many new projects at home, sleeps about 2 to 4 hours per night, and has not been taking his medications. Per the old medical chart, the patient has carried multiple prior diagnoses including bipolar disorder, schizoaffective disorder, substance-induced psychotic disorder, and substance-induced mood disorder. On past urine toxicologies, the patient has tested positive for cocaine. He admits to using cocaine "occasionally" but is rather vague and not forthcoming about the details. What is your initial management in the emergency room?
  A. Hold off on management until you can clarify the diagnosis.
  B. As the patient is not suicidal, his civil liberties and demands should be respected and he should be discharged.
  C. The patient should be restarted on his home medications immediately as they were previously effective but he stopped taking them, leading to the current symptoms.
  D. The patient's symptoms clearly meet criteria for and are explained by acute mania.
  E. Ensure the safety of the patient, other patients, and hospital staff, and consider medicating the patient if any of these is in question.

34. Which medication has the best evidence for its use in preventing depressive relapse in bipolar disorder?

A. Tricyclic antidepressants
B. SSRIs
C. Lithium carbonate
D. Divalproex sodium
E. Olanzapine

35. A 58-year-old woman is admitted to the hospital for evaluation of a 20-lb weight loss and vague GI complaints including mild pain. She has no significant medical history beyond mild hypertension. She is 5'4" and 110 lbs. A thorough medical workup, including an evaluation for malignancies, thyroid dysfunction, and GI pathology, has been negative. Despite reassurance from her internist she remains convinced that she has "some serious disease" and asks for a second opinion. She does concede that perhaps her fears are exaggerated but refuses tosee a psychiatrist. Which of the following accurately describes this condition?

A. A prevalence of 1% in general medical patients.
B. It is more common in women.
C. Medical work ups should generally be avoided in these patients.
D. Such preoccupations may occur secondary to an axis one disorder
E. There is usually a family history of this disorder

36. Ms. R is a 45- year-old woman being treated for borderline PD. At her most recent presentation to the ER, she described a few days of mildly depressed mood, severe anociety, irritability, and auditory hallucinations. What likely accounts for her psychotic symptoms?

A. Borderline personality disorder
B. Major depressive disorder with psychotic features
C. Generalized anxiety disorder with psychotic features
D. Schizophrenia
E. Schizoaffective disorder

37. A 23-year-old woman with no psychiatric history presents to the psychiatrist with complaints of 3 months of paroxysmal and unexpected shortness of breath, chest tightness, palpitations, dizziness, a fear of going crazy, and an uncontrollable fear that she is dying. She has been to numerous medical emergency rooms and all tests have been negative. She has begun to sit on the aisle of movie theaters just in case she has to leave to "get some air." What is the best treatment for her condition?

A. As-needed alprazolam
B. Standing clonazepam
C. Lithium carbonate
D. Referral to a medical specialist (e.g., pulmonologist, cardiologist)
E. SSRI

38. An 81-year-old woman is brought to her internist by her family because of their concern about her cognitive decline. On cognitive examination she is forgetful and apathetic. She has been falling, particularly when trying to get up a curb or climb stairs, and her gait is somewhat wide-based. The family also notes that she has been having more difficulty making it to the bathroom on time and has been having urinary "accidents." She is sent for a CT scan, which shows ventricular enlargement out of proportion to sulcal atrophy. The most appropriate next step would be to

A. Start a cholinesterase inhibitor
B. Start an NMDA receptor antagonist
C. Do a spinal tap to evaluate for treponemal antibodies
D. Evaluate for shunt placement
E. Do an MRI to evaluate for stroke

39. A 24-year-old woman has been out of work since graduating from an Ivy League college. She attributes her unemployment to multiple medical problems including blurry vision, inability to recall familiar objects around her house, arm tingling, chronic weakness, headache, gas, diarrhea, chest tightness, hair loss, disc disease, urinary frequency, urinary hesitancy, abdominal pain at menses, inability to focus, and cold clammy hands. All evaluations have been negative except for the presence of a urinary tract infection 18 months ago. What is her likely primary diagnosis and which personality disorder likely accompanies it?

A. Conversion disorder, Cluster B personality disorder
B. Somatization disorder, Cluster A personality disorder
C. Somatization disorder, Cluster B personality disorder
D. Conversion disorder, Cluster A personality disorder
E. Somatization disorder, Cluster C personality disorder

40. Ms. O. is a 22-year-old woman who acutely was unable to move her arm after the sudden death of her sister in a freak shark attack, in which her sister's arm was bitten off, and she exsanguinated before she could be rescued. Which of the following is most consistent with a diagnosis of conversion disorder?

A. The symptom is intentionally produced.
B. Pain or sexual dysfunction are a primary features.
C. Involuntary motor or sensory symptoms are a key feature.
D. The symptom does not correspond to known physiological patterns.
E. It cannot be diagnosed if the patient has a pre-existing brain injury.

41. A 23-year-old medical student who has two doctors as parents develops a pain in his right upper quadrant. He presents to his internist with the complaint that his "liver hurts." Lab tests and ultrasonography are negative, and he is prescribed a proton pump inhibitor which controls his symptoms for 3 weeks. When his symptoms recur, he returns to the doctor who orders a CT scan and upper endoscopy, which are negative, and his symptoms again remit for a few weeks. Upon returning to his doctor for a third time, he should be offered

A. Referral to a gastroenterologist
B. Referral to a psychiatrist
C. Referral to a surgeon
D. An evaluation for depression or anxiety
E. Referral to his parents who are both doctors

42. A 45-year-old man presents to the emergency room with a complaint of auditory hallucinations commanding him to "harm myself and others." He reports experiencing this symptom for 2 days, and it "nearly caused me to walk into traffic." He has a long history of psychiatric hospitalizations, but neither follows up after discharge nor takes his medications. He is homeless but not disheveled; noted are poorly executed tattoos on both forearms. On exam, he reports nine out of nine depressive symptoms, feelings that people are after him, and auditory hallucinations as above, but does not appear distracted. What is the likely diagnosis?

A. Major depressive disorder with psychotic features
B. Schizophrenia
C. Factitious disorder
D. Malingering
E. Bipolar disorder

43. A 35-year-old man with schizophrenia has failed adequate treatment trials with risperidone, olanzapine, and haloperidol. You believe he has treatment resistant schizophrenia and want to start him on a new medication. What life-threatening side effect would you be most worried about with this new treatment?

A. Neuroleptic malignant syndrome
B. Dystonic laryngospasm
C. Torsades de pointes
D. Agranulocytosis
E. Suicide

44. Mr. Z. is a 26-year-old male with narcissistic personality who comes to a psychiatric clinic for an intake after moving to a new city. The attending turns to the resident who is about to interview the patient and asks what is the most frequently diagnosed DSM-IV axis I disorder in persons with Cluster B personality disorders?
A. Schizophrenia
B. Generalized anxiety disorder
C. Borderline personality disorder
D. Bipolar disorder
E. Major depressive disorder

45. A 21-year-old college student experiences a "bad trip" on mushrooms (psilocybin). When he smokes marijuana 2 weeks later, he re-experiences a subset of his prior trip in an attenuated form and starts to panic; these symptoms respond to 2 beers. For the next few years, he experiences occasional panic attacks whenever he smokes marijuana such that he will smoke only when he is sure that alcohol is at hand or when he has already been drinking. The only symptoms he manifests when not high are a mild discomfort when feeling "out of it" and anxiety whenever he is dizzy, but he has not limited his activities nor is his functioning impaired. He comes to your office following a presentation to the psychiatric emergency room for panic experienced when high. What is the correct diagnosis for this patient?
A. Panic disorder
B. Cannabis-induced anxiety disorder
C. Anxiety disorder NOS
D. Posttraumatic stress disorder
E. Alcohol dependence

46. A 12-year-old girl is brought in by her mother who has concerns about her behavior. Though she is a very compliant child who gets good grades in school and who helps out and takes charge of many things around the home, notably cooking elaborate meals for the family, she refuses to eat with the family. She will occasionally eat the white foods that they eat (e.g., three florets of plain cauliflower), but she always says, "I'll get something later." This has been going on for 9 months, and she has taken to wearing layers of baggy clothes. On exam she is 62 lb and 5 feet tall, with a body mass index (BMI) of 12.7. What might you see on physical exam?

    A. Parotid enlargement

    B. Tachycardia

    C. Dental caries

    D. Lanugo

    E. Hyperthermia

47. Ms. A. comes in for an evaluation of depressed mood, anhedonia, and decreased energy, appetite, and concentration. Ms. P. has the same symptoms but also describes a history of symptoms consistent with borderline PD. Compared with Ms. P., Ms. A. is more likely to

    A. Have a better response to treatment

    B. Have more unstable relationships

    C. Have comorbid substance abuse

    D. Report precipitating stressors

    E. Have nonserious suicide attempts

48. A 35-year-old woman was the victim of repeated childhood sexual assaults by close family members, all orchestrated by her mother. Diagnosed with PTSD, she has been maintained on risperidone and supportive psychotherapy for the past 6 years with good effect on her affective instability, though she remains unable to function in a work environment. When her mother unexpectedly died on Mother's Day a few days ago, the patient missed her appointment, threw out all her belongings, did not sleep, and isolated herself in her house fearing harm by people on the street. On admission to the hospital, she believed her doctor of the past 6 years had been replaced by an impostor because he was unable to recall her mother's age. What is the additional likely diagnosis?

    A. Schizophrenia

    B. Bipolar disorder, manic episode

    C. Only PTSD

    D. Brief psychotic disorder

    E. Delusional disorder

49. A 45-year-old woman with schizophrenia is discharged from an inpatient psychiatric unit on chlorpromazine, to go live at her group home. Three weeks later she returns to the emergency department with an acute exacerbation of her psychosis. The most likely explanation for her relapse is

A. Cigarette smoking
B. Argument with peers
C. Nonadherence to medications
D. Drug use
E. Medical comorbidities

50. Mr. Q. is a 37-year-old man who has an aunt and a brother with schizophrenia. Upon examination, you find that he is suffering from a personality disorder. Which of the following is genetically linked to schizophrenia?
    A. Schizoid personality disorder
    B. Schizotypal personality disorder
    C. Borderline personality disorder
    D. Multiple personality disorder
    E. Schizophrenia personality disorder

51. A 22-year-old man experiences shortness of breath, chest tightness, dizziness, nervousness, and a feeling of detachment from his surroundings and intense fear whenever he attempts to stop washing his hands and get on with his day. He has come to expect this feeling but notes that he has no control over it. He is preoccupied with cleanliness, fearing invisible germs even when others mock him, and he feels "ridiculous" throughout the course of washing his hands. The likely diagnosis is
    A. Panic disorder
    B. Panic disorder and obsessive compulsive disorder
    C. Obsessive-compulsive disorder
    D. Delusional disorder
    E. Obsessive compulsive disorder, special type with panic attacks

52. Mr. T. is a 42-year-old man who has a narcissistic personality disorder and has never sought treatment. He disregards all confrontations by co-workers and acquaintances about his hurtful and unempathic demeanor. The inability for most patients with personality disorders to acknowledge their pathological symptoms is termed
    A. Ego-alien
    B. Ego-syntonic
    C. Ego-dystonic
    D. Ego-boundaried
    E. Ego-dysphoric

53. A 15-year-old girl refused to join her tour group on their trip to the top of the Empire State Building, stating that she had already seen it and would only be bored. She did not reveal that not only had she had never been to New York but that she had a lifelong fear of elevators which had impacted her ability to be with her group and experience many sites on this school trip. When the tour leader did not allow her to stay behind for safety's sake, she developed palpitations, shortness of breath, a feeling of being outside of herself, and an impending fear of death. Which of the following is the correct diagnosis?

A. Agoraphobia
B. Specific phobia
C. Social phobia
D. Panic disorder
E. Specific phobia with panic disorder

54. A 55-year-old lawyer arrives in town for his father's funeral. He shares a limo with his sister and brother in-law, and the whole ride to the cemetery describes in great detail the celebrities whom he has represented. He does not seem to realize the social inappropriateness of his statements, but of note, it is not any different from his usual commentary. This is an example of which disorder?

A. Schizoid personality disorder
B. Narcissistic personality disorder
C. Borderline personality disorder
D. Histrionic personality disorder
E. Dependent personality disorder

55. A 30-year-old man comes into the emergency room extremely agitated, believing that the CIA is following him, and he wants asylum. He is disorganized and disheveled. His laboratory results and urine toxicology were all normal. Schizophrenia can be differentiated from bipolar disorder by which of the following?

A. The presence of psychotic symptoms
B. The presence of mood symptoms
C. The age of onset
D. The course of the illness
E. Symptoms present on a cross-sectional mental status exam

56. Mr. P. and Mr. S. both avoid the company of others. One is diagnosed with avoidant personality disorder and the other with schizoid personality. What is the major difference between these two disorders

A. Magical thinking
B. Identity diffusion
C. Perfectionism
D. Avoidant of activities that involve significant interpersonal contact
E. Desire to be with others

57. A 75-year-old retired lawyer comes in to the neurologist's office because of concerns about his memory. He reports that his "mind is a sieve," he has trouble remembering what he has read, and often will have to reread a paragraph a number of times. He is not interested in anything, has no motivation, and is very worried that he is developing a dementia. His appetite is poor. His wife says that she noticed a significant change in him over the past month. His neurologic exam is nonfocal, and his MMSE is 23/30 (–2 on orientation to time, giving an approximate date a few days off from the correct one; –2 on delayed recall, stating "I just don't know"; he remembers both words when given a category hint; –3 on spelling world backwards). His laboratory tests, including thyroid function and B_{12}, are unremarkable. What would most likely be the most effective intervention?

  A. Evaluate for ventriculo-peritoneal shunt
  B. Start donepezil
  C. Start sertraline
  D. Start lithium
  E. Arrange for a lumbar puncture

58. A 26-year-old man in the psychiatric emergency room was brought in by ambulance after he was found trying to walk in front of traffic. He describes the acute onset of suicidal ideation, appears highly dysphoric, and denies all psychotic symptomatology. Over the next few hours, he is seen either lying asleep or when awake, asking other patients for their food. On physical exam the only notable finding is a dry cough. What is the most likely explanation for his behavior?

  A. Schizophrenic relapse
  B. Major depressive disorder
  C. Heroin withdrawal
  D. Heroin intoxication
  E. Cocaine withdrawal

59. As a child a 24-year-old man experienced multiple episodes of strep throat as well as frequent bouts of abdominal pain so severe that his mother had to pick him up from school. He is just beginning business school, and throughout the first semester, he has been presenting to his internist's office every few weeks with complaints of sore throat for which no medical cause can be found. He is resistant to the idea that he may be experiencing increased stress in his new capacity. In which of the following ways should somaticizing patients be managed by an internist?

A. They should initially be referred to a psychiatrist.
B. They should be scheduled at regular and frequent intervals with the idea that new symptoms are not required for them to see a physician.
C. They should be seen only when new symptoms develop.
D. It doesn't matter, but when patients are seen, a psychiatrist should always be present.
E. For yearly check-ups.

60. Due to concerns over stepping in the wrong place, having to count all his movements, and not being able to tolerate accidentally touching anything, a 45-year-old man has been housebound for the past 3 years. He has failed trials of clomipramine, fluvoxamine, risperidone, behavior therapy, and long-term psychodynamic psychotherapy. The best treatment at this point is
A. Electroconvulsive therapy
B. Cingulotomy
C. Lorazepam
D. Monoamine oxidase inhibitor
E. Clozapine

61. A 35-year-old MD-PhD immunologist presents to the psychiatrist with complaints of shyness and insecurity. All his life, he has been inhibited, anxious, and feared rejection by others, but he desperately wants relationships, both friendly and romantic. He believes that he is socially inept and inferior to others, and as such tries to refrain from engaging in any activities that will involve interpersonal contact. What do you expect the course of his illness to be?
A. Chronic and without change
B. Chronic but significantly fluctuating based on discrete stressors
C. Chronic but somewhat ameliorated by SSRIs
D. Exacerbations and complete remissions
E. Improving drastically as he ages

62. A 32-year-old dental hygienist arrives for an intake evaluation at a local clinic. As the psychiatrist begins to delve more deeply into the patient's anxiety 20 minutes into the session, the patient suddenly goes quiet and begins to stare into space; a few minutes later, she begins talking about rivers and hair and is not responsive to the psychiatrist's voice or presence. Dissociative disorders are most commonly linked to
A. Schizophrenia
B. Bipolar disorder
C. Posttraumatic stress disorder
D. Major depressive disorder
E. Malingering

63. A 39-year-old man is brought into the psychiatric emergency room by EMS after attempting suicide by trying to jump off a large bridge. The police found him hanging from the cables and pulled him down. On interview, the patient is acutely suicidal and also demands to be given the 100 mg of methadone that he takes every day. As it is Sunday morning, you are not able to confirm the dose with the clinic. What is your best option?

- A. Give him a lower dose of methadone, e.g., 30 to 50 mg, to prevent opiate withdrawal.
- B. Treat him symptomatically for withdrawal.
- C. Offer supportive counseling about how he may be uncomfortable during the next several days, but that opiate withdrawal is not life threatening and this is a good opportunity to taper off methadone.
- D. Assess the patient's reliability through the psychiatric interview, and if he is found to be reliable, give him his normal dose of 100 mg.
- E. Give him as-needed low-dose opiates, such as meperidine or acetaminophen with codeine, until you can confirm the dose.

64. A 47-year-old patient with PTSD called his psychiatrist and left a cryptic message on the answering machine, "You got him in trouble. He's in trouble. You gotta help him." At the patient's next visit, the psychiatrist replayed the message, but the patient was truly dumbfounded, convinced he did not leave it. Earlier that week, in his closet he found a half-made model airplane; a type of toy he had not played with since he was 10, the year his mother died of an aneurysm. He denied any memory of having made it. This is an example of

- A. Dissociation
- B. Seizure disorder
- C. Malingering
- D. Factitious disorder
- E. Repression

65. Mr. P. has a recurrent major depression, with two previous suicide attempts by overdosing on his medications. Which of the following is the safest in overdose?

- A. Lithium carbonate
- B. Selective serotonin reuptake inhibitor
- C. Tricyclic antidepressant
- D. Acetaminophen
- E. Monoamine oxidase inhibitor

66. Ms. G. reports periods of feeling "mechanical . . . like I'm separated from my own thoughts and emotions," while at the same time maintaining intact reality testing. This is known as
   A. Psychosis
   B. Anxiety
   C. Panic
   D. Depersonalization
   E. Dissociation

67. Mr. L. is a 37-year-old man with a 2-year history of spontaneous panic attacks that have left him fearful of leaving the house, in fear of having an attack while in the street or on public transportation. You decide to start him on an SSRI. What is the expectation of dosage for patients with panic disorder compared to those with major depression?
   A. Higher initial and end doses because panic is less responsive to treatment
   B. Lower initial dose but equivalent end dose because SSRIs initially tend to exacerbate anxiety
   C. Lower initial and end doses because higher dose SSRIs tend to exacerbate anxiety throughout treatment
   D. High initial dose but lower end dose because as the condition is treated, the medication requirements decrease
   E. Initial and end doses equivalent to those used in the treatment of major depression

68. A 35-year-old employed, relatively reclusive man with a few friends and without a psychiatric history has recently hired his 50th maid. After putting her through an arduous screening process, he insists on being present for the first five times she cleans his house. While cleaning his closet, she coughs, and he gets upset believing that she is making a statement about the bad odor in his closet. He is able to restrain himself until she makes a comment that a stain in his carpet is difficult to get out, at which point he flies into a rage, screaming that she is just trying to get him upset so he will leave and then she can steal his money. This patient is likely suffering from which disorder?
   A. Schizophrenia
   B. Borderline personality disorder
   C. Paranoid personality disorder
   D. Delusional disorder
   E. Schizoid personality disorder

69. A 15-year-old boy is held down by his brother's friends while his brother forces a hose down his throat, causing the boy to gag and aspirate. This is only one event of a number of similar tortures inflicted by the brother. When you see the patient in your office 20 years later, he reports vomiting first thing every morning for many years after this event following being woken up by night-mares. In which PTSD symptom cluster would this symptom fit?

A. Exposure to traumatic event
B. Avoidance phenomena
C. Hyperarousal phenomena
D. Numbing phenomena
E. Re-experiencing phenonema

70. A 40-year-old man who married into money is having an affair. When his wife finds out, she threatens to divorce him. He carefully calculates the financial losses he would sustain, and decides that it would be advantageous to pay for her to be murdered than go through with a divorce. He asks his sister-in-law for her opinion. This is an example of which personality disorder?

A. Borderline
B. Obsessive-compulsive
C. Dependent
D. Antisocial
E. Paranoid

71. A 47-year-old man reports being molested by the dentist at the age of 12. He has not been to the dentist for the past 5 years and finds he needs his bridge repaired. Which of the following is the most time-effective appropriate initial treatment?

A. Cognitive therapy
B. Behavior therapy
C. Psychoanalysis
D. Antidepressant medication
E. Antipsychotic medication

72. A 20-year-old man has been diagnosed with schizophrenia and is attending a resident-run clinic. He is adherent to his medica-tion (risperidone) and to his appointments, and his symptoms are limited to low-volume auditory hallucinations and fairly well-sys-tematized delusions which only very minimally impact his behav-ior. For the past few months, his major complaint has been feelings of isolation, loneliness, poor self-esteem, and a desire to be more social despite his intense insecurity and ambivalence around peo-ple. To this end, he has begun using alcohol when he is to be around others, stating that it helps him socialize. What is the cor-rect course of action in the treatment of this patient?

A. Prescribe more antipsychotic medication.
B. No change; he is using alcohol as a social lubricant.
C. Prescribe an antidepressant medication for major depression.
D. Address the motivations behind his use of alcohol and, if required, prescribe an antidepressant medication to help with symptoms of anxiety and depression.
E. Address his use of alcohol and prescribe a benzodiazepine for his symptoms of anxiety.

73. A 26-year-old college graduate has a well-paying job and is advancing rapidly in his chosen field. For the past few years, he has been drinking a six-pack of beer on a nightly basis with binges on the weekends. While continuing to remain productive and trusted at work, he has fallen out of favor with many of his friends, getting into fights and acting rowdy on the street (e.g., throwing bottles at people). What pathology is this patient manifesting?

A. Alcohol abuse
B. Alcohol dependence
C. Normal alcohol consumption by a man in this age range
D. Substance-induced explosive disorder
E. Behavior consistent with antisocial personality disorder

74. A 14-year-old girl is 85% of her ideal body weight. She no longer menstruates and is convinced that her thighs and buttocks are fat, such that when she sits, she sits at the edge of seats to minimize the size of her thighs. She eats a very restricted diet of apples, carrots, and oat cereal, will not lick stamps for fear of the calories, and exercises at least 3 hours a day. Approximately twice a month she will vomit food if she feels that she has overeaten. What is her most likely diagnosis?

A. Bulimia nervosa
B. Anorexia nervosa
C. Specific phobia (food)
D. Eating disorder NOS
E. Psychotic disorder NOS

75. K. is a 10-year-old boy with mild mental retardation. His parents describe a delay in his language development and report that he is somewhat distractible and impulsive. He is initially shy with poor eye contact but soon warms up and is extremely friendly, becoming "overly chatty." On physical exam he has a long jaw, high forehead, narrow face, and large, long, protuberant ears. What is the most likely diagnosis of this child?

A. Down syndrome
B. Klinefelter syndrome
C. Fragile X syndrome
D. Noonan syndrome
E. Turner syndrome

76. A 20-year-old woman is admitted to the hospital after ingesting 10 tablets of acetaminophen in an apparent suicide attempt. This is the third such attempt she has made, and both were in the context of the end of a relationship with a boyfriend. Her history is replete with physical abuse, explosive emotionality, vague depressive symptoms consistent with dysthymic disorder, and continuing to live in her parent's house despite good grades in school and all her friends leaving for college. The psychotherapeutic intervention for this patient that has been empirically shown to reduce deliberate self-harm and suicide attempts is

A. Psychodynamic psychotherapy
B. Dialectical behavioral therapy
C. Body-focused psychotherapy
D. Eye movement desensitization and reprocessing
E. Systematic desensitization

77. A 65-year-old man has been diagnosed with major depressive disorder with a significant anxiety component a few months after receiving a diagnosis of cancer. He has lost a great deal of weight, is frequently nauseated, and exudes a profound despondency. What is the best treatment for this individual?

A. Clonazepam
B. Fluoxetine
C. Mirtzapine
D. Nortriptyline
E. Buproprion

78. L., a 2-year-old girl who recently immigrated with her parents to the United States, is brought in to the pediatrician's office for evaluation. She is not yet walking, and she has significantly delayed language development. On exam you note that she is a pale, blond, blue-eyed child, with mild microcephaly and eczema. What is the most important initial treatment?

A. IV glucocerebrosidase
B. Phenylalanine-free diet
C. Oral beta-hexosaminidase A
D. Penicillamine
E. Zinc acetate

79. A third-year medical student is going in to begin the evaluation of a new patient in the personality disorders clinic. The attending tells the student that the most important part of the psychiatric history in making a diagnosis of a personality disorder is
  A. The elucidation of symptoms in the history of present illness
  B. The social history
  C. The medication history
  D. A history of substance abuse
  E. The review of psychiatric symptoms

80. A 28-year-old man without a psychiatric history presents with symptoms suggestive of a major depressive disorder. For how long should he be treated with an antidepressant?
  A. 2 months
  B. 2 to 6 months
  C. 9 to 12 months
  D. 5 years
  E. Indefinitely

81. A 13-month-old girl is brought into the pediatrician's office for a check-up. Her exam at 6 months of age was normal, and she was grasping at objects and sitting unassisted. At this visit she is not doing as well, and her parents report that she has been having more difficulty grasping objects, her movements are less coordinated, she seems less interested in the social environment, and she is babbling less. Her head circumference, which had been on a normal curve, has now decelerated. What other features is this child likely to manifest as she develops?
  A. Normal gait
  B. Hand wringing
  C. Impaired expressive but normal receptive language
  D. Extreme friendliness
  E. Hemiballismus

82. A 23-year-old man is brought by police to the psychiatric emergency room after he was found running naked through his neighborhood. He is carrying no identification and looks as if he has not shaved for several days. He is quite agitated and uncooperative with an exam, but after receiving a haloperidol and lorazepam injection, he is calmer and gives blood and urine for testing, all of which are negative (including urine toxicology). When he again becomes agitated, he is put into a seclusion room and appears to be talking to himself and yelling about how the "President of the Federated European Union of States" is on his way for an important meeting with the patient. Which of the following is the least likely diagnosis?

A. Bipolar disorder, manic episode
B. Delusional disorder
C. Schizophrenia
D. Bipolar disorder, mixed episode
E. Schizoaffective disorder

83. A 22-year-old woman is being evaluated for psychiatric treatment. Her only presenting symptom is an intense fear of dogs such that she has intense difficulty walking down the street for fear of encountering even a leashed canine. What would make her disorder delusional rather than phobic?

A. Inability to acknowledge that her fear is possibly too extreme
B. Ability to tolerate dogs if she had to
C. Belief that she will be attacked if she comes within a few feet of a dog
D. Belief that dogs are dirty germ-carriers
E. Recognition that she is unduly afraid of dogs but inability to alter her behavior in light of this

84. A 9-year-old boy is brought in to the pediatrician's office for an onset of intermittent grunting which has been going on for a "couple of months." On questioning, the parents report that for the past year and a half, he has been having some "movements" including blinking, movements of the neck and head, and occasional shrugging, all of which have been increasing in frequency. What is most likely true about this disorder?

A. The usual age of onset is between 12 and 15 years.
B. Vocal tics usually precede motor tics.
C. Individuals cannot suppress tics temporarily.
D. Hand clenching is the most common motor tic.
E. Obsessive-compulsive disorder is a common comorbidity.

85. Mr. G. comes in for a psychiatric evaluation and admits to a history of early childhood abuse. Which personality disorder is he at higher risk of demonstrating?

A. Schizotypal
B. Borderline
C. Narcissistic
D. Schizoid
E. Paranoid

86. An 83-year-old woman has been increasingly forgetful over the past year. She lives in a two-family home with her son, and he notes that she has been having increasing difficulty managing her finances and keeping her once-immaculate home in order. On exam you notice that she has some difficulty with word finding and memory (she remembered 0/3 words at 5 minutes). Otherwise she is able to manage her activities of daily living (ADL), and she cooks for herself, and often for her son and his family. Her lab studies are within normal limits, and her MRI only shows atrophy. Which of the following is the most appropriate pharmacologic management?

A. Sertraline
B. Donepezil
C. Memantine
D. Benztropine
E. Clopidogrel

87. A 9-year-old boy was evaluated by you 6 months ago for hyperactivity, impulsivity, and distractibility which significantly interfere with his making friends at school and succeeding at his class work. You started him on methylphenidate and noted a good response in his symptoms, but unfortunately he has had significant trouble with maintaining his weight and complains of a decreased appetite. Which of the following is a reasonable treatment to try?

A. Fluoxetine
B. Phenylzine
C. Chlorpromazine
D. Desipramine
E. Atomoxetine

88. Ms. T. is a 37-year-old woman who has experienced an episode of mania with elevated mood, insomnia, increased spending, flight of ideas, pressured speech, and delusions of grandeur. She has never suffered from depression. What is her diagnosis?

A. Bipolar disorder not otherwise specified (NOS)
B. Bipolar I disorder
C. Bipolar II disorder
D. Manic disorder
E. Mood disorder not otherwise specified (NOS)

89. An 83-year-old man, in town visiting his nephew, presents to the walk-in section of the ER complaining of confusion, fatigue, and weakness. He did not bring his medications, but he says he takes something for his pressure and something for his mood. You draw labs. What findings might suggest that his symptoms may be due to a medication side effect?

A. MAOI; leucocytosis
B. SSRI; hyponatremia
C. Lithium; leucopenia
D. Clozapine; leucocytosis
E. TCA; hyperkalemia

90. A 16-year-old girl admits to "being bulimic." She eats very little during the day, but at night she consumes thousands of calories and then purges. She also purges if she happens to eat during the day. Which of the following are correctly associated in bulimia?

A. Dental caries; excessive sugar intake
B. Vomiting; hyperchloremic metabolic acidosis
C. Ipecac; cardiomyopathy
D. Bingeing; Mallory-Weiss tear
E. Laxatives; hyperkalemia

91. An 8-year-old boy has recently refused to go to his new summer camp. He has complained of "stomach aches" or not feeling well when getting ready to go to camp, and he became extremely clingy when his dad attempted to put him on the bus. He is also very anxious at night, constantly asking if it is Friday or if he can go to work with his dad instead of going to camp. His energy and appetite are good, and when he is with his parents his mood is bright. Which of the following pairings would be consistent with the symptoms and diagnosis?

A. Someone at camp is bullying him, and he has separation anxiety disorder.
B. He is afraid that something bad will happen to him or to his parents, and he has separation anxiety disorder.
C. He is unable to sleep without his parents in the room, and this is a normal developmental phase.
D. He constantly worries about being kidnapped and never seeing his parents again, and he has early onset major depression.
E. He is having hallucinations telling him not to go to camp, and this is early onset schizophrenia.

92. Mr. R. is a 57-year-old Vietnam veteran who comes to the VA ER with pressured speech, flight of ideas, and irritability. He has no history of bipolar disorder. He is a combat veteran who has chronic symptoms of PTSD (flashbacks, avoidance, and hyperarousal), but has never been to see a psychiatrist. He also has had no medical care since "my Army admit physical." He has been traveling around the country on his motorcycle "since 'Nam." He is noted on physical exam to have a somewhat unsteady gait, and he is thin and pale with some temporal wasting. He has old track marks on his arms. His short-term memory and concentration are impaired. What would be the most important test to order in this man?

A. TSH
B. B_{12}
C. HIV
D. RPR
E. Ceruloplasmin

93. A 52-year-old woman has no past psychiatric history. Her social history is significant for having been a sex worker for 10 years, starting in her twenties. She has been divorced twice and currently lives with her boyfriend of 5 years. She presents with a history of poor concentration, mild confusion, irritability, short-term memory problems, a tremor of the fingers and lips, and mild headaches. Her boyfriend reports that she has become disinterested in her personal appearance and hygiene, and has been showing poor judgment. On physical exam she is noted to have decreased proprioception and vibratory sense, and her pupils are more reactive to accommodation than to light. What is the most likely etiology or neuropathology of her symptoms?

A. Amyloid beta
B. Treponema pallidum
C. Alpha-synuclein inclusions
D. Prion
E. Fungi

94. A 38-year-old woman presents with continuous symptoms of isolation, anxiety, nightmares, refusal to return to work, feelings of detachment, and intense irritability after being raped at work 2 months ago. Which of the following psychotherapeutic interventions is indicated?

A. Psychoanalysis
B. Debriefing
C. Interpersonal psychotherapy
D. Dialectical behavioral therapy
E. Exposure therapy

95. A 2-year-old boy is brought to the walk-in ER because he is refusing to walk. His mother says that he slipped in the bathroom and banged his leg. On physical exam he is a quiet child who doesn't speak much. You notice that he has bruises on his back and upper arm. An X-ray of his leg reveals a femoral fracture. After you call orthopedics to cast the leg, what is the appropriate next step?

A. Give pain medications PRN, arrange for followup with orthopedics, and discharge home.
B. Reinterview the family as a group to understand the circumstances of the fall.
C. Arrange for developmental testing as an outpatient because he isn't speaking much.
D. Order a complete skeletal survey.
E. Call the police.

96. A 10-year-old boy presents with paroxysms of obsessions and compulsions in the context of fevers and sore throat. What is the best treatment for the psychiatric symptoms?
A. Antipsychotic
B. Selective serotonin reuptake inhibitor
C. Antibiotics
D. Plasmaphoresis
E. Benzodiazepines

97. A 23-year-old man presents to the psychiatrist at the request of his mother who notes that he has always been "a bit reclusive." The patient himself denies anything out of the ordinary and is content and functional as a puzzle maker, living in his cabin in the woods and not keeping up to date with fashion. His mother's main complaint is that he never seemed interested in other people, and she notes that he would leave the house whenever she threw dinner parties to get him to interact. He most likely suffers from which disorder?
A. Schizophrenia
B. Schizotypal personality disorder
C. Avoidant personality disorder
D. Antisocial personality disorder
E. Schizoid personality disorder

98. A 65-year-old woman, brought to the psychiatrist's office by her sister, is convinced that her neighbors are putting voodoo hexes on her and sending fumes through the vents in her apartment. Five months ago she had moved because of similar complaints regarding the neighbors, but now she believes that her former neighbor has followed her to her new apartment building. Her sleep and appetite are normal, as is her mood, though she describes feeling upset about the neighbors. She denies experiencing auditory or visual hallucinations, and she does not appear to be responding to internal stimuli. She continues to participate in her church activities, and she is cognitively intact, has no significant medical problems, and her neuroimaging and labs were unremarkable. Her most likely diagnosis is

A. Major depression with psychotic features
B. Delusional disorder
C. Schizoaffective disorder
D. Brief psychotic disorder
E. Psychosis due to a general medical condition

99. Which of the following is the best initial treatment for obsessive compulsive disorder?
A. Nortriptyline
B. Low-dose clomipramine
C. High-dose clomipramine
D. Low-dose sertraline
E. High-dose sertraline

100. Mrs. G., a middle-aged single woman hospitalized for a non-healing leg wound, was found by the nursing staff to be putting blood and feces into her wound. Which of the following best describes patients with factitious disorder?
A. Aware of both their role in producing the signs and symptoms of illness and their motivation.
B. Unaware of both their role in producing the signs and symptoms of illness and their motivation.
C. Aware of their role in producing the signs and symptoms of illness but usually unaware of their motivation.
D. They intentionally feign illness to get out the military, to receive financial compensation, or to secure a bed in the hospital to get off the street.
E. Their illness is not intentionally produced.

Answers and Explanations

1. C	**26.** B	**51.** C	**76.** B
2. B	**27.** C	**52.** B	**77.** C
3. C	**28.** E	**53.** B	**78.** B
4. D	**29.** A	**54.** B	**79.** B
5. B	**30.** C	**55.** D	**80.** C
6. A	**31.** B	**56.** E	**81.** B
7. C	**32.** B	**57.** C	**82.** B
8. D	**33.** E	**58.** E	**83.** A
9. B	**34.** C	**59.** B	**84.** E
10. E	**35.** D	**60.** B	**85.** B
11. C	**36.** A	**61.** C	**86.** B
12. B	**37.** E	**62.** C	**87.** E
13. D	**38.** D	**63.** B	**88.** B
14. D	**39.** C	**64.** A	**89.** B
15. B	**40.** D	**65.** B	**90.** C
16. B	**41.** D	**66.** D	**91.** B
17. C	**42.** D	**67.** B	**92.** C
18. E	**43.** D	**68.** C	**93.** B
19. A	**44.** E	**69.** E	**94.** E
20. C	**45.** B	**70.** D	**95.** D
21. B	**46.** D	**71.** B	**96.** C
22. B	**47.** A	**72.** D	**97.** E
23. C	**48.** D	**73.** A	**98.** B
24. D	**49.** C	**74.** B	**99.** E
25. A	**50.** B	**75.** C	**100.** C

1. (C) Schizophrenia may be diagnosed by the presence of two or more of the symptom categories listed in this question. The first two (hallucinations and delusions) are considered positive symptoms and reflect a loss of reality testing or being able to distinguish between one's own thoughts and those that he or she obtains by observing the external world. Hallucinations are perceptions experienced in the absence of an external stimulus, and while they may occur in any sensory modality, in schizophrenia they are most commonly auditory. Delusions are false fixed beliefs that the person maintains despite their being contrary to the person's cultural background. Disorganization symptoms involve speech and thinking (illogicality, loose association) and behavior (catatonia, mannerisms, inappropriate social behavior). Many patients can live and function, albeit with much hardship, while suffering from hallucinations or delusions and disorganization, but it is the presence of negative symptoms (alogia, affective flattening, avolition, anhedonia, attentional impairment) that produces the most functional impairment and is the hardest to treat. Negative symptoms may be seen as reflecting a deficiency of mental functioning that is normally present, while positive symptoms reflect the addition of processes and content not normally experienced. In this vein, it is much easier to treat positive symptoms by reducing the excess than it is to treat negative symptoms by adding what is not there.

2. (B) Substance abuse and dependence are commonly comorbid with certain personality disorders, specifically antisocial, borderline, and avoidant PD (though the latter is frequently limited to the socially lubricating use of alcohol). Both antisocial and borderline patients manifest limited impulse control and excessive aggressive tendencies, making them at risk for substance abuse. Borderline patients may be seen as trying to fill themselves up with an externally rewarding substitute for their internal feelings of emptiness. Substance abusers with antisocial PD engage in more risky behaviors and are more likely to be infected with HIV than those without this disorder. It is important to remember that when a patient is in the grips of a substance (either addiction, intoxication or withdrawal), it is difficult, if not impossible, to diagnose a personality disorder.

3. (C) Patients with psychogenic nonepileptic seizures, or pseudoseizures, are not infrequently encountered in both psychiatric and neurological clinics. Importantly, these patients are commonly found to be suffering from true seizures as well as the psychogenic variant; this does not preclude the diagnosis of conversion disorder. Conversion disorder is a condition marked by the presence of one or more symptoms or deficits that affect voluntary motor or sensory function, suggesting a neurological condition, but not explained by medical findings (e.g., double vision, blindness, deafness, loss of touch, paralysis, ataxia, aphonia). The symptom is frequently precipitated or exacerbated by psychological stress, but the symptom itself is not intentionally produced or feigned (as in factitious disorder or malingering). Patients may present with *la belle indifference*, but their symptom(s) nonetheless significantly impairs their functioning. Frequently, presentations resemble the patient's preexisting pathology (e.g., patients with epilepsy who have pseudoseizures) and are difficult to tease out. Conversion disorders are common, occurring in up to 33% of female psychiatric patients with female to male ratios ranging from 2:1 upto 10:1, and run an acute and episodic course with a 20% to 25% chance of recurrence in 1 year. Somatization disorder is discussed in question 27. Hypochondriasis involves an excessive and pervasive preoccupation with fears of having or a belief that one has a serious illness; the patient does not respond to reassurance. It is marked by a greater focus on the cognitive processes and anxiety (i.e., fears), rather than limited to the presentation of a physical symptom. Hysteria is an older term for conversion disorder, no longer used in common psychiatric parlance. Pseudoneurologica fantastica does not exist.

4.(D) This patient is likely suffering from generalized anxiety disorder (GAD), marked by chronic and excessive worry about multiple factors in one's life. It is not uncommon for patients with GAD to "own" their symptoms and to experience them as healthy or at the very least normal. One of the theories underlying GAD is that the constant worry serves as a shield to, in effect, protect the patient from actually experiencing overwhelming anxiety; thus they focus on the cognitive aspects rather than the emotional and affective feel of their stress. While many people can turn their worry into action, in patients with GAD, eventually the anxieties and worries build up such that the person becomes increasingly impaired interpersonally, occupationally, or otherwise. This patient experiences poor sleep and muscle tension and is unable to enjoy many aspects of her daily life; she thus deserves treatment with either an SSRI or cognitive behavioral therapy (CBT).

5.(B) This patient is likely intoxicated with phencyclidine (PCP, angel dust), a compound originally developed as an anesthetic but pulled from the market due to frequent postoperative dysphoria, confusion, delirium, and psychosis. Since that time, it has become a drug of abuse and dependence (with users developing tolerance and withdrawal), but one with a reputation of causing significantly unpleasant psychological symptoms approximately 50% of the time. The time course of intoxication varies as well, lasting from 6 to up to 48 and even 72 hours. PCP has unique effects on behavioral pharmacology, producing amphetamine-like stimulant effects together with benzodiazepine/barbiturate-like depressant effects. At low to moderate doses, PCP induces a small increase in respiratory rate, a pronounced rise in blood pressure and pulse rate, flushing, profuse sweating, generalized numbness of the extremities, and loss of muscular coordination. At high doses, blood pressure, pulse rate, and respiration decline precipitously and are accompanied by garbled speech, delusions, hallucinations (auditory and visual), formal thought disorder, vomiting, blurred vision, vertical and rotatory nystagmus, ataxia, seizures, coma, and death (though death more often results from accidental injury or suicide during PCP intoxication). High doses can cause symptoms that mimic schizophrenia. Additionally, PCP may cause an analgesic effect in users leading to significant injuries, even death.

6. (A) This case is reminiscent of a common occurrence in inpatient psychiatry: the difficult patient with borderline personality disorder who manifests splitting. Splitting, common in borderline PD, is a defense mechanism in which a person or thing is seen as all good or all bad and is employed in the context of emotional conflict or internal or external stressors; essentially, the patient compartmentalizes opposite affect states and fails to integrate the positive and negative qualities of the self or others into cohesive images. Borderline patients have difficulty tolerating ambiguity and feeling emotional shades of gray; they become so wrapped up in their current mood state that they forget what it is like to be in another emotional frame. The idealization ascribed to one object (the intern in this case) is not permanent and frequently shifts into devaluation when the intern frustrates the patient (on a daily or momentary basis). Patients with borderline PD also have difficulty with object constancy, reading each action of people in their lives as if there were no prior context and not being able to form an integrated and whole view of another. Similarly, they manifest an inability to self-soothe or experience the presence of a loving feeling when a loved one is absent. Projective identification is another defense common in borderline PD in which the patient deals with emotional conflict or internal or external stressors by attributing to another his or her own feelings, impulses, or thoughts; importantly, the patient induces these very feelings in others, making it difficult to clarify who did what to whom first. Borderline patients defend against their own angry feelings by inducing anger in the therapist which justifies their being angry in return. Reaction formation is a defense mechanism in which an unacceptable impulse that would cause anxiety (e.g., being angry with one's wife) is converted and experienced as the opposite (e.g., bringing her flowers). Identity diffusion is one of the criteria for borderline PD and consists of a fragmented view of the self, with contradictory character traits, temporal discontinuity in the self, and feelings of emptiness. While splitting is an emotional inability to attribute concepts of good and bad onto the same object, multiple personalities exist as wholly different selves, occasionally with different physiological traits (e.g., skin conductance, heart rate variability).

7. (C) Normal grief is characterized by minor sleep disturbances, sadness, possible weight loss, possible guilt about the deceased, normal attention to hygiene, and illusions. An example of an illusion would be "thinking she hears her husband voice," or after the death of a pet, seeing a shadow or something on the floor and fleetingly thinking it is the pet. Complicated grief is usually associated with severe symptoms lasting more than two months with multiple symptoms of major depression (e.g., significant sleep disturbance, weight loss, worthlessness or hopelessness, hallucinations or delusions, suicidal ideation or attempts and poor attention to hygiene). This could be called complicated grief or a major depressive episode (in the context of a loss). This patient is not psychotic, so neither schizophrenia nor brief psychotic disorder would be appropriate.

8. (D) SSRI discontinuation syndrome is a well-established clinical entity that is directly mediated by the half-life of the specific medication used. Of the drugs listed, fluoxetine has the longest half-life (>1 week), as it has a highly active metabolite nofluoxetine. Sertaline and citalopram and are both intermediate (26 and 35 hours, respectively), and paroxetine and venlafaxine are significantly shorter (~20 and <12 hours, respectively). After a few days of abrupt cessation of treatment with either of these shorter half-life medications, a syndrome characterized by dizziness, insomnia, nervousness, nausea, agitation, malaise and flu-like feelings, electric shocks in the extremities, functional impairment, and occasionally disorientation may emerge. Thus, all of the SSRIs, save for fluoxetine, need to be tapered before they are discontinued.

9. (B) Patients with obsessive-compulsive personality disorder (OCPD) are preoccupied with rules, authority, details, and perfectionism to such an extent that they frequently lose the forest for the trees. They have difficulty recognizing emotional salience in their environment, and they usually focus on rational arguments rather than the intuitive feel of things; it is not that they do not care and cannot love, rather they prioritize level-headedness which manifests as being cold. Their inflexibility is apparent to those around them, as is their preoccupation with impossible standards, and they frequently become despondent and occasionally frankly depressed when perfectionism is not attainable. The "anal-retentive" person is the classic OCPD patient. OCPD entails a rigid system of rules and judiciousness to which the patient ego-syntonically adheres, while OCD is marked by ego-dystonic and anxiety-inducing obsessions combined with anxiety-reducing compulsions with which the patient has a daily struggle. Narcissistic PD may be similar to OCPD in a desire for perfection and achievement, but they differ in what drives them, specifically the narcissist's need for recognition and the obsessive's need to fulfill his or her internal idealized standards. While patients with OCPD may be impersonal in interpersonal settings ("relate to your family"), patients with schizotypal PD typically have difficulties with close relationships, cognitive or perceptual distortions and eccentric behaviors.

10. (E) Between 4% and 13% of people with schizophrenia commit suicide and between 25% and 50% make a suicide attempt. Schizophrenia takes an enormous toll on quality of life and subjective and objective sense of well-being. Risk factors for suicide in schizophrenia include previous suicide attempts, depression, hopelessness, substance abuse, and male gender. High premorbid functioning, insight into having a serious mental illness, and less severe cognitive impairment are also associated with increased risk for suicide; however, they are also associated with improved functional outcome if suicide does not occur.

11. (C) The most common and effective treatments for Tourette syndrome (TS) are the antipsychotic agents haloperidol (Haldol), pimozide (Orap), and risperidone (Risperdal). Other agents that are somewhat less efficacious but have fewer side effects include α_2-adrenergic agonists (e.g., clonidine) and benzodiazepines (clonazepam). Nonpharmacologic behavior modification strategies such as positive reinforcement programs can also be effective.

12. (B) This patient most likely has a chronic subdural hematoma. He is an alcoholic (possibly the etiology of his pancreatitis) and may well have had a small fall or trauma that he does not remember. Chronic subdural hematomas most typically occur in elderly persons on anticoagulants or in alcoholics with some brain atrophy. Common symptoms include headache (80%), fatigue or decreased alertness, and focal neurologic signs contralateral to the subdural. Examples include mild weakness, hyperreflexia, and Babinski sign. If the hematoma enlarges, the headache worsens and the level of consciousness decreases. CT or MRI should be done as part of the diagnostic workup. The treatment is often burr holes with drainage, which leads to marked improvement in 80% to 90% of cases. He does not have evidence of an acute bacterial infection and CNS fungal infections are rare, mostly seen in significantly immunocompromised hosts. Prions are responsible for bovine spongiform encephalitis and Creutzfeldt-Jakob disease, in which memory deficits, EEG changes, myoclonus, and often ataxia are prominent, along with a rapidly progressive course. Plaques and tangles together in high density are pathognomonic for Alzheimer disease.

13. (D) Schizophrenia is a chronic illness, beginning in early life (adolescence) with months to years of prodromal symptoms of social withdrawal, strange ideas, subtle and nonspecific changes in behavior and emotional responsiveness. Following the acute initial episode or psychotic break (usually between 15 to 25 years for men, slightly older for women), the course is marked by acute exacerbations and remissions of both positive (hallucinations and delusions) and negative symptoms (apathy, anhedonia, avolition), and a progressive functional decline. The patient with schizophrenia never fully returns to his or her prior level of functioning. This progressive and active phase usually lasts through middle age until it generally develops into a residual phase marked by the prominence of negative symptoms with fewer positive symptoms.

14. (D) Patients with antisocial personality disorder manifest a wanton neglect for the rights of others and experience no remorse when these rights are violated. While they may be charming and charismatic, their motivation is predatory, to "put one over" on other people who they see as weak. Illegal activities, substance abuse, lying, deceit, and assaultive behavior are common in this population, and this diagnosis is highly overrepresented in prisoners (up to 75% of prison inmates have antisocial PD). It is difficult to treat, the most common method being imprisonment where external agents can fill in for the patients' moral failings. Mistrust of the motives of others is common in paranoid PD. Social anxiety is descriptive of avoidant PD, although it may be seen in self-conscious narcissistic patients as well. Patients with OCPD manifest overly deliberate planning and tend to be hypermoral. Constricted affect is present in schizoid and schizotypal PD as well as OCPD.

15. (B) This patient is likely suffering from an acute depressive episode, and should be treated with either psychopharmacology or psychotherapy, or optimally a combination of the two. It is important to remember, though, that most patients with bipolar disorder more frequently present with depressive episodes than manic episodes, and the prescription of an antidepressant medication can induce a manic episode in these patients. Therefore checking for prior manic symptoms can avert this crisis. As her symptoms clearly point to a diagnosis of a depressive episode (either bipolar or unipolar). A family history may help clarify the diagnosis and point one toward a treatment that worked for a genetically related family member. If the patient denies a history of mania, a family history of bipolar disorder would also warrant caution in prescribing. Assessing whether her problems at work are in fact her fault is fruitless, because it is not the events or trauma themselves but rather her reaction to them that is important; this is beside the fact that her guilt-ridden symptoms are part of a syndrome. Taste testing has no role here.

16. (B) This boy meets criteria for conduct disorder. He is aggressive to people (aggression to animals is also possible), steals, lies, and manifests a serious violation of rules (running away, being truant). He has not destroyed property (e.g., fire setting), which is another common behavior seen in conduct disorder. It is unlikely that he is psychotic, as the "voices" seem more like an excuse for his behavior. Thus schizophreniform disorder is unlikely (meeting the criteria for schizophrenia but for <6 months). Oppositional defiant disorder is a pattern of negativistic, hostile, and defiant behaviors lasting at least 6 months, with symptoms like frequently losing one's temper, actively defying rules, blaming others for mistakes, and being spiteful; however, it is less overtly hostile, aggressive, and destructive than conduct disorder. Antisocial PD is only diagnosed in people over 18, but evidence of conduct disorder is generally required for a later diagnosis of antisocial PD. Though children may at times be aggressive and flaunt authority, the pervasiveness of the symptoms and the clinically significant impairment in social, academic, or occupational functioning marks the behavior in conduct disorder as outside of normal development.

17. (C) Manic patients are notorious for their difficulty in sticking to one subject; they manifest rapidity of thought, flight of ideas, and pressured speech, and when interrupted frequently become irritable and angry. While letting them talk initially provides you with mental status findings and diagnostic clues, after a point their energy and seemingly endless logorrhea are no longer meaningful. Efforts to interrupt these patients will frequently fail and will only provoke their ire, however, there is no need to prematurely terminate the interview. Like many other patients, explaining the reason behind your interruptions in a meaningful and empathic way can avert some of these problems and allow for a more complete evaluation. Reflecting on the process—commenting that the patient has a lot to say and seems energetic, commenting on her affect (angry, joyous, etc.)—can convey to her your understanding. Finally, interviews are fruitless only if the interviewer lacks understanding of the patient's internal world.

18. (E) This patient is presenting with symptoms characteristic of histrionic personality disorder (HPD), prominent features of which are omnipresent preoccupation with appearance and receiving attention, frequent emotional outbursts, excessive emotionality, and impressionistic speech lacking details. These patients tend to be provocative and dramatic. They believe their relationships to be more intimate than they actually are, and at their core are viewed by others as vain and superficial. Cognitively, these patients tend to see and experience things in an impressionistic style (think of Monet), highly influenced by their emotional state. This is in contrast to the person with OCPD who misses the forest for the trees (think of a close-up of a Seurat pointillist piece). Patients with HPD respond to psychodynamic psychotherapy which helps them to clarify their emotional responses and provides greater structure to their cognitions. Dialectical behavioral therapy is useful for those with borderline PD. Medications are useful in HPD only for comorbid axis I disorders. Treatment would be quite helpful to this patient whose illness has impaired her social functioning.

19. (A) Patients with obsessive-compulsive disorder (OCD) are tormented by recurring thoughts and images which, by definition, are anxiety-inducing, while disturbing recurrent thoughts (e.g., someone will die, my hands are dirty) are well known and popularized examples of obsessions, intrusive images, and unwanted impulses are equally disturbing obsessions in their own right and are experienced by just as many patients. Importantly, these impulses and images, while recognized as a product of one's own mind (i.e., not a thought insertion), are not in keeping with one's sense of self; they are ego-dystonic (i.e., seen as foreign and unwanted). Frequently, patients with OCD have a hypermoral character and are highly disturbed by the frequently aggressive and sexual images and urges that pop into their mind's eye. During these experiences, which are instantaneous, patients are conscious of themselves, able to attend fully to the world around them, and able to describe their personal histories and the nature of their images (i.e., not a dissociative experience). Finally, they recognize the unreality of the image and its production in their mind (i.e., not a hallucination), akin to thinking of a pink elephant but with a significantly loaded emotional tone and urge. It is highly uncommon for patients to act on these impulses and images.

20. (C) Approximately two-thirds of depressed patients will respond to an initial trial with an antidepressant. In those who don't respond, approximately one-third will respond to a change in medication. Of note, the placebo-response rate in uncomplicated major depression can approach and surpass 50%; however, it must be noted that these patients frequently relapse within a few weeks of starting the placebo, while those treated with a medication maintain their euthymic state.

21. (B) Treating nicotine dependence, and any form of substance abuse for that matter, involves a multistep approach. Initially, a complete substance abuse history should be elicited, including the success of previous approaches (e.g., nicotine patch, nicotine gum, therapy, "cold turkey") to help guide current and future options. A key element in the patient's success is her or his motivation to quit, and thus developing collaborative, attainable treatment goals is essential (e.g., decrease consumption to X cigarettes per week, plan a stop date after which no cigarettes will be smoked). In this case the patient had already tried reasonable first choice options, including the patch and gum. As a general rule, a medication that worked before may well work again, and this supports restarting buproprion, although only after completing the steps mentioned above. By some reports, buproprion is less likely to precipitate mania than are the SSRIs, although the jury is still out. The time course for smoking cessation is similar to that for its antidepressant effects (i.e., 4 to 6 weeks), and thus the patient should be warned not to expect an immediate response. Given its past tolerability in this patient, it is reasonable to use buproprion again; however, especially with bipolar patients, one should monitor closely for any emerging side effects, including mania.

22. (B) Because of the high prevalence of unipolar depression, a depressive episode likely forecasts a depressive disorder. However, a small number of these patients go on to develop bipolar disorder. While there is no identifier for this group, a family history of bipolar disorder is a significant marker; of those depressed patients with a close family history of bipolar disorder, 30% to 50% will eventually develop a manic episode and therefore bipolar disorder. Of note, a family history of bipolar disorder also places one at increased risk for unipolar depression. Remember that patients with bipolar disorder frequently first present with one or more depressive episodes.

23. (C) This patient has a constellation of symptoms consistent with obsessive-compulsive disorder (OCD). OCD is frequently first manifest in adolescence, and initial symptoms may appear spontaneously.

While the anxious and behavioral symptoms of OCD may be somewhat responsive to high dose serotonergic medication (i.e., SSRIs), they usually never totally remit. The general course of the illness is one of attenuated symptoms throughout most of the person's life, though they are exacerbated by stressful situations. Deterioration, likewise, is not the norm. Frequently, patients with OCD develop a major depressive disorder superimposed on their OCD; whether this results from OCD-specific neurobiology or from the stress of living with chronic symptoms is unknown, but both are likely involved in the depressive pathogenesis.

24. (D) This patient is suffering from a major depressive episode with mood-congruent psychotic features. While each of the listed medications may be used, no single treatment is reported to be as effective in isolation as electroconvulsive therapy (ECT) for a psychotic depression. The standard of care for this severe disorder includes either ECT or both an antidepressant and an antipsychotic. In this elderly patient, concerns over his substantial and rapid loss of weight point to the use of a treatment with rapid results (i.e., ECT). ECT is safe to use is the elderly population, in relative contrast to tricyclic antidepressants, which have cardiac conduction and anticholinergic side effects.

25. (A) The anxiety associated with obsessive thoughts (grandmother will die) is frequently unbearable to patients with OCD and leads to the formation of compulsions (rereading directions) which serve to decrease this anxiety. However, this anxiety is attenuated for only a brief period before the cycle starts again. A hallmark of OCD is that the person recognizes the senseless nature of his or her thoughts and frequently labels them as ridiculous, but the anxiety can be so powerful that the person caves in to the compulsion even though he or she knows it makes no sense. Part of the therapy for this condition is exposure and response prevention: she has the thought that her grandmother will die, and she is prevented from acting out the compulsion to ward against the anxiety associated with this thought; multiple rounds of this lead to a habituation to the thought and an extinction of the pathological behavior. Delusions are false beliefs that are held with great conviction and influence one's behavior. Overvalued ideas are beliefs held firmly but without the conviction of delusions or the anxiety and intrusive nature of obsessions; they also influence one's behavior (e.g., superstitions). Loss of ego boundaries refers to the difficulty that psychotic patients have in determining whether stimuli exist inside of outside of themselves.

26. (B) Bupropion has been associated with seizures, especially in high doses and in bulimic patients (who may already have a reduced seizure threshold due to electrolyte abnormalities). Paroxetine has a very short half-life and is therefore not thought to be as good in a patient who may vomit up a dose. Fluoxetine is recommended because of its long half-life. MAOIs are not good because a bingeing bulimic might inadvertently eat a tyramine-containing food resulting in a hypertensive crisis. TCAs are not safe in overdose because they can cause cardiac conduction abnormalities.

27. (C) This patient is likely suffering from alcohol withdrawal delirium (delirium tremens [DT]). Symptoms may develop a few hours after abrupt cessation of drinking and peak at 48 to 72 hours, but the window of risk frequently extends to 7 days. Symptoms include irritability, insomnia, tremors, hallucinations (frequently visual and lilliputian or small objects), seizures, autonomic hyperactivity, disorientation, severe agitation, and fluctuating level of consciousness. Five percent of patients with ethanol withdrawal progress to DT; the untreated syndrome may be fatal in up to 35% of patients. As DT is a medical emergency, it should be treated with IV lorazepam, IV thiamine, and admission to a medical unit. A main goal of treatment is in attenuating CNS excitotoxicity with benzodiazepines, which can then be slowly tapered over days. Naltrexone is an opiate antagonist and has no use in acute alcohol withdrawal.

28. (E) This patient is manifesting some symptoms of OCPD, a syndrome marked by lifelong rigidity, perfectionism, and frequent unemotionality; this is in contrast to OCD which includes true obsessions and compulsions. Additionally, patients with OCPD frequently state that their behaviors are adaptive and in keeping with their persona (i.e., ego-syntonic), while those with OCD are bothered by their symptoms and feel they are not in keeping with their personalities (i.e., ego-dystonic). However, it has yet to be determined if this patient suffers from OCPD; one needs to know the chronicity and severity of his symptoms as well as whether they are present in multiple contexts (e.g., not just at work). It is most likely that this patient's presentation is a marker for a dysfunction in the marriage rather than the development of an anxiety or personality disorder. True, he may have OCPD traits, but the relative isolation of his symptoms and his overall functionality make a diagnosis of disorder less likely. Something has withered in the communication between husband and wife, and in these cases the overt chief complaint is frequently the product of ill-informed pop psychology.

29. (A) Schizophreniform disorder is diagnosed when the patient meets all criteria for a diagnosis of schizophrenia save for the time component. For this diagnosis, all symptoms including prodromal, active, and residual phases must last between 1 and 6 months; so if even residual symptoms are present after 6 months, the diagnosis changes to schizophrenia. There have been few and conflicting studies about the long-term outcome of schizophreniform patients. Prodromal symptoms of schizophrenia are those that occur before the initial onset of psychosis. These symptoms are nonspecific and the length of this phase may vary from days to many years. Most commonly, observable and experiential changes in behavior, thinking, and feelings occur along with attenuated psychotic symptoms like attentional or perceptual distortions. For example, the patient may become increasingly preoccupied with religious, spiritual, or philosophical pursuits and may seclude him or herself from friends and family. Suicidality may be present but is far less prominent, as the individual does not generally experience this change as threatening or painful. The other answers listed are all in the psychotic realm.

30. (C) In response to a significant loss, people often respond with grief or bereavement-related depressive symptoms (e.g., sadness, insomnia, poor appetite, decreased interest in the world), and they tend to see these symptoms as a normal reaction. However, even in normal bereavement, the individual may seek help for associated symptoms such as insomnia. While the duration of normal bereavement varies between sociocultural groups, the DSM-IV defines a "normal" reaction as less than 2 months of serious depressive symptoms. In addition to this time component, the presence of certain severe symptoms is also useful for identifying pathology. These include excessive feelings of worthlessness, guilt about things other than actions taken or not taken by the survivor at the time of the death, thoughts of death other than feeling that he or she would be better off dead or should have died with the deceased person, marked psychomotor retardation, prolonged and marked functional impairment, and hallucinatory experiences other than thinking that he or she hears the voice of, or transiently sees the image of, the deceased person. Thus, without the presence of these symptoms, and within 2 months, grief reactions are normal. The patient in this example is not psychotic; rather, she is emotionally distraught and likely manifesting amygdalar hyperactivity making her transiently re-experience the presence of her husband. She should be offered reassurance.

31. (B) In its natural history, a major depressive episode may last 6 months. However, as a depressive disorder progresses over the course of time, with more and more depressive episodes, the length of each episode increases and the symptom-free period between them decreases. While early in the course of the illness, a patient's refusal of treatment may entail suffering for 6 months, an increasing amount of data shows that duration of untreated episodes may have a lasting effect on the brain. With medication treatment, most episodes fully remit within 4 to 6 weeks.

32. (B) According to epidemiological studies PTSD is an under-diagnosed illness, perhaps due to the failure of many practitioners to specifically inquire about a history of trauma or symptoms specific to PTSD. These patients may be ashamed by their symptoms and may not volunteer this information. Most studies of medications in PTSD have shown SSRIs to be fairly effective, and they are recommended as the first-line psychopharmacological treatment. Fewer studies, if any, have been done for SNRIs and NDRIs. TCAs may be effective, but given their increased side effect burden and lethality in overdose, they are generally considered second- or (more commonly) third-line agents. Antipsychotics may be useful for more complicated presentations or in those for whom SSRIs are not entirely effective.

33. (E) In the acute setting of the psych ER, the actual diagnosis is less important than is the management of presenting symptoms. Given his agitation and potential for violence, this patient may need to be restrained and provided with calming medications (e.g., intramuscular haloperidol, lorazepam, and diphenhydramine) before an interview is possible. It should be mentioned that the symptom complex with which this patient is presenting is not only disturbing to staff and other patients, but is likely a manifestation of the distress being experienced by the patient himself. Once he is able to be interviewed, a diagnostic differential can be further developed, but for the time being, the patient presents with an agitated psychosis that must be treated. In the psych ER, cocaine-induced psychotic disorder, mania, and an exacerbation of schizophrenia may appear identically. However, outside of the psych ER, cross-sectional diagnoses in psychiatry are inappropriate and severely limited, as the time course of the illness is crucial in establishing a correct treatment.

34. (C) While the seeming cardinal symptom of bipolar disorder is mania, most patients with this illness actually spend the majority of their time mildly to moderately dysthymic. Mania can facilitate one's financial ruin, the acquisition of a sexually transmitted disease, and legal difficulties, but it is arguably the time spent depressed that most significantly impacts the patient's quality of life. However, while there is much research along the lines of preventing depressive relapse in bipolar disorder, an older medication, lithium, has the most evidence to support its use in this respect. Lithium is the prototypical mood-stabilizing medication, and it is safe and effective as an acute as well as maintenance treatment for bipolar disorder. There is not as much evidence to support the use of divalproex or olanzapine to treat bipolar depression; however, both are effective for manic mood-stabilization, and divalproex is frequently used for prophylaxis of mania. It is not usually recommended that a patient with bipolar disorder be maintained on an antidepressant (e.g., TCA, SSRI) long-term, as this may increase the risk of rapid cycling or precipitate a manic episode.

35. (D) Hypochondriasis is an unrealistic interpretation of physical symptoms or sensations as abnormal thus leading to a preoccupation with fears of having a serious disease. It has lifetime prevalence between 1-5% and may reach 9% in general medical patients. It is equally common in both genders. Hypochondriasis may occur secondary to depression, which should be the initial focus of treatment. Hypochondriasis may reach delusional intensity in either depression or schizophrenia. The peak age of onset is in 20's and 30's. Patients with this disorder tend to doctor shop and alliances with these patients may be tenuous at best. Unnecessary medical work-ups should be avoided but underlying medical causes of these symptoms must be ruled out (e.g. neurological, endocrine, autoimmune disorders or occult neoplasms). Once established it tends to follow a chronic course and may be very disabling. Although the family lives of these patients can be severely impacted due to the limitations imposed by this disorder, family history itself per se is not associated with an increased risk of this disorder. Group therapy and antidepressants may be helpful.

36. (A) Micropsychotic episodes are included in the diagnostic criteria for borderline personality disorder. These episodes, lasting minutes to days, are usually precipitated by psychosocial stressors (e.g., abandonment, interpersonal conflict) and can include auditory hallucinations to kill oneself, paranoid feelings of persecution or jealousy, and severe depersonalization. Interestingly, the experience of auditory hallucinations in BPD often occurs without loss of insight, in contrast to patients with schizophrenia who do not recognize that a hallucination is imaginary. Though these psychotic symptoms are usually self-limited, many borderline patients are (perhaps inappropriately) put on high-dose antipsychotics for months at a time, hoping to target these symptoms. This patient is not likely suffering a psychotic depression, as her depressive symptoms are mild and have been present for only a few days. Additionally, psychotic symptoms due to a major depression usually consist of delusions of guilt or bodily dysfunction, rather than auditory hallucinations. Other than auditory hallucinations, she has no psychotic symptoms suggestive of schizophrenia or schizoaffective disorder.

37. (E) This patient is suffering from panic disorder, which is diagnosed when some of the panic attacks are "spontaneous" and "out of the blue," and when the patient develops a fear of having a panic attack in and of itself. As she is young, it is unlikely that her symptoms represent a nonpsychiatric entity, but thyroid function should be tested, especially if she were to have a family history. Given that she was worked up in multiple ERs, these tests (including urine toxicology and cardiac function) were likely done, and the reports should be available to you. In your office, she should be screened for excessive caffeine intake (which exacerbates panic disorder), as well as for depression (which frequently accompanies panic disorder). The degree to which her work and social functioning have been impaired must be assessed as well. Finally, the best treatment for panic disorder is either cognitive behavioral therapy or antidepressant medication (e.g., SSRIs); it should be her choice. She should be told that SSRIs take 2 to 4 weeks to work, and she may experience increased anxiety initially. Standing or as-needed benzodiazepines are useful in patients who cannot tolerate the initial activating effects of an SSRI. However, clonazepam is a better choice than alprazolam, as the latter has a rapid onset and offset, thus increasing its abuse potential as well as rebound anxiety. Lithium is not used for the treatment of panic disorder.

38. (D) This woman has the classic triad of cognitive decline, gait disturbance, and incontinence which is seen in normal pressure hydrocephalus (NPH). Her CT scan is consistent with NPH. The definitive treatment for NPH is a ventriculo-peritoneal shunt, but unfortunately not all patients will benefit; the earlier the process is diagnosed, the more likely the person will benefit from the shunt. Other evaluative measures include a "therapeutic" spinal tap in which fluid is drained, and then the patient is evaluated to see if this improves his or her symptoms. Cholinesterase inhibitors are primarily used for mild to moderate Alzheimer disease. NMDA antagonists (e.g., memantine) are indicated for moderate to severe dementia. Fluorescent treponemal antibodies are found in the CSF of patients who have neurosyphilis. This woman does not have focal findings suggestive of a stroke.

39. (C) Somatization disorder is chronic and is characterized by multiple, clinically significant somatic complaints not accounted for by medical findings, resulting in impairment of function or frequent use of medical services. To be suffering from somatization disorder, a patient must present with four pain symptoms, two non-pain-related gastrointestinal symptoms, one sexual symptom, and one pseudoneurological symptom. It is thought that, while the symptoms are neither intentionally produced nor feigned, the major motivation behind them is apparently to communicate significant distress. A patient with somatization disorder may have difficulty differentiating between somatic and emotional symptoms; witness patients who describe a highly dramatic history, frequently without specific information, other than details related to their physical symptoms. They are clearly suffering, but they appear blind as to the actual nature of their pain. Somatization disorder is more common in women, nearly all of whom have a comorbid cluster B (dramatic) personality disorder. Conversion disorder is marked by the presence of one or more symptoms or deficits affecting a voluntary motor or sensory function suggesting a medical or neurological condition; again the symptom is not able to be accounted for by a medical investigation. It can be distinguished from somatization disorder by the patient's frequent *la belle indifference* as well as its more episodic and acute course.

40. (D) See question 3 for a thorough description of conversion disorder. Patients with conversion disorder can, and frequently do, have pre-existing neurological disorders, oftentimes similar to the symptom of conversion itself. Their conversion symptoms are not intentionally produced, are not manifest by primarily pain or sexual symptoms, and affect voluntary motor or sensory function. Importantly for the diagnosis of conversion disorder, the symptom cannot correspond to known physiological or neurological patterns. Thus, this patient may complain of an inability to move her arm, but it is likely that upon examination, her "paralyzed" arm will not fall onto her head when dropped, or in other cases, nystagmus is still evident in conversion "blindness." Hypotheses behind the development of conversion symptoms include the following: (i) a solution to an unconscious conflict (i.e., if the patient was very angry with her sister before she died); (ii) cortico-cortical miscommunication; (iii) may be an element of dissociation (patients with conversion symptoms have higher levels of hypnotizability). Conversion disorder is more common among patients with a history of childhood abuse and those from rural and lower socioeconomic areas.

41. (D) This patient is presenting with a somatoform disorder that can be diagnosed as either hypochondriasis or undifferentiated somatoform disorder. The nervous stomach that many people experience occasionally becomes a true somatoform disorder in the presence of anxiety and depressive disorders and in the context of a high degree of stress. It is not uncommon for medical students to experience such symptoms, but again, they reach the level of clinical significance when their help-seeking behaviors impair their daily functioning. This patient has responded to a placebo effect mediated first by the proton pump inhibitor and then again by the negative CT scan and upper endoscopy. It is unlikely that a healthy medical student has some other physical pathology that has yet to be discovered by new and more invasive testing, and it is much more likely that he is experiencing depression, anxiety, or merely despondency in the context of medical school. The fact that both of his parents are physicians is important in that he probably has a high degree of expected success and being frustrated and upset in medical school is not an option, thus his symptoms present somatically.

42. (D) Malingering is the intentional production of false or exaggerated symptoms motivated by external incentives, such as obtaining compensation or drugs, avoiding work or military duty, or evading criminal prosecution. Malingering should be considered when there is a marked discrepancy between the claimed distress and the objective findings (e.g., complaining of auditory hallucinations but not manifesting distraction or internal preoccupation; note that persons malingering psychotic disorders often exaggerate hallucinations and delusions but cannot mimic formal thought disorders, and they usually cannot feign blunted affect, concrete thinking, or impaired interpersonal relatedness); lack of cooperation during evaluation and in complying with prescribed treatment (though this is highly nonspecific and common in clinical populations); or in the presence of an antisocial PD. This patient apparently knows exactly what to say to be taken seriously, at least initially, by espousing his experiencing command auditory hallucinations to "harm myself and others." This is rarely reported as such by symptomatic patients, but it is nonetheless important to take quite seriously until a formal evaluation can be made. The poorly executed tattoos on his forearms are likely "prison tats," or markings obtained in prison by using a "bic" pen attached to a needle. It is noteworthy that malingering is not considered a mental illness per se; however, the person who is malingering certainly does appear to be suffering. While his or her presenting symptoms may not be the true nature of the suffering, they are produced for a reason.

43. (D) Treatment-resistant schizophrenia may be defined as an inadequate response from one adequate trial of a typical antipsychotic medication and two of the atypical antipsychotics, excluding clozapine criteria which this patient meets. Studies have shown clozapine, the first atypical, to be effective for one-third of treatment-resistant schizophrenic patients. However, this efficacy comes with a risk of agranulocytosis (1%) such that weekly (and occasionally biweekly) blood counts need to be obtained throughout the course of treatment. Other side effects of clozapine include orthostatic hypotension, weight gain, sedation, diabetes mellitus, seizure, sialorrhea, cardiomyopathy, and transient autonomic dysregulation. Clozapine is less likely than the typical antipsychotics to cause neuroleptic malignant syndrome (NMS), and it also does not carry an increased risk of torsades de pointes over other antipsychotics. One would not be concerned about dystonic laryngospasm, as clozapine has been shown to produce minimal, if any, acute dystonic reactions. In fact, clozapine is a treatment for tardive dyskinesia. Finally, clozapine has been shown to reduce the risk of death by suicide in patients with schizophrenia.

44. (E) Major depressive disorder is frequently found comorbid with cluster B (and other) personality disorders, such that approximately 60% of patients with borderline PD will experience an episode of depression at some point in their lives. While the figures are not as high for the other personality disorders, major depression is the most commonly encountered axis I disorder in this wide-ranging and diverse population. One may look at a personality disorder as a type of emotional retardation, such that with each disorder, different types of emotional situations provoke intense stress, anxiety, and despondency (i.e., abandonment for borderline PD, social contact for avoidant PD, failure for narcissistic PD, interpersonal intrusion for schizoid PD). Generalized anxiety disorder is not as common in these patients; rather they tend to suffer from a nonspecific form of anxiety related to their idiosyncratic emotional fears, as above. It is difficult to diagnose a personality disorder in the presence of schizophrenia, as the latter is such an all-consuming and severe illness that takes over most of the person's life; however, it is not impossible, and schizotypal PD is more common in persons with a family history of schizophrenia and is believed to lie on a schizophrenia spectrum. Of note, while one may diagnose an axis I disorder atop a personality disorder, one should try and refrain from making a personality disorder diagnoses in the midst of an acute axis I condition, as symptoms may be better accounted for by the latter.

45. (B) This rather complicated presentation fits the diagnostic criteria for substance-induced anxiety disorder. In this syndrome, further specified by the discrete substance, the manifest symptoms are clearly the direct physiological effects of a substance, and the anxiety symptoms are both in excess of those usually associated with the intoxication syndrome (i.e., impaired motor coordination, euphoria, anxiety, sensation of slowed time, impaired judgment, social withdrawal, conjunctival injection, increased appetite, dry mouth, tachycardia) and are sufficiently severe to warrant independent clinical attention (i.e., presenting to the psych ER). This patient's symptoms clearly fit each of these criteria, and while marijuana is a well-known cause of anxiety and mild paranoia, discrete panic attacks and anxiety leading to clinical presentation are indicative of a further impairment. Panic disorder is diagnosed in the context of recurrent unexpected panic attacks with persistent concern about having additional attacks and change in behavior related to the attacks; this patient's symptoms fit these criteria only when he is high. While theoretically one may say he was traumatized by his bad trip and additional panic attacks when on marijuana, thus conditioning him to fear the sensations, the pathological symptoms occur to a clinically significant extent only when high. The time course of symptom onset as well as pre-existing anxiety symptoms are crucial to assess when evaluating a patient in whom you suspect a substance-induced anxiety disorder.

46. (D) This girl most likely suffers from anorexia nervosa (AN). Diagnostic criteria for AN include a body weight of less than 85% of the minimal ideal weight for age; she is at 82%. She is also below the 15th percentile for BMI (in her age group this represents <5% of BMI). The physical findings associated with AN include lanugo (a layer of fine, downy-soft hair that usually begins on the face and then progresses to the extremities, and is seen in sustained severe starvation), loss of subcutaneous fat, dry skin, and hypercarotenemia (often associated with increased consumption of high carotene foods like carrots). The cardiovascular exam is usually significant for bradycardia, hypotension, and loss of cardiac muscle with "floppy" mitral valves. Patients with anorexia may have a functional mitral valve prolapse with a mid-systolic click, despite an anatomically normal valve. Some people with anorexia have peripheral edema, although the cause is unknown. Hypothermia and difficulty with temperature regulation, which is thought to be hypothalamically mediated, is also common. Over time, osteoporotic changes due to increased cortisol and decreased estrogen are common, and may lead to significant morbidity.

47. (A) Patients without comorbid illnesses tend to manifest a better response to treatment, whether psychotherapeutically or psychopharmacologically. Personality disorders are no exception, such that an acute axis I condition—likely major depression in this case—will be less amenable to treatment in the presence of borderline personality disorder. Other complicating factors in the treatment of major depression include comorbid substance abuse, dysthymic disorder, chronic medical illnesses, psychotic symptoms, and a history of prior episodes. Patients with borderline PD frequently manifest turbulent relationships (e.g., rapidly falling for someone and investing everything they have in that person in an idealized way, then realizing that person is not perfect and will not be there for them indefinitely, leading to devaluation and serious emotionally laden arguments; this cycle repeats itself many times throughout the course of a single relationship). Comorbid substance abuse is also common in borderline PD, as is a history of nonserious suicide attempts. Finally, as in most personality disorders, patients with borderline PD are exquisitely sensitive to certain emotional stressors and cite these as precipitating their episodes of depression.

48. (D) Despite seeming stability, it is not uncommon for patients with PTSD to experience an exacerbation of their illness at the anniversary of or in the context of reminders of the original traumatic event. This exacerbation is usually manifest by a worsening of their symptoms, rather than the onset of a new constellation of symptoms which is what this patient is experiencing. While psychotic symptoms such as hallucinatory flashbacks, dissociative phenomena, and some degree of paranoia are common in PTSD, the gross disturbance of behavior and the extension of paranoia to her trusted doctor (an example of delusional misidentification or Capgras syndrome) make this a manifestation of a psychotic disorder. Brief psychotic disorder is diagnosed when psychotic symptoms follow an obvious stressor and are present for 1 day to 1 month. These patients tend to be more labile, volatile, and confused than other patients with longer lasting psychotic symptoms, and also tend to have prior histories of personality disorders or trauma. Frequently, hospitalization is the treatment of choice, combined with antipsychotic medications (in the short term, as these symptoms by definition resolve on their own in a matter of time) and psychotherapy to help the patient develop greater coping skills for future stressors.

49. (C) Nonadherence to medications and undertreating (time or dose) are the two most common reasons for lack or loss of therapeutic efficacy. This patient was likely adherent to her treatment (inpatient) and initially showed a response, but it is most likely that she failed to continue taking her medications upon discharge. However, while not the most likely explanations, each of the other answers may also contribute to her relapse. Cigarette smoking decreases the bioavailability of many antipsychotic medications; patients are prohibited from smoking in the hospital and thus may experience an effective dose reduction upon discharge when they begin smoking again. Social distress, stress from medical comorbidities, and drug use can each independently lead to a psychotic relapse.

50. (B) Schizotypal personality disorder (SPD) is included in the odd cluster (A) of the personality disorders, along with paranoid PD and schizoid PD. It is marked by perceptual, behavioral, and cognitive symptoms, such that patients with SPD frequently appear and act eccentric, being preoccupied with the occult and other magical-like beliefs. While they may have ideas of reference, frequent illusions, and paranoia together with social discomfort, they maintain intact reality testing and do not manifest formal thought disorders. When stressed or significantly decompensated, these patients may evince brief reactive psychoses. There is substantial evidence that this illness is genetically linked to schizophrenia, and the two frequently run together in families and exist along a schizophrenic spectrum. Endophenotypes (biological markers between genotype and external phenotype that may indicate susceptibility to or manifest as early signs of a disorder) exist for this spectrum and are present in both SPD and schizophrenia impaired: prepulse inhibition, P50 suppression, antisaccade paradigms, and working memory impairments.

51. (C) This patient is suffering from OCD. While he experiences symptoms consistent with a panic attack, they are necessarily in the context of an obsession/compulsion dyad and therefore are not symptomatic of a primary panic disorder. Importantly for the diagnosis of OCD, this patient's obsessions are ego-dystonic or ego-alien (as opposed to ego-syntonic), meaning that they are experienced as incompatible with the individual's ego or self-concept. Thus, he feels "ridiculous" having to carry out the compulsions (which serve to neutralize the anxiety produced by the contamination obsession), as he knows that the perceived presence of germs is a product of his own mind. Were he to firmly believe, beyond a shadow of a doubt and in the presence of evidence to the contrary, that he would suffer a severe illness were he to be prevented from washing his hands, he might be diagnosed with the much more rare delusional disorder. OCD is a common illness, affecting approximately 2% to 3% of the population, and frequently first occurring in one's mid-twenties.

52. (B) The person with a personality disorder usually does not believe that he or she is manifesting pathology. Ego-syntonic refers to aspects of a person's thoughts, behavior, and attitudes that are viewed as acceptable and consistent with one's self-concept. For example, a patient with histrionic or borderline PD may exclaim that they are merely sensitive and emotional and complain that their suffering is the fault of others. Usually, patients with ego-syntonic symptoms come to treatment only when developing an ego-dystonic axis I disorder, or when it becomes painfully clear that their relationships and functioning are impaired by something that they are doing. The goal of psychotherapy with these patients is to make ego-alien what was previously ego-syntonic. Ego-alien and ego-dystonic are synonymous. Ego-dysphoric does not exist as a term. Ego boundary refers to the demarcation between what is self and what is not self.

53. (B) Specific phobias (e.g., fear of insects, blood exposure, heights) are among the most common psychiatric illnesses, with a lifetime prevalence of 10%. They frequently first present in childhood. This patient is suffering from a fear of elevators that impairs her ability to sight-see on a school trip, to the extent that she makes excuses to avoid encountering the situation. It is not stated here, but she does recognize that her fears are excessive and unreasonable, but her anxiety is all too real. As is common in phobias, her ultimate exposure to the feared situation results in a so-called situational panic attack. Benzodiazepines on an as-needed basis are useful to decrease phobic anxiety and facilitate exposure (i.e., before a plane flight); while cognitive behavioral therapy involving exposure and desensitization offers more comprehensive and persistent benefits. Agoraphobia is the fear of crowds (from the Greek root meaning "marketplace"), and social phobia is the fear of being exposed to public scrutiny or being embarrassed.

54. (B) Patients with narcissistic personality disorder are overly preoccupied with their own importance, lack empathy for others, and frequently act in an exploitive manner to get to the top. However, despite their exaggerated (and pathological) self-absorption, at their core lies a hypersensitive and fragile individual exquisitely attuned to issues of self-esteem. They tend to react aggressively, with extreme emotion, and are significantly traumatized when slightly criticized. Their autonomous exterior belies their deeply dependent interior. Occasionally, these individuals are highly functional, rising to the top of corporations and on people along the way; however, their frequent dismissal of other's needs impairs their ability to maintain romantic and other social relationships.

They can be differentiated from borderline patients' diffuse sense of self, greater impulsivity, and more chaotic lives. Histrionic patients need to be the center of attention, but are more focused on their appearance than is described in this case; this patient's focus is on his own importance, and he seems oblivious to decorum. Dependent patients need love and will do anything to get it, but are far more passive and submissive toward others than is the narcissist. Of note, cluster B personality disorders frequently co-occur in the same individual.

55. (D) Most of the diagnoses in DSM-IV include a time specifier, such that on cross-sectional evaluation, it is impossible to come to a definitive conclusion regarding a specific disorder. Whatever symptoms the patient presents—mood, anxiety, or psychotic—it is the course of those symptoms and the disorder as a whole that allows one to arrive at a diagnosis. No single symptom is pathognomonic for either bipolar disorder or schizophrenia. While both disorders generally appear during early adulthood and both are characterized by exacerbations and remissions, patients with schizophrenia manifest a progressively deteriorating course, such that after each psychotic episode, they never fully regain their prior level of functioning. Bipolar patients, however, usually return to their functional baseline.

56. (E) Both patients with avoidant PD and those with schizoid PD avoid social contact. However, beyond this simple behavioral manifestation, the core features of these disorders differ drastically. Schizoid patients are hermits, wanting nothing to do with other people, even family members. An example is an affectively flat, socially withdrawn, unfashionably dressed, and absent-minded scientist working night hours alone in his laboratory. Avoidant PD exists as the extreme end of the shyness spectrum with social phobia somewhere in the middle. These patients crave social contact, but are terrified of ridicule, embarrassment, and humiliation. Their exceptionally low self-esteem frequently precludes their engaging in satisfying relationships; however, given a safe and caring environment, marriage and family are not out of the question. Magical thinking is common in schizotypal PD. Identity diffusion is manifest in borderline PD. Perfectionism is characteristic of OCPD.

57. (C) He is most likely suffering from a "pseudodementia" of depression. He is anhedonic, has trouble concentrating, and has poor appetite and energy. The items that he misses on his MMSE are concentration ("world" backwards), the date (although he is close to correct), and delayed recall (saying "I just don't know," but getting the correct answer with a hint.) People with Alzheimer disease are more likely to not even remember that you asked them to remember three words! Additionally, patients with Alzheimer disease very infrequently say "I don't know," and instead they may try to make something up. In addition, depression may have a relatively quick acute or subacute onset, but Alzheimer disease is usually quite insidious and delayed and a lawyer would probably not have an MMSE of 23 for a number of years after developing symptoms. Of note, some studies suggest that patients who present with pseudodementia of depression have a greater incidence of becoming demented in the subsequent 5 years. He has no evidence of a bipolar disorder, so lithium would not be indicated. He does not likely have Alzheimer disease, so donepezil, a cholinesterase inhibitor, would not be appropriate. A VP shunt would be used for normal pressure hydrocephalus (magnetic gait, incontinence, and cognitive impairment). An LP could be used, for example, to look for a CNS infection or to evaluate for NPH. Sertraline, an SSRI, would be a first-line treatment for depression in this individual.

58. (E) This patient is manifesting the classic presentation of cocaine withdrawal. A rule of thumb is that withdrawal effects from a substance are opposite of intoxication effects. In this case, as cocaine causes agitation, euphoria, autonomic hyperactivity, anorexia, and psychosis, this patient is presenting with dysphoria, fatigue, and hyperphagia; transient suicidality not uncommonly accompanies acute cocaine withdrawal, especially in a patient with a long history of use. His cough is likely due to the bronchial irritation induced by smoking crack (a crystallized form of cocaine, much cheaper than the powder). His constellation of symptoms is not indicative of schizophrenia, most notably his neurovegetative symptoms and his interacting with other patients. Major depressive disorder rarely presents acutely. Heroin intoxication is manifest by euphoria, sedation, analgesia, and pinpoint pupils. Heroin withdrawal presents with vomiting, abdominal cramps, diarrhea, anorexia, muscle aches, sweating, and a flu-like syndrome. Both cocaine and heroin withdrawal are not life-threatening and are managed supportively.

59. (B) Somatization is the expression of psychological distress in a physical form, ranging from a preoccupation with a normal bodily function (e.g., peristalsis), to a belief that one has a life-threatening illness (e.g., cancer). The function served by this physical manifestation of negative affect is manifold; for example, it can be used as an intrapsychic defense (against forbidden aggressive or sexual impulses), a communication of suffering and deserving care (especially when psychiatric principles are not culturally avowed), or an acting out of a recalled illness when one was cared for in the past. It is important to recognize that the person generally lacks insight into the psychological nature of his or her symptoms, and if such insight is present, it is generally of a superficial degree and influences his or her behavior only to a limited extent. Thus, the patient may view referral to a psychiatrist as unwarranted and may even take it as a sign of hostility. Prior to their developing greater insight, patients with these disorders respond well to frequent visits to their general practitioners—sort of check-ins—underscoring the idea that the presentation of physical symptoms is not required for them to receive care. Only after a good relationship is established with the patient should the primary care physician attempt a discussion of the psychological nature of the symptoms and a possible referral for psychiatric treatment.

60. (B) While we do not know for sure what this patient is experiencing in these various phenomena, his illness behaviors manifest a symptom profile consistent with OCD. As he has failed trials of first-, second-, and third-line treatments for this condition, he may be a candidate for cingulotomy, a neurosurgical procedure that has been shown to be beneficial in one-third to one-half of patients with treatment-refractory OCD. ECT is frequently used for treatment- resistant depression or mania or for psychotic depression. Clozapine is used for treatment-refractory schizophrenia or mania. MAOIs may be useful as a third-line treatment for major depression. Benzodiazepines are generally not effective for the core symptoms of OCD.

61. (C) This patient appears to be suffering from an illness on the social anxiety spectrum, specifically social phobia or avoidant personality disorder. Both of these conditions are chronic and involve intense anxiety at the prospect of humiliation or social rejection, with avoidant PD patients manifesting more pervasive pathology. Social phobia can be effectively treated by beta-blockers, benzodiazepines, and antidepressants such as SSRIs and MAOIs (TCAs are generally not effective). Avoidant PD, like most personality disorders, is more effectively treated with psychotherapy, but it may show a limited response to SSRIs given its significant anxiety component.

62. (C) Dissociative identity disorder (DID), previously called multiple personality disorder, is the extreme end of a series of dissociative disorders (dissociative amnesia, fugue, NOS, and depersonalization disorder). While more common than previously thought, DID is still rare; however, nonspecific dissociative phenomena are quite prevalent in inpatient psychiatric populations (e.g., hallucinatory experiences, thought insertion, losing time and amnesia, other cognitive disturbances, depersonalization). Traumatic experiences are usually thought to underlie the development of many of the dissociative disorders, and a common clinical experience is that the earlier in childhood the trauma occurs, the more likely it is to engender dissociative phenomena, though nearly all patients with DID have comorbid PTSD. Dissociation is a means of dealing with experiences engendered during a severe trauma, and is manifest by information about one's self being compartmentalized or split off from the rest. For example a person may have the circumstances of a trauma dissociated from his or her current sense of self, resulting in an escape from the pain of the trauma and amnesia surrounding the experience. This disruption in memory leads to an altered sense of identity and personal history and a lack of connection in a person's thoughts, memories, feelings, and actions.

63. (B) It is not uncommon for patients to demand that they be given their standing dose of methadone when they are brought to the psych ER. However, it is not safe to administer the usually high doses of this long-acting opioid without first receiving official confirmation, as doses greater than 20 mg can be fatal to an opioid-naïve individual. As is the case with most substances, the time course of withdrawal from opioids is dependent on the specific agent involved; methadone's long half-life produces a withdrawal syndrome which may take 2 to 4 days to emerge versus heroin's 6 to 12 hours. When combined with the nonfatal nature of opioid withdrawal (i.e., dysphoric mood, nausea or vomiting, muscle aches, lacrimation, rhinorrhea, pupillary dilation, piloerection, sweating, diarrhea, yawning, fever, insomnia), this leads to a fair amount of flexibility in one's clinical management of the situation presented. Clonidine, a central α_2-agonist, is useful in treating many of the symptoms mentioned above but does nothing to attenuate cravings; antiemetics are also useful, as are nonopiate pain medications. Finally, if withdrawal symptoms become severe, treatment with 20 mg or less of methadone is an option.

64. (A) It is not uncommon for patients with PTSD to suffer from episodes of dissociation. In its simplest form, a dissociative state is a trance-like episode in which one's actions, thoughts, memory, and feelings are detached from one's consciousness and hence one's self-identity. Dissociation as a symptom is also a core feature of a group of disorders called, not surprisingly, dissociative disorders; however, in these the dissociative episodes account for the majority of the pathology suffered by the patient. In PTSD, on the other hand, dissociative episodes can occur frequently or rarely. Importantly, the patient usually does not remember his or her experiences while in a dissociated state, and these experiences are frequently reminiscent of elements of the original traumatic situation. While a presentation similar to dissociation may occur in a complex partial seizure disorder, the content of the episode in this case as well as the clear association between PTSD and dissociation make a seizure disorder far less likely. There is no stated reason why this patient would malinger. Likewise, nothing in the case points to factitious disorder other than the patient's refusal to acknowledge he left the message; factitious disorder is marked by a patient's need to be in the sick role rather than determined by purely behavioral manifestations. Repression is a psychodynamic defense in which painful or unacceptable memories are excluded from conscious awareness; in effect, nothing unwanted gets through, and there is no choice but to have "objectionable" material filtered out.

65. (B) Among the newest of the antidepressants, selective serotonin reuptake inhibitors (SSRIs) are now the most commonly used treatments for depression. While they arguably are no more effective than earlier treatments (e.g., tricyclics and monoamine oxidase inhibitors), they have become so widespread due both to their reduced side effects and to their low likelihood of causing death in overdose. Each of the other options produces a toxidrome which can be lethal. Lithium overdose is manifest by incoordination, tremors, weakness, diarrhea, vomiting, drowsiness, obtundation, coma, stupor, seizures, and death and is treated by hemodialysis. Tricyclic overdose results in anticholinergic symptoms (dry mouth, blurred vision, mydriasis, urinary retention, constipation, pyrexia), hypotension, drowsiness, coma, seizures, and most importantly, cardiac conduction effects (delayed propagation of depolarization through both myocardium and conducting tissue and prolongation of the QRS complex and the PR/QT intervals with a predisposition to cardiac arrhythmias); the cardiac effects are the dreaded and lethal outcome in many cases. Acetaminophen is normally metabolized by the liver, and when taken in excess, the liver calls upon a second processing system which turns the acetaminophen into a toxic compound that damages the liver. Symptoms include initial nausea and vomiting followed by nothing for approximately 24 to 48 hours, and then jaundice, confusion, liver failure, kidney failure, coma, and death. Monoamine oxidase overdose is manifest by severe and malignant hyperthermia, tachycardia, tachypnea, muscular rigidity, confusion, seizures, cardiorespiratory collapse, and death. Note that acute overdose usually does not result in a hypertensive crisis unless the patient provokes the interaction.

66. (D) Depersonalization is most frequently experienced in the course of an anxiety disorder, most commonly panic disorder. It is an experience in which patients feel as though they are outside of themselves, but it is not quite an out-of-body experience per se. In other words, patients retain intact reality testing but feel detached from their actions, feelings, and thoughts, *as if* they were outside looking in. It is a feeling of a loss of connection with oneself, and one's actions are experienced as mechanical and rote. This symptom frequently coexists with one termed derealization, which is marked by a feeling that one is living in a dream and nothing seems real. In derealization, the normal emotional feel one would receive from an object in the environment is absent, such that things feel *relatively* fake. Both of these symptoms are present in many panic attacks and anxiety, and may account for some of the anxiety suffered by psychotic patients. However, a crucial difference between depersonalization and psychosis is that psychotic patients tend to fully uphold their symptoms, to not complain of them as pathological or disturbing, and by definition have a marked impairment in reality testing. Dissociation entails the patient's losing touch with himself, such that he does not feel "like I'm separated from my own thoughts and emotions," but rather *is* separated.

67. (B) The effective dose of an SSRI needed to treat panic disorder is similar to that used for major depression, and both are equally responsive to treatment. However, the treatment of panic disorder requires starting with a lower dose, as the SSRIs tend to initially exacerbate anxiety before making it better. Patients with panic disorder have a high *anxiety sensitivity*, meaning that they become anxious about physical sensations and do not respond well to the jitteriness and initial anxiogenic effects of SSRIs. In fact, patients with high anxiety sensitivity react to hyperventilation and other somatic challenges with more fearful thoughts and negative emotions. This is played out neurobiologically, as the initial burst of serotonin eventually settles into a downregulation of serotonin receptors and a calm steady state. Occasionally, such patients benefit from the co-prescription of an antianxiety agent, such as a benzodiazepine, during initial SSRI titrations. After approximately 1 to 2 weeks, panic disorder patients do not usually experience any increased anxiety and start to respond to the medication.

68. (C) Pervasive mistrust of people is the core feature of paranoid personality disorder and is manifest in patients' misreading neutral actions and cues as slights. They feel chronically exploited and constantly search the environment for confirmation of these fears. They are litigious and bear grudges, but when feeling threatened, may decompensate into psychosis or manifest intense anger and rage. Defense mechanisms manifest by these patients include primarily projection and rationalization. This patient is the proto-type of someone suffering from paranoid PD. Delusional disorder is quite rare and is marked by impaired reality testing; this patient is not psychotic but is overreading actions and statements made by the maid and interpreting them according to his pathology. Schizophrenia would manifest by a greater impairment in life prior to age 35 in a man. While patients with borderline PD are certainly rageful, nothing else in his history points to this diagnosis. Schizoid patients tend neither to have friends nor to wish to be present when someone else is around.

69. (E) This is an example of a reexperiencing phenomenon (i.e., intrusive thoughts, nightmares, flashbacks, and psychological dis-tress and physical reactivity to reminders or subliminal cues remi-niscent of the trauma). Patients with PTSD have basically developed a hair-trigger response to their environment, such that they are always, at least subliminally, on the lookout for threats. Impor-tantly, such threats can come from the external world as well as from interoceptive senses, including bodily functions and feeling states. While we may not know exactly what it was that triggered this patient's specific symptomatology each morning, we can safely say that a nightmare induced a physiological reaction reminiscent of the original trauma; patients with PTSD describe their re-experi-encing phenomena as including all of the symptoms initially expe-rienced in the index trauma—the body doesn't forget.

70. (D) Patients with antisocial PD can be engaging and charis-matic con artists, but at their core, they lack concern for others. They have an exaggerated sense of self-worth and believe the world is such that if they do not push people around, they will never get what they deserve. They actually see breaking laws and social rules as desirable traits and see working within these laws as limited to the weak. In this case, the patient's confiding in his sister-in-law (who by definition also married into the family) shows his general-ization of this belief. In describing these patients, the terms "psy-chopathy," "sociopathy," and antisocial personality disorder are often used interchangeably. This disorder has a strong genetic etiol-ogy. It is also marked by the frequent occurrence of suicide, homi-cide, somatization, and substance abuse. Importantly, for a diagnosis of antisocial PD, the patient must have had an onset of conduct disorder before age 15.

71. (B) While we cannot for certain say that this patient's avoid-ance of the dentist is consistent with PTSD, a dental phobia, or another syndromal pathology, we can nonetheless provide him with a symptom-based initial treatment. However, it is important to note that the best symptom-based approaches also take into account the under- or overlying disorder of which the symptom is a part. That being said, behavioral therapy is the most time-effective approach to overcoming phobic avoidance. Essentially there are two types of exposure-based behavior therapy: systematic desensitization and flooding. In the former, the patient is slowly exposed to increasing amounts of the feared stimulus while simultaneously being provided with concurrent relaxation exercises. Flooding, on the other hand, entails the patient being immersed in the feared situation until the fear fades; some phobic reactions are so intense that flooding must be carried out in one's imagination prior to engaging the phobic stimulus itself. Each of the other listed treatments may also be effective for this patient (with the caveat that antidepressant medications, while effective for PTSD, are relatively ineffective for simple phobias), but they are not the most time-efficient initial treatment for a phobic symptom.

72. (D) It is not uncommon for patients with schizophrenia to feel out of place in the world, especially when their psychotic symptoms dematerialize. Both during times of improvement and during distressing psychotic experiences, these patients not uncommonly turn to alcohol or drugs as a means of coping with a changed and threatening world. One may argue that they are self-medicating adaptive anxiety and demoralization, but the use of substances poses a significant risk to the patient with poor coping skills and psychotic symptoms. While it is not inherently pathological to use alcohol as a social lubricant, its self-prescribed use for particular symptoms easily morphs into abuse. In fact, a common comorbidity of social phobia is alcohol abuse and dependence. When a patient with a psychiatric illness begins to use a drug, one must be vigilant for the development of abuse or dependence symptoms and must ascertain whether the use can be understood as self-medicating discrete symptoms (in which case the treatment to date is substandard), whether one is addicted to the drug in question, or whether one is merely using in a social or experimental way as is common. Even if the latter is determined, in patients with limited resources, this should be discouraged.

73. (A) Based on the information given, this patient fits criteria for alcohol abuse, a syndrome characterized by continued use of the substance despite the development of alcohol-related problems (e.g., failure to fulfill major obligations, recurrent use in physically dangerous situations [e.g., DUI], recurrent legal problems, interpersonal problems). Additionally, the patient must never have met criteria for alcohol dependence. The latter requires physiological tolerance and withdrawal, as well as use for longer periods than intended, unsuccessful attempts to cut down, spending a great deal of time obtaining, using, or recovering from alcohol, giving up important activities due to alcohol, or continuing use despite knowledge of the problems caused. Essentially, abuse is manifest as a behavior and dependence as a loss of control. Substance-induced explosive disorder is not a real diagnosis, but clearly alcohol can induce behavioral disinhibition. While alcohol abuse is prevalent among patients with antisocial PD, we know nothing about this patient's character over his lifetime or within different spheres (necessary to diagnosis a personality disorder), or whether he had a history of conduct disorder as a child (necessary to diagnose antisocial PD in adults).

74. (B) This girl meets criteria for anorexia nervosa (AN). She displays a refusal to maintain body weight at or above a minimally normal weight for age and height (e.g., body weight less than 85% of expected), and despite being underweight, she has an intense fear of gaining weight or becoming fat, manifesting a disturbance in the way in which she experiences her weight or shape. She has amenorrhea, defined as the absence of at least three consecutive menstrual cycles. There are two subtypes of anorexia: restricting type in which weight is maintained through restricting intake, and binge-eating/purging type in which the person regularly engages in binge-eating or purging behaviors (e.g., self-induced vomiting, laxatives, diuretics, enemas). One cannot meet criteria for AN and concurrently be diagnosed with bulimia nervosa. This patient does not meet the frequency criteria for bulimia in which the binge eating and inappropriate compensatory behaviors both occur, on average, at least twice a week for 3 months. Patients with bulimia typically have normal weights, or are slightly overweight.

75. (C) Fragile X, found particularly in boys, is the leading inherited cause of developmental disabilities and mental retardation. Fragile X is caused by a mutation of the X chromosome, and thus the full phenotype is uncommon in girls. The physical characteristics common to patients with fragile X syndrome, in addition to those described in this case, include hyperextensible joints and macro-orchidism (large testicles in postpubertal boys). Down syndrome is the most common cause of mental retardation and occurs from maternal nondisjunction during meiosis, leading to trisomy of the 21st chromosome. Common features include moderate to severe mental retardation (IQ 20 to 85; mean approx 50), microcephaly, sloping forehead, up-slanting palpebral fissures, bilateral epicanthal folds, Brushfield spots (speckled iris), hypoplastic nasal bone and flat nasal bridge, small ears, and an open mouth with a tendency to tongue protrusion. Congenital heart defects are common in Down syndrome (40% to 50%), with the most frequent being endocardial cushion defects (43%) and ventricular septal defects (32%). Klinefelter syndrome (47-XXY) affects 1 in 1000 newborn boys, and is caused by meitotic nondisjunction. The following characteristic findings usually become apparent after puberty: tall and thin, with long legs, gynecomastia, small testes, small phallus, frequent infertility, and frequent learning problems with a normal to borderline IQ (mean 90). Noonan syndrome may be autosomal dominant, with some affected persons having a mutation on chromosome 12q. The clinical manifestations include short stature, webbed neck, shield chest, pectus excavatum, characteristic facies (epicanthal folds, ptosis, down-slanting palpebral fissures, low-set ears), cardiac abnormalities, and mental retardation (in approximately 25% of cases). Turner syndrome (45-X0) is only seen in females, with an incidence of 1 in 2500 live female births. Characteristic features include a triangular face, small mandible, prominent ears, webbed neck, shield chest, short stature, absent secondary sexual characteristics in adults (with amenorrhea and ovarian dysgenesis), and cardiac defects (30% to 50% with bicuspid aortic valve, and 10% to 20% with coarctation of the aorta). Intelligence is usually normal.

76. (B) This patient's history is highly consistent with borderline PD, an illness that has been shown to respond well to treatment with dialectical behavioral therapy (DBT). Specifically, DBT is effective at reducing parasuicidal (self-injuring) and life-threatening behaviors, behaviors that interfere with the therapy process, and behaviors that affect the client's quality of life. Patients with borderline PD react abnormally to emotional stimulation, manifesting a rapid hyperarousal and a significant delay before returning to baseline. The emphasis in DBT is on teaching patients how to manage emotional trauma, and the therapist actively teaches and reinforces adaptive behaviors, especially as they occur within the therapeutic relationship. Through weekly individual and group sessions, DBT targets behaviors in a descending hierarchy, beginning with decreasing suicidal behaviors, then behaviors that interfere with therapy, quality of life, respect for oneself, and so on. Psychodynamic psychotherapy is effective for BPD, but has not been as empirically validated, especially for suicidal behaviors, as has DBT. Eye movement desensitization and reprocessing is a takeoff on cognitive behavioral therapy used in the treatment of PTSD. Systematic desensitization is effective for phobias. Body-focused psychotherapy has been used for PTSDs but has not been validated.

77. (C) A diagnosis of a severe medical condition is not a justification for someone to experience symptoms consistent with a major depressive disorder. While the weight loss and anergia may be secondary to the neoplastic component, his anhedonia and despondency are psychiatric symptoms that he deserves to have treated. That being said, among the medications listed above, mirtazapine is the best option for ameliorating his symptoms. Mirtazapine works by blocking central presynaptic α_2-adrenergic receptors, resulting in an increased release of norepinephrine and serotonin; it also blocks serotonergic (5-HT2 and 5-HT3) and histaminic H1 receptors and weakly blocks peripheral α_1-adrenergic and muscarinic receptors. Based on this neurotransmitter profile as well as clinical experience, it is an effective antidepressant and relative anxiolytic without adverse gastrointestinal side effects (nausea, diarrhea), sexual side effects (anorgasmia), or insomnia. In fact, mirtazapine is frequently used in cancer patients as it is sedating and calming, but most importantly it promotes weight gain. Clonazepam is a benzodiazepine and has no antidepressant properties. Fluoxetine (SSRI) possesses GI and sexual side effects and is stimulating, thus not a good choice for an anxious depressed person. Nortriptyline (TCA) is a second-line treatment with a number of side effects (anticholinergic, cardiac, lethal in OD). Buproprion (NDRI) lacks the sexual and most of the GI side effects of the SSRIs, but is activating, less effective in anxious patients, and does not promote weight gain.

78. (B) This child has the classic symptoms of phenylketonuria (PKU). PKU is usually caused by a deficiency of phenylalanine hydroxylase which results in an accumulation of phenylalanine. It is the most common inborn error of amino acid metabolism (~1/11,000 live births). All states in the United States now test for this enzyme deficiency within 48 hours of birth. If untreated, eventual symptoms include failure to walk or talk, mental retardation, seizures, hyperactivity, tremor, microcephaly, failure to grow, and IQ of below 50. Phenylalanine is indirectly involved in the production of melanin, thus children with PKU often have lighter complexions than their unaffected siblings. Treatment consists of institution of a low phenylalanine diet. Glucocerebrosidase is the enzyme that is mutated in Gaucher disease. Glucocerebroside accumulates in the liver, spleen, and marrow and results in pain, fatigue, jaundice, anemia, and death. In the general public, Gaucher disease affects approximately 1 in 100,000 persons. In 1991, enzyme replacement therapy became available. The glucocerebrosidase enzyme is given via IV and can halt or reverse the symptoms. Beta-hexosaminidase A is mutated in Tay-Sachs disease, an autosomal recessive disease in which GM2 ganglioside accumulates in neurons and causes progressive neurodegeneration and death. Both penicillamine and zinc acetate are used to treat copper accumulation in Wilson disease, a rare autosomal recessive disorder of copper transport. In this disease copper accumulates and causes toxicity to the liver and brain; usually the liver is affected first. Kayser-Fleischer rings (deep copper-colored rings at the periphery of the cornea) are seen. Neuropsychiatric symptoms of Wilson disease include tremor, rigidity, drooling, difficulty with speech, abrupt personality change, grossly inappropriate behavior, and unexplained deterioration of school work. Psychotic symptoms may also be seen.

79. (B) Personality can be defined as a persisting pattern of perceiving, relating to, and thinking about the environment. When disordered, this pattern becomes increasingly rigid such that the person is unable to flexibly alter his or her style to adapt to novelty or stressors, thus becoming overwhelmed. It can be seen as a type of emotional retardation analogous to the intellectual impairments seen in mental retardation when a person becomes overwhelmed when asked to complete a task outside the realm of his or her abilities. Patients with personality disorders must manifest their discrete symptomatologies in multiple situations, at home and at work, in love and in play, for a majority of their adult life (i.e., older than 18 years). Thus, cross-sectional symptoms, while helpful, are less important than the patient's social and relationship history—a marker of the person's interactions with the world.

80. (C) Essentially, for a first episode of uncomplicated (e.g., without psychosis or comorbid eating disorder, etc.) major depression, the initial treatment of choice is an SSRI, and the specific SSRI chosen is distinguished by the individual's history and symptoms. That is, one would choose a more sedating medication if the patient were suffering from a more agitated depression, or a more activating drug were he or she to feel too withdrawn; family history, drug interactions, etc. are also important in this regard. However, ultimately all antidepressants (TCAs, SSRIs, MAOIs) are equally effective. An adequate trial of an antidepressant typically lasts 4 to 6 weeks at an adequate dosage, and this acute phase of treatment generally lasts 12 weeks until a full remission is attained. Following this acute phase of treatment is the continuation phase (4 to 6 months) during which treatment should be maintained at the original effective dose, as there is a high risk for relapse during this period. It is not uncommon for an initial episode of depression to be treated for 9 to 12 months, and earlier withdrawal of treatment is associated with an increased risk of relapse. Longitudinal studies have demonstrated that a history of three or more episodes place the patient at a greater than 80% risk for recurrence, thus necessitating longer term and sometimes indefinite treatment.

81. (B) This child has the classic symptoms of Rett syndrome. Found almost exclusively in girls, it is characterized by normal early development followed by a loss of purposeful use of the hands, distinctive hand movements, slowed brain and head growth, gait abnormalities, seizures, and mental retardation. At sometime between 5 months and 4 years, head circumference decelerates and previously achieved milestones are lost. Eventually these girls develop characteristic hand wringing stereotyped behaviors. Also found are truncal and gait incoordination, severe problems in receptive and expressive language, and often profound mental retardation. Retts is seen in 3.8 per 10,000 girls and is caused by a defect in the MECP2 gene. Since this genetic discovery, variants have been reported in males who have mutations of MECP2, with some overlap in symptomatology. Extreme friendliness may be seen in fragile X. Hemiballismus is a violent, involuntary movement on one side of the body, usually caused by damage to the contralateral subthalamic nucleus, often due to strokes.

82. (B) When seen in cross-section each of these disorders may look alike, and a time frame (e.g., >1 month) is required for diagnosis. However delusional disorder may be separated from the rest even on cross-sectional analysis. It is rare, tends to affect people in middle to late adult life, and does not commonly present with an acute episode. Rather, the person is generally self-supporting and employed and retains reality testing in areas outside of his or her specific delusion; bizarre delusions, grossly disorganized behavior, or prominent hallucinations are not present, and mood disorders are brief relative to the duration of the delusion. Types of delusional disorder include erotomanic (belief that a person is in love with the patient), grandiose, jealous, persecutory, somatic, mixed, and unspecified. Delusional disorder responds poorly to treatment.

83. (A) Important in the diagnosis of a phobia is the patient's ability to recognize the excessive nature of his or her fears. Even with this intellectual insight, however, phobic patients have great difficulty actually coming into contact with their feared objects or situations and actually changing their behaviors without therapy. While they may not acknowledge it at first blush, many phobic patients retain irrational beliefs about their feared objects or situations (e.g., all dogs are mean and bite), but understand that such beliefs are out of proportion to the actual threat involved. Delusions, on the other hand, are held with unwavering belief, with the patient's inability to acknowledge that his or her fear is possibly too extreme. Additionally, delusional beliefs are frequently systematized, such that patients have constructed a world far beyond the specific feared object or situation.

84. (E) Tourette syndrome is a chronic tic disorder, characterized by both motor and vocal tics, with onset in childhood, usually between 6 and 10 years of age. The motor tics usually precede the vocal tics. With concentration, individuals can usually suppress tics for minutes, or even hours (e.g., at work or school), but will often have a flurry of tics when they get home and relax their vigilance. A buildup of anxiety precedes the motor act of the tic which, when carried out, effectively but temporarily reduces this anxiety (i.e., like scratching an itch). The most common motor tics are facial. Both ADHD and OCD are commonly comorbid.

85. (B) Early childhood abuse is a significant risk factor for the development of both child and adult psychopathology, including depressive disorders, stress disorders, anxiety disorders, and borderline PD. These patients may grow up with a skewed perspective as to what constitutes a safe environment; to whom can they can turn if fearful or hurt when their protectors (those they trust) are the ones perpetrating the abuse? Rather than developing a non-specific paranoia (or paranoid PD) regarding the world at large, these patients tend to manifest ambivalent and conflicted relationships, both looking for closeness but fearing it nonetheless as they find it leads to eventual abandonment. There is evidence that early abuse affects and sensitizes the hypothalamic-pituitary-adrenal axis such that responses to future stressors are abnormal and maladaptive. While one prominent antecedent to borderline PD is a history of early childhood abuse, especially sexual abuse, it is not required for a diagnosis.

86. (B) This woman probably has mild stage Alzheimer disease. Donepezil is an acetylcholinesterase inhibitor FDA approved for mild to moderate Alzheimer disease, whereas memantine is an NMDA antagonist approved for moderate to severe disease. Sertraline is an SSRI and can be used in the treatment of depression or anxiety co-occurring with Alzheimer disease. Benztropine is an anticholinergic agent that is used to treat extrapyramidal symptoms associated with antipsychotic use. It should be avoided in Alzheimer disease, as the anticholinergic and antihistaminergic properties of the drug can increase confusion in cognitively impaired patients. Clopidogrel is an antiplatelet agent used in stroke prevention.

87. (E) Atomoxetine is a selective inhibitor of the presynaptic norepinephrine transporter. Atomoxetine is thought to increase both norepinephrine and dopamine in the prefrontal cortex, and is the first nonstimulant medication approved for the treatment of ADHD. Desipramine (a tricyclic antidepressant) is a second- or third-line medication. SSRIs (e.g., fluoxetine), MAOIs (e.g., phenelzine), and antipsychotic medications (e.g., chlorpromazine) do not have an evidence base in the treatment of the core symptoms of ADHD. Bupropion affects norepinephrine and dopamine levels in the brain and is also used as a second- or third-line medication.

88. (B) A diagnosis of bipolar I disorder requires only the presence of a manic episode. While the presence of sequential and interspersed major depressive episodes is the rule rather than the exception in bipolar disorder, it is not required for a diagnosis. Bipolar II disorder is marked by the presence of both hypomanic and depressive episodes (nonconcurrently), and by the absence of manic or mixed episodes. There is no such thing as manic disorder (though a "manic episode" is a part of bipolar I disorder, as above). NOS denotes an illness that does not heed the current syndromal nomenclature.

89. (B) SSRIs can be associated with hyponatremia secondary to the syndrome of inappropriate antidiuretic hormone secretion (SIADH), in which water is preferentially reabsorbed by the kidneys, overly diluting the sodium in the blood. The symptoms of fatigue, confusion, and weakness could all be due to hyponatremia. Other symptoms include nausea, vomiting, headache, obtundation, and eventually seizures, coma, and respiratory arrest if plasma sodium falls below about 115 meq/L. Of note there are case reports of all classes of antidepressants (SNRI, MAOI, TCA, bupropion) being associated with hyponatremia. Carbamazepine has also been implicated. Lithium is associated with a mild leucocytosis, thought to be due to demargination of neutrophils. Clozapine may be associated with agranulocytosis. Hyperkalemia due to medications may be due to potassium sparing diuretics, such as aldactone or nonselective beta-blockers.

90. (C) Ipecac abuse may cause cardiomyopathy. Though dental caries can be caused by excessive sugar, in bulimics erosion or caries are from excessive exposure to stomach acid upon purging. Bingeing can cause gastric dilatation and rarely rupture. Vomiting may cause esophagitis, Mallory-Weiss tears, and rarely esophageal rupture. Vomiting can also cause hypochloremic metabolic alkalosis from the loss of HCl from gastric fluid. Potassium is lost through emesis or laxative or diuretic abuse, but most is lost from increased renal excretion because of metabolic alkalosis. Hypokalemia leads to skeletal and smooth muscle weakness and to cardiac conduction abnormalities, arrhythmia, and cardiac arrest. Chronic metabolic alkalosis can be associated with hypokalemic nephropathy and renal failure.

91. (B) With separation anxiety disorder, the child has excessive and developmentally inappropriate anxiety concerning separation from home. This is characterized by being frantically afraid of separation, becoming highly anxious when it happens or is anticipated, and using various behaviors to avoid it (e.g., tantrums, school refusal), and is accompanied by symptoms of autonomic arousal when separation has occurred or is anticipated. This can be associated with inability to sleep without major attachment figures around and worrying that something will happen to himself or a major attachment figure that would cause true lasting separation and loss. One of the first concerns is whether there is an environmental stressor at camp which might account for his behavior; if this were so than separation anxiety disorder would not be the diagnosis. A new inability to sleep without his parents in the room is indicative of a problem. Childhood onset schizophrenia is an extremely rare disorder, and he has no other symptoms suggestive of a psychotic process. He has no other symptoms of depression.

92. (C) This man presents with symptoms consistent with AIDS dementia complex (ADC). He has HIV risk factors (IV drug use), and he has some physical symptoms of AIDS/chronic illness (weight loss, temporal wasting). Patients with ADC most often present with a classic subcortical dementia: the triad of cognitive, motor, and behavioral symptoms. However, patients with ADC can initially present solely with psychiatric symptoms such as depression, mania, or psychosis. ADC is most common in patients with late stage disease, and patients with low CD4 counts (e.g., under 200) are at increased risk. Certainly many of the other tests mentioned in the answer list are important to evaluate as well, but for this patient, the most important and likely concern is whether or not he has HIV.

93. (B) This woman most probably has general paresis, a form of tertiary syphilis (due to *Treponema pallidum*) that usually presents 10 to 20 years after initial infection in approximately one-tenth of patients with untreated syphilis. In general paresis there is cortical atrophy, particularly in the frontal and temporal lobes. Ventricular dilation is common, and on autopsy, there is an abundance of microglia and astrocytes, and spirochetes can be seen in the brain parenchyma. In the pre-antibiotic era, general paresis was the most common cause of dementia. After WW II, the use of penicillin caused a near eradication of neurosyphillis, but since AIDS, there has been resurgence. There may be associated mood symptoms (depression or mania) and psychotic symptoms (hallucinations, delusions). As the dementia progresses, seizures are common (50%), as is dysarthria, dysnomia, dysgraphia (handwriting deteriorates), and facial musculature may lose its tone giving the patient a vacant look. Argyll-Robertson pupil is often present (pupils are sluggishly reactive to light, but briskly to accommodation, and are often small and unequal). There may be a coarse tremor in fingers, hands, lips, and tongue. The gait becomes unsteady, and eventually a "general paresis" occurs, with profound widespread weakness of all voluntary muscles. Eventually the patient becomes bed-bound and vegetative. Tabes Dorsalis, another manifestation of tertiary syphilis due to degeneration of the posterior columns of the spinal cord, causes the loss of vibratory sense and proprioception seen in this patient. Prions are the infectious agents associated with bovine spongiform encephalitis, kuru, and Creutzfeldt-Jakob diseases. Aggregated alpha-synuclein inclusions are seen in Parkinson disease. Beta amyloid is a hallmark of Alzheimer disease. Fungi may cause focal deficits, particularly in the brains of immunocompromised patients.

94. (E) While symptoms consistent with PTSD are experienced by ~90% of people within the first week after a traumatic event, the disorder itself is only diagnosable when the symptoms have been continuously present for at least one month. Even after that period, a significant minority of people (now with PTSD) experience spontaneous remission of their symptoms; however the curve generally plateaus after 1 month, and the presence of symptoms necessitates treatment. Unfortunately, this patient falls into that latter category, as she is still experiencing significantly impairing symptoms 2 months out. The best studied treatment for PTSD is exposure therapy, the goal of which is disrupting the link between trauma-related cues and anxiety or avoidance. Essentially, the patients are taught to modify their responses to their memories, feel more in control of their world, and master their fear, all with the idea that once-threatening traumatic cues no longer anticipate a real life threat. Formal psychoanalysis is inappropriate so soon after a trauma when the patient is in such a raw state, but exploratory or supportive psychodynamic psychotherapy may be helpful. Debriefing is used immediately after the traumatic event to give the participants a forum to discuss and emotionally process their experiences. It has been shown effective with firefighters and other noncivilian personnel, but may increase the risk of developing PTSD in civilians and those not yet ready to process their feelings. Interpersonal psychotherapy is effective for depression and dialectical behavioral therapy is a treatment of choice for borderline personality disorder.

95. (D) A skeletal series should be ordered in nearly all cases of suspected child abuse, especially in a preverbal child or in one who may have a developmental delay. This child has multiple bruises in uncommon places (back, upper arm) as well as a femoral fracture. The issue of potential child abuse needs to be investigated, and it would be inappropriate to simply discharge the family. It is also important to interview each member of the family separately to better understand the circumstances of the event. Inconsistent or changing stories and extremely vague or evasive answers may be seen in cases of abuse. It is important to also look through the hospital ER records to see if there are previous instances of suspicious injuries. The most common manifestations of abuse are burns, bruises (in unusual locations), cuts, fractures, head trauma, and abdominal injuries. There are an estimated 4 million cases of child abuse reported yearly in the United States, though underreporting is the norm, accounting for 2000 to 5000 deaths annually. Over 50% of abused children are less than 5 years old.

96. (C) Pediatric autoimmune neuropsychiatric disorder associated with streptococcus (PANDAS) is a syndrome marked by the development of OCD-like symptoms in the context of strep infection. Autoimmune effects on the basal ganglia have been implicated in the pathogenesis of PANDAS, similar to that in Sydenham chorea and analogous to poststreptococcal glomerulonephritis and acute rheumatic fever. The symptoms of PANDAS are indistinguishable from OCD but are treated by treating the strep throat. Occasionally, when it is not treated, a child with multiple bouts of this illness may develop the general syndrome of OCD, but PANDAS may also simply run its course, responding to antibiotics.

97. (E) Schizoid personality disorder is typified by the loner seeming to lack a connection with other people. These patients tend to be indifferent to the social world around them, with little desire for even familial relationships; contrast with the person with avoidant PD, who intensely desires but is terrified of social contact. Their hobbies and other pursuits are frequently solitary and are marked by impersonal themes, and they manifest clear thinking and intact reality testing; contrast with the oddness and magical thinking common in schizotypal PD and the gross thought disorder and loss of reality testing in schizophrenia. Patients with schizoid PD are asocial and indifferent, tending to be kind but withdrawn, as opposed to antisocial patients whose goal is to dominate and "put one over" on another person. Psychotherapy is the best treatment for schizoid PD, but it should be noted that these patients infrequently present to a psychiatrist's office, and usually only in the context of a comorbid axis I disorder.

98. (B) This woman has a new onset paranoid persecutory psychosis at age 65. It is marked by the isolated symptom of fixed false beliefs (delusions) which, though affecting her behavioral choices, do not affect her general functioning in that she still actively participates in her church activities, manages her ADLs, and is cognitively intact. She has no evidence of major depression or mania, and thus meets criteria neither for MDD with psychotic features nor for schizoaffective disorder. Brief psychotic disorder is defined as the presence of at least one of the following symptoms: delusions, hallucinations, disorganized speech (e.g., frequent derailment or incoherence), and grossly disorganized or catatonic behavior. Brief psychotic disorder lasts between 1 day and 1 month, followed by full return to premorbid level of functioning, and is most often seen in response to a significant identifiable stressor. This patient's symptoms have clearly lasted for more than a month. She has no evidence of a general medical condition that could cause her symptoms.

99. (E) At this point in our understanding and pharmacologic toolbox, the treatment of OCD most commonly includes high dose serotonin reuptake inhibitors (SRIs). Of the medications listed, both sertraline and clomipramine are functionally SRIs, but while sertraline is a true SSRI, clomipramine is a tricyclic antidepressant specifically selective for serotonin reuptake and has all the disadvantages of TCA treatment (i.e., greater side effect burden and lethality in overdose). Nortriptyline is a TCA without a serotonin-specific mechanism of action. In theory any of the SRIs should be effective in the treatment of OCD, but only a few companies have paid for the studies required to obtain an FDA indication for this disorder. Important in OCD treatment is both the use of high doses as well as giving the medication a longer time to work, such that 12 weeks is considered an adequate trial.

100. (C) Factitious disorder is an illness characterized by the intentional production of physical or psychological symptoms with the goal of assuming the sick role. Importantly, these symptoms are produced voluntarily and do not exist as unconscious factors as in somatoform disorders (answer B). Nonetheless, patients with factitious disorder are not aware of their wish or motivation, and this illness is differentiated from malingering (answers A and D) by the latter's distinct awareness of their reasons behind producing their symptoms (e.g., to obtain some real external incentive). In factitious disorder, the only apparent objective is to assume the role of the patient. Feigned fever can account for up to 5% to 10% of hospital admissions, and perhaps not surprisingly, this condition is more common in healthcare workers. These patients have many times been the victim of early childhood abuse, and their production of current symptoms is frequently a means of coping with rejection, need for love, identification with a sick figure from one's past, or masochistic gratification from undergoing painful surgical procedures.

Index

Page numbers followed by *f* or *t* indicate figures or tables, respectively.